Barkley's Curriculum Review for Pediatric Nurse Practitioners

Thomas W. Barkley, Jr., PhD, ACNP-BC, ANP, FAANP
President, Barkley & Associates
Los Angeles, California
and
Professor
Director of Nurse Practitioner Programs
California State University, Los Angeles
School of Nursing

Barkley & Associates
www.NPcourses.com

www.NPcourses.com
P.O. Box 69901
West Hollywood CA 90069

BARKLEY'S CURRICULUM REVIEW FOR PEDIATRIC NURSE PRACTITIONERS
NATIONAL CERTIFICATION ISBN 978-0-9864021-5-9

Notice

Knowledge and best practices are subject to change, as new research and further experience expand knowledge. Changes in practice, treatment, and drug therapy may be warranted or appropriate. It is recommended that readers verify the most up-to-date information regarding procedures featured or check the manufacturers of administered products, so as to verify the recommended dose, formula, methods of administration, and contradindications. It is the duty of practitioners, relying on their experience and knowledge of the patient's circumstances, to determine dosages and the best treatment for each patient, while taking all safety precautions. To the fullest extend of the law, neither the Publisher nor the Editor, Contributors, or Reviewers assume any liability for any injury and/or damage to persons or property arising out of or related to any use of the content in this book.

The Publisher

International Standard Book Number: 978-0-9864021-5-9
Printed in the United States of America

Managing Editor: Taylor Spining
Staff Coordinator: Christopher Cudé
Cover Design: Andres Morgan
Contributing Writers: Andrey Gordienko, Roberto A. Rael, Justin R. Searles, Kaitlyn C. Sullivan

Preface

Barkley's Curriculum Review for Pediatric Nurse Practitioners is a long-overdue resource in advanced practice nurse practitioner education. The text is written at a level appropriate for pediatric nurse practitioner (PNP) students, faculty, and practicing nurse practitioners.

For students and faculty, the text can be strategically utilized in several ways to enhance nurse practitioner curricula. First, the text can be used as an excellent culminating work to review key subject areas of the entire PNP curriculum prior to national certification.

For most faculty who adopt a modular approach to systems and special topics learning, the book can be extremely valuable throughout the PNP student's entire course of studies. Assigning chapter by chapter, in conjunction with course topical outlines, serves to reinforce classroom lectures and other learning activities as either pre- or post-class assignments.

For the certified PNP, a comprehensive review of the PNP curriculum is always rewarding to assist in revisiting those "not-so-commonly seen" patient diagnoses in individual practice. Whether being used by student, faculty, or certified nurse practitioner, *Barkley's Curriculum Review for Pediatric Nurse Practitioners* is an outstanding asset.

In light of the varied needs of the readers, the text is designed for both practicality and flexibility. *Barkley's Curriculum Review for Pediatric Nurse Practitioners* is essentially two books in one, comprising a Practice Question/Rationale Section and a comprehensive Discussion Section. Extensive question rationales feature not only why the correct answer is correct, but also why all other answer choices are either incorrect or not the best answer. After the Practice Question Section in each chapter, an extensive Discussion Section includes the following: Overview (incidence/predisposing factors), Presentation (signs and symptoms), Workup (laboratory/diagnostic tests), and Treatment (management options) for all common diagnoses presented in the chapter. Further, the book is supplemented with relevant figures, tables, and diagrams in color.

As editor, I sincerely thank the Distinguished Reviewers of this text who represent some of the most exceptional nurse practitioner experts in the country. In addition, I am extremely grateful to the talented staff of Barkley & Associates, Inc. who tirelessly produced this work with never-ending enthusiasm. I trust that you will find *Barkley's Curriculum Review for Pediatric Nurse Practitioners* to be an invaluable educational tool.

Thomas W. Barkley, Jr., PhD, ACNP-BC, ANP, FAANP
Editor

Acknowledgments

We gratefully acknowledge the combined efforts of the staff of Barkley & Associates whose knowledge and dedication provided the foundation for this review guide. We would additionally like to thank the outstanding contributors and reviewers of this text. Without the expertise of these scholars, this work would not have been possible.

We also thank the following people:

Pediatric Content Experts: Sharyn Flavin, Molly K. Rothmeyer, Joetta D. Wallace, Stacey A. Warner
Managing Editor: Taylor Spining
Staff Coordinator: Christopher Cudé
Cover Design: Andres Morgan
Contributing Writers: Andrey Gordienko, Roberto A. Rael, Justin R. Searles, Kaitlyn C. Sullivan

whose combined efforts have produced what we believe is a state-of-the-art, evidence-based, excellent resource for the profession.

Reviewers

Sharyn Flavin, APRN, DNP, AGNP, CPNP
Long Beach Memorial & Miller Children's Hospital
Long Beach, CA

Donna Susan Freeborn, PhD, FNP
Assistant Professor, Coordinator FNP Program
Brigham Young University
Provo, UT

Jane T. Garvin, PhD, RN, FNP-BC
Assistant Professor of Nursing
Georgia Regents University
Augusta, GA

Gay L. Goss, PhD, APRN-BC
Professor
Cal State University Dominguez Hills
Carson, CA

Paula Gray, FNP/DNP, CRNP, NP-C
Clinical Assistant Professor of Nursing, Director Family (Individual Across the Lifespan) CRNP Program
Widener University, School of Nursing
Chester, PA

Yvonne L. Joy, MBA, MSN, APRN
Assistant Professor of Nursing
University of Saint Joseph
West Hartford, CT

Vanessa M. Kalis, DNP, PNP-AC, ACNP-BC, CNS, RN
Assistant Professor, Director Acute Care DNP Programs: Pediatric and Adult-Gerontologic
Brandman University
Irvine, CA

Pamela L. King, PhD, FNP, PNP, FAANP
MSN Program Director
Spalding University, School of Nursing
Louisville, KY

Deborah Lee-Ekblad, MSN, FNP, ACNP-BC
Clinical Instructor, Acute Care Nurse Practitioner Program
University of Michigan, School of Nursing
Ann Arbor, MI

Denise M. Linton, DNS, FNP-BC
Assistant Professor and Nurse Practitioner Coordinator
University of Louisiana at Lafayette, College of Nursing and Allied Health Professions
Lafayette, LA

Ildiko E. Monahan, MS, ANP-C, FNP
Instructor
SUNY Institute of Technology, College of Health Sciences and Management
Utica, NY

Martha J. Morrow, PhD, FNP-BC, CNE
Associate Professor Graduate Nursing Program
Shenandoah University, Eleanor Wade Custer School of Nursing
Winchester, VA

Mary B. Neiheisel, BSN, MSN, EdD, FNP-BC, CNS-BC, FAANP, FNAP
Professor
University of Louisiana at Lafayette
Lafayette, LA

Michelle Pardee, DNP, FNP-BC
Clinical Assistant Professor
University of Michigan, School of Nursing
Ann Arbor, MI

Gloria M. Rose, PhD, NP-C, FNP-BC
Assistant Professor, Coordinator of FNP Program
Prairie View A&M University
Prairie View, TX

Molly K. Rothmeyer, DNP, APRN, FNP-BC, CPNP-AC
Assistant Professor
University of Alaska
Anchorage, AK

Sharon L. Stager, DNP, FNP-BC
Assistant Professor of Nursing
Salve Regina University
Newport, RI

Twila Sterling-Guillory, RN, FNP-BC, PhD
Associate Professor
McNeese State University
Lake Charles, LA

Joetta D. Wallace, RN, MSN, NP-C
Program Coordinator
Pediatric Palliative Care Service
Miller Children's and Women's Hospital
Long Beach, CA

Frankie Wallis, DNP, RN
Associate Professor
Samford University, Ida V. Moffett School of Nursing
Birmingham, AL

Stacey A. Warner, RN, MSN, CPNP
Assistant Professor
California State University, Los Angeles
Los Angeles, CA

Ann Weltin, DNP, FNP-BC, CNM
Assistant Professor of Nursing, DNP Program Coordinator
Clarke University
Dubuque, IA

Johnnie Sue Wijewardane, PhD, APRN, FNP-BC
Associate Professor
Mississippi University for Women
Columbus, MS

Mary Ellen Wilkosz, RN, FNP-BC, BSN, MSN, PhD
Director FNP Program
Sonoma State University
Rohnert Park, CA

Alyssa N. Wislander, MS, BSN, APN, RN, ACNP, CPNP
University of Illinois at Chicago, Quad Cities Regional Campus
Moline, IL

Carmen Wycoff, DNP, MBA, ARNP, CPNP
Pediatric Nurse Practitioner, Assistant Professor of Nursing
Clarke University
Dubuque, IA

Table of Contents

1. Growth and Development 3
2. Immunization Recommendations 25
3. Genetic Evaluation 34
4. Prenatal Assessment/Screening 43
5. Infant Health and Issues 61
6. Toddler/Preschool Health and Issues 73
7. School Age Health and Issues 87
8. Adolescent Health and Issues 104
9. Cardiovascular Disorders 115
10. Gastrointestinal Disorders 128
11. Dermatological Disorders 143
12. Eye, Ear, Nose, and Throat Disorders 170
13. Respiratory Disorders 187
14. Musculoskeletal Disorders 199
15. Neurologic Disorders 213
16. Hematologic and Oncologic Disorders 227
17. Endocrine Disorders 243
18. Genitourinary Disorders 253

PEDIATRIC
Curriculum Review

Chapter 1

Growth and Development

QUESTIONS

1. The mother of a 2-month-old patient says that their family is relocating to Japan to pursue a long-term business opportunity. You know that the majority of Japan does not practice water fluoridation. You recommend that the mother incorporate fluoride supplementation of 0.25 mg/day into her child's diet, starting at what age?

   a. Three months

   b. Six months

   c. One year

   d. Three years

2. When treating a child prone to seizures, a nurse practitioner should primarily keep which childhood anatomical feature in mind?

   a. Smaller circulating blood volume

   b. Large tongue compared to the oropharynx

   c. A thin cranium

   d. Large head in comparison to body proportion

3. A newborn is born weighing 9 lb. After 2 weeks, what would be the expected weight of the newborn?

   a. Eight lb

   b. Eight lb 5 oz

   c. Nine lb

   d. Nine lb 10 oz

4. The Denver II assessment test commonly measures a child for all of the following <u>except</u>:

   a. Personal-social development

   b. Language

   c. Fine motor development

   d. Intelligence

5. Kasey, age 7 months, is brought to the clinic by her concerned parents. They have been talking to other parents in their parenting group and need reassurance that Kasey is keeping up developmentally. As you observe Kasey, you notice that she responds to her name, consistently babbles, crawls around on the floor, and is able to pick up objects. Which of the following additional milestones would also be expected in a child her age?

   a. Supports weight on feet

   b. Holds head steady

   c. Equal coordination of hands

   d. Plays independently

6. Isaac, age 6 months, has been brought to your practice by his parents for a routine check-up. As you enter the interview phase, you would know all of these methods would be well-suited for the interview <u>except</u>:

   a. Carefully phrasing potential health and safety concerns to respect the cultural practices of Isaac's parents

   b. Breaking from the assessment regularly to ensure the parents have accurately expressed their concerns

   c. Phrasing your questions in an open-ended fashion to ensure a non-judgmental approach

   d. Using play to keep the patient engaged, regularly putting the assessment on hold to ensure to a proper response

7. Which of the following does <u>not</u> commonly impact temperature stability and regulation in a child?

   a. Increased subcutaneous tissue with increased evaporative heat loss

   b. Decreased body surface area to mass ratio

   c. Thinner skin

   d. Increased energy expenditure

8. You ask Samuel, a toddler, to point to one body part and he points directly to his elbow. Samuel's mother states that he just started correctly pointing to body parts last week. If Samuel is properly reaching expected developmental milestones, he would most likely be:

   a. About 13 months old

   b. About 18 months old

   c. About 20 months old

   d. About 2 years old

9. Holly, age 4, is at a well-child visit. During the visit, her weight is recorded as being 40 lb. Assuming expected growth parameters, how much will Holly most likely weigh in 2 years?

   a. Sixty lb

   b. Fifty-two lb

   c. Forty-five lb

   d. Forty-two lb

10. All of the following accurately reflect the typical well-child care visit except:

   a. After age 4 years, a child should have a well-child care visit yearly.

   b. Children on ADHD medication should see a physician or nurse practitioner every 6 months.

   c. Well-child care visits are arranged around immunization schedules, which are the key purpose of the visit.

   d. If the parents are experienced, their newborn does not commonly need to have a check-up until 1–2 weeks after birth.

RATIONALES

1. b

The American Academy of Pediatrics recommends that in areas with little to no water fluoridation, children should be started on fluoride supplementation at 6 months, with a daily dose of 0.25 mg. Supplementation is not required for the first 6 months of life, meaning 3 months of age is too early to introduce fluoride. By 1 year of age, the patient should already be receiving 0.25 mg/day. From 3 to 6 years of age, children should receive 0.50 mg/day of supplementary fluoride.

weight
5 months doubled
1 year tripled
2 year 4x birth weight

2. b

Developmentally, the tongue of a child is often comparatively larger than the oropharynx, which can potentially cause obstruction during a seizure and may lead to severe repercussions attributed to oxygen loss. Children have a smaller circulating blood volume in absolute terms, but this is primarily a concern in cases of blood loss or bacterial infection, not seizures. Children have thinner craniums, which would place them at a greater risk of head injury if the skull is penetrated; this may present a concern during convulsions, but is less of a concern than the risk of obstruction. Lastly, a child's large head, in comparison to the child's body, accounts for a smaller body surface area when compared with an adult, but this does not greatly influence potential complications from seizures.

3. c

The normal weight gain progression of an infant indicates that, at the 1–2 week mark, the weight will be approximately the same as it was at birth. The infant will typically lose 10% of the birth weight in the days after birth, weighing a little over 8 lb, and then gain that weight back within 7–14 days. By 5 months, the infant's weight should be doubled. The weight will usually be tripled by the first year and will be four times the birth weight by the second year.

4. d

Although the Denver II assessment test measures several aspects of child development, it is not an intelligence test. The Denver II measures the fields of language, personal-social development, and fine and gross motor development.

5. a

A child exhibiting the milestones of a 6–9 month old, as evidenced by crawling, babbling, picking up objects, and responding to her name, is likely to be able to support her weight on her feet. The ability to hold her head steady is an age milestone that typically occurs around 2–5 months; as such, the patient should already be able to do this. At around 10–12 months, she should be able to play independently and exhibit equal coordination in her hands.

6. c

Although a non-judgmental approach should be utilized at all times during the interview, questions should be directed and purposeful, not open-ended, to ensure that key details of the patient's history are not missed. Other proper techniques to utilize during an interview include ensuring cultural sensitivity, ensuring accurate perception of the parents' concerns, using play to enhance the patient's comfort, and pausing to allow adequate time for a response.

7. a

Temperature stability in children is commonly impacted by their limited, not increased, subcutaneous tissue with evaporative heat loss, as well as a smaller body surface area to mass ratio, thinner skin, and increased energy expenditure. Due to the fact that more energy is needed to facilitate proper growth, less energy is available for thermoregulation. These factors are important because they put children at an increased risk of hypothermia.

School age
gain about 5-7lb annually

8. b

A properly-developing toddler would be expected to point to his body parts at 15–18 months old. A 13-month-old can typically walk and understand a few words, but would not be expected to point to body parts. A 20-month-old and a 2-year-old would already be expected to be able to properly indicate parts of their body.

9. b

School-age children typically gain around 5–7 lb annually, so a 40 lb, normally-developing child would often weigh between 50 and 54 lb in 2 years; as such, 52 lb is the only answer choice that falls within that range. Gaining only 5–8 lb within 2 years, as indicated by a final weight of 45 lb or 48 lb, may suggest a developmental deficiency or malnutrition. A child who gains 16 or more pounds within 2 years exceeds the normal weight gain progression, and may indicate obesity in later childhood.

10. c

Well-child care visits commonly include physical exams to assess the physical well-being of a child; preventative care (i.e., immunizations), communication with the parents, developmental tracking, and personal family issues are all equally important aspects of a well-child care visit. If there are no complications in development, a child should have a well-child care visit yearly after the age of 4. However, a child taking medication for ADHD should see a health care professional every 6 months. After a baby is born, it is recommended that the newborn receive a check-up within 2–4 days; however, if the parents have experience with newborns, they may not need to see a health care provider for 1–2 weeks.

DISCUSSION

Overview

A child's growth and development progresses across four stages: infancy, preschool, school age, and adolescence.[1] Knowing the major growth and development landmarks for each stage will allow the nurse practitioner (NP) to determine a patient's expected developmental progression, in addition to providing anticipatory guidance measures. Moreover, being knowledgeable about the various stages will help to identify developmental warning signs or red flags in a child's development.[2]

A child's growth and development is monitored during regular health maintenance visits. Developmental surveillance occurs in three main domains: physical, cognitive, and psychosocial. Primary guidelines for growth and development are contained in the American Academy of Pediatrics' (AAP) *Bright Futures: Guidelines of Health Supervision of Infants, Children, and Adolescents*.[3]

The Physical Domain

Overview

Physical growth occurs in an orderly sequence. Children progress at different rates through this sequence depending on a number of factors, such as genetics, culture, nutrition, and individual variability.[2] Serial measurements are important for assessing a pediatric patient's physical growth. The Centers for Disease Control and Prevention (CDC) recommend assessing the patient's growth using standardized growth charts. The World Health Organization (WHO), in conjunction with the CDC and the National Center of Health Statistics, have created standardized growth charts that allow health care providers to collect serial growth data in order to develop an overall clinical impression of the child's growth and development.[4]

Nutritional Factors

Caloric requirements for children vary according to the child's age. From birth to 6 months of age, children should consume 120 kcal/kg/day. Some sources suggest 110 kcal/kg/day through 1 year of age, with a decrease to 100 kcal/kg/day from 1 to 3 years of age. The daily caloric requirement decreases to 100 kcal/kg for children 7 months to 1 year of age. Children 2–10 years of age may consume a daily caloric intake from 70 to 100 kcal/kg. Lastly, adolescents should consume 45 kcal/kg daily.[2]

Typical weight gain progression consists of rapid decelerating growth, followed by consistent growth. Neonates may initially lose 5%–10% of their weight within the first few days of life, and then regain their birth weight by 14 days.[2] An infant's weight usually doubles by 6 months of age, triples by 1 year of age, and quadruples by 2 years of age. Furthermore, young children tend to grow 2.5 inches and gain about 4 lb annually from 3 years of age to school age, and school-age children commonly grow 2 inches and gain 6.5 lb annually.[7]

Breastfeeding is the evidence-based standard for infant feeding, as breast milk is the best source of nutrition during the first 6 months of a child's life.[5,6] The AAP recommends, in its policy statement on breastfeeding, that women with no health problems should breastfeed infants for a minimum of 6 months.[7] During these 6 months, infants should be exclusively breastfed on demand.

Furthermore, the AAP recommends that breastfeeding continue for the first 12 months of life, if possible. Breastfeeding offers numerous health benefits for both mothers and children, such as improving gastrointestinal function and decreasing the incidence of acute illnesses.[2,8] Breastfeeding may also decrease the risk of allergic diseases and prevent inflammatory diseases.[6] Additionally, breastfeeding may help prevent childhood problems of being overweight or obese, regardless of parental education or socioeconomic status. Consequently, the longer the mother breastfeeds, the less likely the child will become overweight. In mothers, potential benefits of breastfeeding include analgesia during painful procedures, more rapid involution of the uterus, and a decreased risk of both ovarian and breast cancer.[2,7,8]

Adequate intake is confirmed by six to eight wet diapers per day in a newborn or young infant, and is associated with satiety and appropriate weight gain. Well-nourished infants may also produce four or more stools per day by 2 weeks of age.[9] The AAP recommends that daily vitamin D supplements of 400 international units (IU) begin a few days after delivery and continue until the child is weaned to whole milk at about 1 year of age.[2,10,11] Mothers of breastfed infants who are vegan or who have vitamin B12 deficiency should receive B12 supplementation to prevent neurological abnormalities in the infant.[12] Term infants typically have sufficient iron stores for up to 6 months. However, breast milk contains little iron, and premature breastfed infants or infants with anemia should receive iron supplementation and multivitamins to ensure proper growth.[12] At around 6 months of age, infants should begin eating iron-fortified, single-grain cereals.[12]

The AAP recommends that fluoride supplements be given to patients over 6 months of age whose local drinking water supply has less than 0.3 parts per million of fluoride; however, supplementation is not needed during the first 6 months of life.[12] For low- to moderate-risk fluoride deficiency, bottled water and toothpaste with fluoride may be recommended. For children who are at high risk for developing dental caries, the dosage of fluoride supplementation depends on the patient's age: Children 6 months to 3 years of age should receive 0.25 mg per day, children 3–6 years of age should receive 0.5 mg per day, and 1 mg per day is recommended for patients 6–16 years of age.[13]

Eruption of the teeth begins with the central incisor, followed by the lateral incisor, canine, first molar, and second molar. This sequence is usually completed by the time the child is 3 years of age (see figures 1.1–1.2).[17]

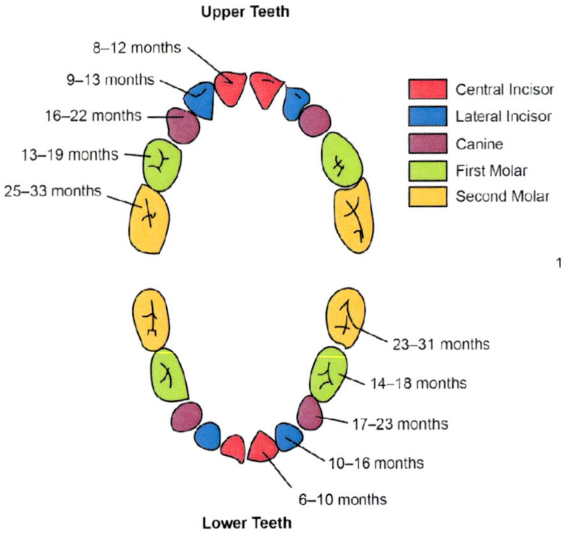

Figure 1.1. Primary teeth eruption.

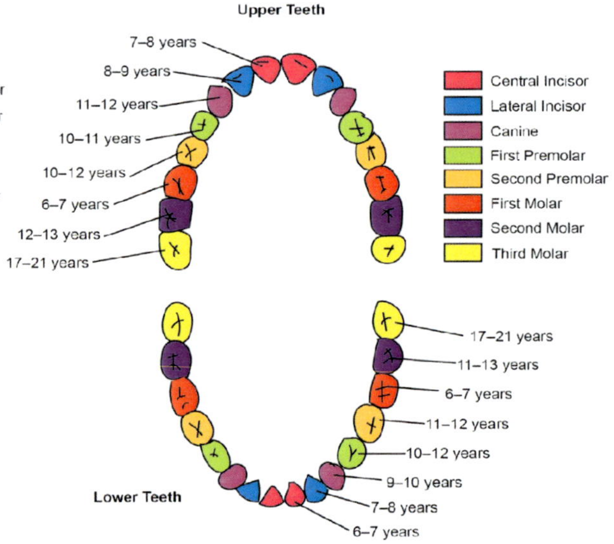

Figure 1.2. Permanent teeth eruption.

Table 1.1 Developmental Milestones and Warning Signs

	What Most Children Do At This Age				
Age	**Social/Emotional**	**Language/ Communication**	**Cognitive**	**Movement/Physical Development**	**Developmental Warning Signs**
2 months	-Begins to smile at people -Briefly calms him or herself -Tries to look at parent	-Coos, gurgling sounds -Turns head towards sounds	-Pays attention to faces -Follows things with eyes, recognizes people at a distance -Begins to act bored if activity doesn't change	-Can hold head up, pushes up when lying on tummy -Smoother arm and leg movement	-Doesn't respond to loud sounds -Doesn't watch things that move -Doesn't smile at people -Doesn't bring hands to mouth -Can't hold head up when lying on tummy
4 months	-Smiles spontaneously -Likes to play with people, cries when playing stops -Copies movements and facial expressions	-Babbles -Copies sounds -Cries in different ways to demonstrate hunger, pain, being tired, etc.	-Lets you know if he or she is happy, sad, etc. -Responds to affection -Reaches with one hand -Uses hands and eyes together -Follows moving things with eyes from side to side -Watches faces closely -Recognizes familiar people at a distance	-Holds head steady when unsupported -Pushes down on legs when feet are on a surface -Roll over from tummy to back -Holds toy, shakes and swings toys -Brings hands to mouth -Pushes up to elbows when lying on stomach	-Doesn't watch things that move -Doesn't smile at people -Can't hold head steady -Doesn't coo or make sounds -Doesn't bring things to mouth -Doesn't push down with legs when feet are on hard surface -Has trouble moving one or both eyes in all directions

Table 1.1 Developmental Milestones and Warning Signs

Age	What Most Children Do At This Age				Developmental Warning Signs
	Social/Emotional	Language/ Communication	Cognitive	Movement/Physical Development	
6 months	-Knows familiar faces and begins to know if someone is a stranger -Likes to play with others, especially parents -Responds to other people's emotions and often seems happy -Likes to look at self in a mirror	-Responds to sounds by making sounds -Strings vowels together when babbling ("ah," "eh," "oh") and likes taking turns with parent while making sounds -Responds to own name -Makes sounds to show joy and displeasure -Begins to say consonant sounds (jabbering with "m," "b")	-Looks around at things nearby -Brings things to mouth -Shows curiosity about things and tries to get things that are out of reach -Begins to pass things from one hand to the other	-Rolls over in both directions (front to back, back to front) -Begins to sit without support -When standing, supports weight on legs and might bounce -Rocks back and forth, sometimes crawling backward before moving forward	-Doesn't try to get things that are in reach -Shows no affection for caregivers -Doesn't respond to sounds around him/her -Has difficulty getting things to mouth -Doesn't make vowel sounds ("ah", "eh", "oh") -Doesn't roll over in either direction -Doesn't laugh or make squealing sounds -Seems very stiff, with tight muscles -Seems very floppy, like a rag doll
9 months	-May be afraid of strangers -May be clingy with familiar adults -Has favorite toys	-Understands "no" -Makes a lot of different sounds -Copies other's sounds and gestures -Uses fingers to point	-Watches the path of something as it falls -Looks for things he/she sees you hide -Plays peek-a-boo -Puts things in his/her mouth -Moves things smoothly from one hand to the other -Picks up things like cereal o's between thumb and index finger	-Stands, holding on -Can get into sitting position -Sits without support -Pulls to stand -Crawls	-Doesn't bear weight on legs with support -Doesn't sit with help -Doesn't babble -Doesn't play back-and-forth games -Doesn't respond to own name -Doesn't recognized familiar people -Doesn't look where you point -Doesn't transfer toys from one hand to the other

Table 1.1 Developmental Milestones and Warning Signs

	What Most Children Can Do At This Age				
Age	**Social/Emotional**	**Language/ Communication**	**Cognitive**	**Movement/Physical Development**	**Developmental Warning Signs**
1 year	-Is shy or nervous with strangers -Cries when mom or dad leaves -Has favorite things and people -Shows fear in some situations -Hands you a book when he/she wants to hear a story -Repeats sounds or actions to get attention -Puts out arm or leg to help with dressing -Plays games such as "peek-a-boo" and "pat-a-cake"	-Responds to simple spoken requests -Uses simple gestures, like shaking head "no" or waving "bye-bye" -Makes sounds with changes in tone (sounds more like speech) -Says "mama" and "dada" and exclamations like "uh-oh!" -Tries to say words you say	-Explores things in different ways, like shaking, banging, throwing -Finds hidden things easily -Looks at the right picture or thing when it's named -Copies gestures -Starts to use things correctly; for example, drinks from a cup, brushes hair -Bangs two things together -Puts things in a container, takes things out of a container -Lets things go without help -Pokes with index (pointer) finger -Follows simple directions like "pick up the toy"	-Gets to a sitting position without help -Pulls up to stand, walks holding on to furniture ("cruising") -May take a few steps without holding on -May stand alone	-Doesn't crawl -Can't stand when supported -Doesn't search for things that he/she sees you hide. -Doesn't say single words like "mama" or "dada" -Doesn't learn gestures like waving or shaking head -Doesn't point to things -Loses skills he/she once had

Table 1.1 Developmental Milestones and Warning Signs

Age	What Most Children Can Do At This Age				Developmental Warning Signs
	Social/Emotional	Language/ Communication	Cognitive	Movement/Physical Development	
18 months	-Likes to hand things to others as play -May have temper tantrums -May be afraid of strangers -Shows affection to familiar people -Plays simple pretend, such as feeding a doll -May cling to caregivers in new situations -Points to show others something interesting -Explores alone but with parent close by	-Says several single words -Says and shakes head "no" -Points to show someone what he/ she wants	-Knows what ordinary things are for; for example, telephone, brush, spoon -Points to get the attention of others -Shows interest in a doll or stuffed animal by pretending to feed -Points to one body part -Scribbles on his/her own -Can follow 1-step verbal commands without any gestures; for example, sits when you say "sit down"	-Walks alone -May walk up steps and run -Pulls toys while walking -Can help undress him/ herself -Drinks from a cup -Eats with a spoon	-Doesn't point to show things to others -Can't walk -Doesn't know what familiar things are for -Doesn't copy others -Doesn't gain new words -Doesn't have at least 6 words -Doesn't notice or mind when a caregiver leaves or returns -Loses skills he/she once had
2 years	-Copies others -Gets excited when around other children -Shows increasing independence -Shows defiant behavior -Plays beside other children, begins to include other children	-Points to things/ pictures when named -Knows names of familiar people and body parts -Says 2–4 word sentences -Repeats words overheard in conversation -Points to things in a book	-Finds things, even when hidden under 2 or 3 items -Sorts shapes and colors -Completes sentences and rhymes in familiar books -Plays make-believe games -Builds towers with 4 or more blocks -May use one hand more than the other -Follows two-step instructions -Names items in a picture book	-Stands on tiptoes -Kicks a ball -Begins to run -Climbs up and down furniture -Walks up and down stairs while holding on -Throws ball overhand -Makes/copies straight lines and circles	-Doesn't use 2-word phrases -Doesn't know what to do with common things (i.e., brush, phone, fork) -Doesn't copy actions and words -Doesn't follow simple instruction -Doesn't walk steadily -Loses skills he/she once had

Table 1.1 Developmental Milestones and Warning Signs

	What Most Children Can Do At This Age				
Age	**Social/Emotional**	**Language/ Communication**	**Cognitive**	**Movement/Physical Development**	**Developmental Warning Signs**
3 years	-Copies adults and friends -Shows affection for friends without prompting -Takes turns in games -Shows concern for a crying friend -Understands the idea of "mine" and "his" or "hers" -Shows a wide range of emotions -Separates easily from mom and dad -May get upset with major changes in routine -Dresses and undresses self	-Follows instructions with 2 or 3 steps -Can name most familiar things -Understands words like "in," "on," and "under" -Says first name, age, and sex -Names a friend -Says words like "I," "me," "we," and "you" and some plurals (cars, dogs, cats) -Talks well enough for strangers to understand most of the time -Carries on a conversation using 2–3 sentences	-Can work toys with buttons, levers, and moving parts -Plays make-believe with dolls, animals, and people -Does puzzles with 3 or 4 pieces -Understands what "two" means -Copies a circle with pencil or crayon -Turns book pages one at a time -Builds towers of more than 6 blocks -Screws and unscrews jar lids or turns door handle	-Climbs well -Runs easily -Pedals a tricycle (3-wheel bike) -Walks up and down stairs, one foot on each step	-Falls down a lot or has trouble with stairs -Drools or has very unclear speech -Can't work simple toys (such as peg boards, simple puzzles, turning handle) -Doesn't speak in sentences -Doesn't understand simple instructions -Doesn't play pretend or make-believe -Doesn't want to play with other children or with toys -Doesn't make eye contact -Loses skills he/she once had

Table 1.1 Developmental Milestones and Warning Signs

	What Most Children Can Do At This Age				Developmental Warning Signs
Age	**Social/Emotional**	**Language/ Communication**	**Cognitive**	**Movement/Physical Development**	
4 years	-Enjoys doing new things -Plays "mom" and "dad" -Is more and more creative with make-believe play -Would rather play with other children than by him/herself -Cooperates with other children -Can't tell what's real and what's make believe -Talks about what he/she likes and is interested in	-Knows some basic rules of grammar, such as correctly using "he" and "she" -Sings a song or says poem from memory -Tells stories -Can say first and last name	-Names some colors and numbers -Understands counting -Starts to understand time -Remembers parts of stories -Understands idea of "same" and "different" -Draws a person with 2–4 body parts -Uses scissors -Starts to copy capital letters -Plays board or card games -Tells you what he/she things is going to happen next in book	-Hops and stands on one foot up to 2 seconds -Catches bounced ball most of the time -Pours, cuts with supervision, and mashes own food	-Can't jump in place -Has trouble scribbling -Shows no interest in interactive games or make-believe -Ignores other children or doesn't respond to people outside of family -Resists dressing, sleeping, using toilet -Can't retell favorite story -Doesn't follow 3-part commands -Doesn't understand "same" and "different" -Doesn't use "me" and "you" correctly -Speaks unclearly -Loses skills he/she once had

Table 1.1 Developmental Milestones and Warning Signs

Age	What Most Children Can Do At This Age				Developmental Warning Signs
	Social/Emotional	Language/ Communication	Cognitive	Movement/Physical Development	
5 years	-Wants to please friends -Wants to be like friends -More likely to agree with rules -Likes to sing, dance, act -Is aware of gender -Can tell what's real and what's make believe -Shows more independence -Sometimes demanding, sometimes cooperative	-Speaks clearly -Tells a simple story using full sentences -Uses future tense -Says name and address	-Counts 10 or more things -Can draw a person with 6 body parts -Can print letters or numbers -Copies a triangle and other shapes -Knows about things used every day (i.e., food, money)	-Stands on one foot for 10 seconds or longer -Hops, may be able to skip -Can do a somersault -Uses fork and spoon -Can use toilet on his/her own -Swings and climbs	-Doesn't show wide range of emotions -Shows extreme behavior -Usually withdrawn, inactive -Easily distracted -Doesn't respond to people or responds superficially -Can't tell what's real or make believe -Doesn't play a variety of games -Can't give first and last name -Doesn't use plurals or tenses properly -Doesn't talk about daily activities or experiences -Doesn't draw pictures -Can't brush teeth, wash and dry hands, or get undressed without help -Loses skills he/she once had

Note. Adapted from: Developmental milestones. CDC. http://www.cdc.gov/ncbddd/actearly/milestones/index.html. Published 2014. Accessed April 2015. Reproduced with permission.

Cognitive Domain

Overview

Jean Piaget's theory of the development of the cognitive domain assigns various stages to the cognitive development of a child. The sensorimotor stage, which lasts from birth to about 2 years of age, is characterized by rapid cognitive growth and learning through trial and error. A primary component of this stage is the concept of object permanence, which consists of an infant understanding that objects exist independently of their own actions or perceptions.[18] Additionally, infants develop greater awareness of their surrounding environment and adapt to the world by relating their actions to the results of those actions.[18]

The preoperational and preconceptual stage lasts from approximately 2 to 4 years of age. During this stage, the child can focus on a single aspect of a situation and begin developing intuitive thought; however, children at this stage are not yet capable of cause-and-effect reasoning. The preoperational stage is also marked by egocentrism, manifested as the inability to see situations from another person's point of view.[18] Additionally, children also exhibit animism, which is the belief that inanimate objects have human feelings.[18] The intuitive and preoperational thinking stage lasts from 4 to 7 years of age and marks the beginning of causation, with the child beginning to make logical assumptions about how one phenomenon produces another.[2]

When children reach roughly 7 years of age, they enter the concrete operational stage, which lasts until about 11 years of age. During the concrete operational stage, the child becomes capable of solving problems logically and gains the ability to conserve numbers and liquid, understanding that quantity may remain the same despite disparities in presentation.[18] Finally, formal operational thought lasts from around 11 to 15 years of age. Children in this stage become capable of thinking abstractly, solving complex problems, and reaching logical conclusions.[18]

Psychosocial Domain

Overview

Erik Erikson's theories of growth and development consist of psychosocial stages in which children mature by resolving social crises and developing a series of life skills.[18] As with all of Piaget's cognitive theories, the age ranges listed are approximate, beginning with the trust versus mistrust stage, which begins at birth and lasts until 18 months of age. During this stage, the infant learns that the world is an uncertain place and seeks some measure of stability from caregivers and the environment. Afterward, the child enters the autonomy versus shame and doubt stage, which lasts until 3 years of age and is characterized by self-assertion and developing confidence in one's own skills and abilities. Next, the initiative versus guilt stage lasts from 3 to 6 years of age, wherein the child begins interacting with peers and develops confidence in his or her ability to make decisions. This is followed by the industry versus inferiority stage, which lasts from 6 to 11 years of age and involves the child learning to be productive in his or her particular competencies. The final Erikson stage before young adulthood is the identity versus role confusion stage, which lasts from 12 to 18 years of age and focuses on defining one's own place in society.[18]

According to Sigmund Freud's psychosexual theory, three components of personalities are developed by experiences in particular stages of a child's development. These three components are the id, the principle of pleasure; the ego, the principle of reality and self-interest; and the superego, the principle of morality or conscience. Freud's stages of psychosexual development begin with the oral stage, which lasts from birth to 18 months of age and is marked by focus on the sensations of feeding, which can lead to the development of a sense of trust and comfort between child and mother. This is followed by the anal stage, which begins at 18 months of age, lasts until 3 years of age, and involves the child developing a sense of independence by mastering control of his or her bodily needs.[19] The phallic stage lasts until the child is 6 years of age and is marked by the development of the ego, love of the opposite sex, and the Oedipus complex, which is characterized by an increased attachment towards the opposite sex parent and resultant jealously towards the same sex parent. The latency stage lasts from 6 to 12 years of age and is marked by socialization, repression of sexual drive, and development of the child's superego and morality. Lastly, the genital stage occurs during adolescence, from 12 to 18 years of age; during this stage, adolescents direct their sexual urges onto their peers.[19]

Growth and Development Landmarks

Overview

Growth measurements are the gold standard by which the NP can assess a child's health and well-being.[20] Individual stages of growth and development, with a comprehensive outline of developmental milestones, follow in the subsequent sections. Assessment of developmental milestones should be determined using corrected age for premature infants; this is especially true when performing the Denver Developmental Screening Test, second edition (Denver II) assessment.[2] The corrected gestational age is the adjustment of developmental expectations for premature infants through 2 years of age, at which point most infants catch up developmentally.[21]

Workup

Every well-child visit requires a physical examination to assess the child's growth in relation to expected growth and developmental milestones. The growth parameters of pediatric patients are measured by growth charts, with norms expressed as percentiles of height, weight, and head circumference in accordance with the patient's age. Serial measurements should be examined; historically, any child whose measurement cross over two or more percentile lines needs further evaluation. Although this remains true, the issue of further workup is much more complex. Other factors to consider for further investigation include, but are not limited to, growth out of proportion to expected norms for ethnicity, body type, and familial trends and nutrition. Body mass index (BMI) uses a baseline of height and weight to measure a patient's body fat. The CDC and AAP recommend BMI screenings for overweight and obese children as early as 2 years of age.[22]

The Denver II test does not measure intelligence, but serves as a generalized assessment tool that can be used from birth to 6 years of age. This test assesses a child's development by measuring his or her growth, use of language, personal-social skills, and gross and fine motor skills.[23] Although normal development is widely variable, any child who is unable to meet the majority of developmental milestones during the well-child visit should be referred for a full developmental assessment.

Growth and Development Milestones (see table 1.1)

Well Child Checks (WCC)

Workup

Well Child Checks (WCCs) are stage appropriate screenings in which specific tools are used to screen the health of children. In the initial screening, a comprehensive health and development history is taken. Subsequent visits include interval histories to update the patient's records. These screenings also consist of a complete physical examination, developmental screening, and questions about the child's well-being.[2] The AAP recommends a screening schedule that begins at birth and continues at regular intervals throughout childhood and adolescence.[24]

A WCC measures a child's health by both objective and subjective data. Subjective data consists of an interval history that evaluates the child's nutrition, appetite, elimination, sleep, and development, among other factors.[25] Furthermore, this stage of the WCC should include discussion of any concerns the child's parents or caregivers may have. Objective data of a WCC includes the physical examination, laboratory testing, and developmental screening, which may include the Ages and Stages questionnaire (ASQ) or the Denver II test. The management plan of a WCC should include health promotion strategies with anticipatory guidance and the initiation of the primary series of immunizations.[2]

The Interview

Overview

The NP's general approach to interviewing a pediatric patient should begin with ascertaining who will be present and ensuring that privacy is maintained. It is important to use a non-judgmental approach during an interview and ensure accurate perceptions of the concerns of the child's parents. Additionally, the NP should phrase his or her questions purposefully, use non-threatening words, convey interest and attention, allow adequate time for response, and employ cultural sensitivity. The NP should play with the child and engage the child, as well as the parents, during the interview process. When seeing an infant or toddler, the conversation will be mostly with the parents; however, as the child grows, he or she should be increasingly included in the interview process. Finally, the child should be kept clothed during an interview until the physical examination or until it is otherwise necessary to remove clothing. In some cases, it is wise to unclothe the child piece by piece during the exam, only removing clothing when an area needs to be examined (e.g., only removing the shirt when the chest needs to be assessed).[2]

Injury Prevention (see table 1.2)

Overview

Injury prevention is particularly important in pediatric patients, as injuries are a leading cause of death in infants and children in the United States and worldwide.[26] Unintentional injury is one of the major types of injuries in children and includes poisonings, motor vehicle accidents, drownings, and falls, among others.[27] To prevent poisoning in children, it is important to have poison control numbers nearby at all times and keep all poisons locked and out of reach.[2] Firearms are another major cause of injury to children; proper storage and safety concerns should be discussed with parents and children when appropriate.[28]

It is important that children be properly placed in adequate restraint systems in passenger vehicles, as motor vehicle accidents are the leading cause of death in children 4 years of age and older.[29] The child's home should likewise be fitted to protect against injuries resulting from fires and other unintentional injuries.[30]

Domestic violence and other types of child maltreatment are a common source of injuries. NPs play a key role in minimizing the risk of child maltreatment by promoting awareness of the issue in the community, engaging in home visits, and educating parents in proper techniques to ensure a positive environment for their child.[31] If child abuse is identified, most states have mandatory reporting statutes that require NPs to report the incident to the proper authorities, such as child protective services, a law enforcement agency, or a state's toll-free child abuse reporting hotline.[32]

Table 1.2	Leading Causes of Unintentional Injury Death Among Children 0–19 Years, by Age Group, United States				
	Age Group (in years)				
Rank	**Younger than 1**	**1–4**	**5–9**	**10–14**	**15–19**
1	Suffocation	MVT-related	MVT-related	MVT-related	MVT-related
2	MVT-related	Drowning	Other injuries	Other injuries	Other injuries
3	Drowning	Other injuries	Fires or burns	Drowning	Poisoning
4	Other injuries	Fires or burns	Drowning	Fires or burns	Drowning
5	Fires or burns	Suffocation	Suffocation	Suffocation	Falls
6	Poisoning	Falls	Falls	Poisoning	Fires or burns
7	Falls	Poisoning	Poisoning	Falls	Suffocation

Note. MVT = motor vehicle traffic. Adapted from CDC childhood injury report: Patterns of unintentional injuries among 0–19 year olds in the United States, 2000–2006. CDC. http://www.cdc.gov/safechild/images/CDC-childhoodinjury.pdf. Published 2008. Accessed April 2015. Reproduced with permission.

Developmental Considerations

During a child's growth and development, the NP must be mindful that children cannot be treated as small adults due to many unique anatomical, physiological, cognitive, and psychological differences.[33]

Anatomic Differences

Size

Because their bodies are not fully mature, children are at increased risk from environmental hazards. Body surface area (BSA) to body mass ratio is highest at birth and diminishes with age.[34] Because children have a higher BSA to body mass ratio, they may absorb larger doses of pollutants than adults.[35]

Small Body Mass

The body mass of a child typically has less fat, less elastic connective tissue, and a closer proximity of the chest to the abdominal organs. Because of these anatomic differences, flying objects, falls, and blunt or blast trauma may result in increased injury to multiple organs.[33] Young children have a very large head size in comparison to their body size, which causes them to be more likely to fall on their head. This predisposes a child to an increased incidence of head injuries. As brain development continues through 20 years of age, any head injuries sustained by children or young adults can have deleterious effects and result in long term sequelae.

Smaller Circulating Blood Volume/Less Fluid Reserve

Blood loss of even a small amount can be considered significant in children. A 5 kg child who has a hemorrhage of 100 ml will lose approximately 10% of their total blood volume.[33]

Skeletal

Children's bones are more susceptible to fractures and offer less protection to the internal organs.[37] Moreover, cervical vertebrae are cartilaginous in an infant and slowly become replaced by bone; thus, childhood cervical spine injuries occur at a higher rate than adult cervical spine injuries. Other injuries are then more likely to result, which may include damage to cartilaginous-osseus structures and surrounding ligaments, as well as spinal cord compression or transection.[37] Due to the increased elasticity of children's bones, they are most prone to having greenstick fractures, which occur when a bone bends before cracking.[38]

Head

Children have larger head-to-body ratios than adults. Because of their larger head sizes, children are more vulnerable to head and spine injuries as well as heat loss and hypothermia.[33] Furthermore, the brain, which typically doubles in size by 6 months and is 80% of adult size by 2 years of age, continues to perform functions such as myelination, synapse formation, neuronal plasticity, and biochemical stability, all of which are at risk for arrest and resultant permanent changes.[2]

Chest

Children's chests are mobile and pliable, and their abdominal walls are relatively thin. Additionally, their small size leads to closer proximity of organs, resulting in an increased likelihood of multiple organs being injured during a given traumatic event.[33]

Airway

The anatomy of the pediatric respiratory system is significantly different from that of an adult. Children have a smaller trachea, smaller lung volumes, a more compliant chest wall, and a smaller forced residual capacity than adults. Thus, they are more vulnerable to respiratory distress during life-threatening injuries.[33,39]

Physiological Differences

Circulatory System

Depending on their stage of development, children may have smaller absolute blood volume, lower systemic vascular resistance, smaller blood vessels, and more subcutaneous tissue than adults.[33] Furthermore, children are vulnerable to certain types of shock, most commonly hypovolemic shock. This occurs from a decreased preload from extravascular or intravascular fluid loss, which subsequently results in decreased cardiac output.[40] A rapid deterioration with little warning may follow.[2]

Temperature Stability and Regulation

Because of their larger head size and increased BSA, children are at increased risk for heat loss and hypothermia.[33] Additional factors that affect the temperature stability and regulation of children include thin skin, evaporative heat loss due to lack of subcutaneous tissue, and increased caloric and energy expenditures. The use of thermal blankets, as well as warmed resuscitation rooms, fluids, and inhaled gases, may be required for treatment while undergoing resuscitative measures.[2]

Ventilation

When managing a child's ventilation, the NP should consider the anatomic differences of pediatric patients' airways when compared to those of adults. For instance, children have a shorter trachea, a larger tongue, and a glottic opening that is anterior and superior to that of an adult.[33] The Broselow-Hinkle measuring tape is recommended for selecting drug doses and equipment sizes during pediatric resuscitation. This tape has drug dosages and equipment sizes printed directly on the apparatus, thus eliminating the need for the practitioner to perform calculations during resuscitation efforts.[41] Meticulous fluid management is critical in pediatric patients, and normal saline or lactated Ringer's solution should be administered to restore intravascular volume.[42]

Glycogen (Energy) Stores

A limited store of glycogen with higher relative metabolism puts children at risk for hypoglycemia. Hypoglycemia is most common in newborns and may also appear in older children as a complication of insulin therapy for diabetes.[43]

Immunologic Differences

An immature immunologic system creates a greater risk of infection for children. As a result, certain conditions can be magnified or are more likely to appear in pediatric patients than adults. One example is eczema, which can manifest over the child's entire body. As children grow older, the manifestation of these conditions becomes more similar to that of an adult.

Developmental Differences

Because of limited verbal abilities, children may not be able to describe symptoms or localize pain. As children are often dependent on caretakers for food, children may be more vulnerable to food source limitations when potential sources are unavailable or contaminated. Children have limited motor skills to escape injury, as well as limited cognitive abilities to conceptualize their way out of danger, follow directions from others, or recognize threatening circumstances. Moreover, children are often emotionally labile due to their developing brain, which is especially taxed during stressful encounters. Reactions to danger and threats may be dictated by the child's developmental stage, and there are additional concerns when the child has special health care needs.[2]

Psychological Differences

Developmental stages alter the child's emotions in specific ways. Hyperactive startle responses may begin to occur during the newborn stage and last up to 2 months of age. A child may begin to cry more around the third month of life, whereas separation anxiety is developmentally appropriate around 9–12 months of age. Toddlers and preschool age children may exhibit regressive behaviors, such as temper tantrums, clinginess, and problems with separation or sleep.[2] These regressive behaviors may be exacerbated by a major change in a child's life.

Mental health problems tend to particularly manifest in late childhood and early adolescence and can have a detrimental impact on school, relationships, and overall health. The WHO suggests that depression is the leading health care concern among children and adolescents.[44] Depression does not have a single cause, but a number of factors may contribute to depression in children, including genetics, stressful situations, and the child's home environment.[45] Furthermore, depression may manifest in the form of risk-taking behaviors such as alcohol and drug use, unplanned pregnancies, and violent behavior.[44]

Figures

Figure 1.1. Primary teeth eruption. Barkley & Associates, Inc. Published 2015.

Figure 1.2. Permanent teeth eruption. Barkley & Associates, Inc. Published 2015.

References

1. Normal growth and development. A.D.A.M. Medical Encyclopedia. http://www.nlm.nih.gov/medlineplus/ency/article/002456.htm. Updated February 26, 2014. Accessed April 3, 2015.

2. Barkley TW Jr. *Pediatric Primary Care Nurse Practitioner Certification Review/Clinical Update Continuing Education Course*. West Hollywood, CA: Barkley and Associates; 2015.

3. Hagan JF, Shaw JS, Duncan P. (Eds.). *Bright Futures: Guidelines for Health Supervision of Infants, Children, and Adolescents, Pocket Guide.* 3rd ed. Elk Grove Village, IL: American Academy of Pediatrics; 2008.

4. United States Department of Health and Human Services, Centers for Disease Control and Prevention. Growth charts. http://www.cdc.gov/growthcharts. Last updated September 9, 2010. Accessed April 3, 2015.

5. Wagner CL. Counseling the breastfeeding mother. In: Rosenkrantz T, ed. Medscape. http://emedicine.medscape.com/article/979458-overview. Updated February 5, 2015. Accessed April 3, 2015.

6. Fleischer DM. The impact of breastfeeding on the development of allergic disease. In: Basow DS, ed. *UpToDate*. Waltham, MA: UpToDate; 2015. http://www.uptodate.com/contents/the-impact-of-breastfeeding-on-the-development-of-allergic-disease. Last updated September 24, 2014. Accessed April 3, 2015.

7. American Academy of Pediatrics. Breastfeeding and the use of human milk. *Pediatrics*. 2012; 129(3): e827–e841. http://pediatrics.aappublications.org/content/129/3/e827.full.pdf+html

8. Schanler RJ. Infant benefits of breastfeeding. In: Basow DS, ed. *UpToDate*. Waltham, MA: UpToDate; 2015. http://www.uptodate.com/contents/infant-benefits-of-breastfeeding. Last updated March 22, 2015. Accessed April 3, 2015.

9. Hellings PJ. Breastfeeding. In: Burns CE, Dunn AM, Brady MA, Starr NB, Blosser CG, Garzon DL, eds. *Pediatric Primary Care*. 5th ed. Philadelphia, PA: Elsevier Saunders; 2013: 186–201.

10. Vitamin D supplementation for infants. American Academy of Pediatrics web site. http://www.aap.org/en-us/about-the-aap/aap-press-room/Pages/Vitamin-D-Supplementation-for-Infants.aspx. Published March 22, 2010. Accessed April 3, 2015.

11. Pettifor JM. Nutritional rickets. In: Glorieux FH, Pettifor JM, Jüppner H. *Pediatric Bone*. 2nd ed. London: Elsevier/Academic Press; 2012: 625–654.

12. Bright Futures. American Academy of Pediatrics. Nutrition supervision. In: Holt K, Wooldridge N, Story M, Sofka D, eds. *Bright Futures: Nutrition*. 3rd ed. Elk Grove, IL: American Academy of Pediatrics; 2011: 17–111. https://brightfutures.aap.org/pdfs/BFNutrition3rdEditionSupervision.pdf

13. Oral health topics: Fluoride supplements. American Dental Association web site. http://www.ada.org/en/member-center/oral-health-topics/fluoride-supplements.

14. Boom JA. Normal growth patterns in infants and prepubertal children. In: Basow DS, ed. *UpToDate*. Waltham, MA: UpToDate; 2015. http://www.uptodate.com/contents/normal-growth-patterns-in-infants-and-prepubertal-children. Last updated March 13, 2014. Accessed April 3, 2015.

15. American Academy of Pediatrics. Physical appearance and growth: Your 2 year old. Healthy Children web site. http://www.healthychildren.org/English/ages-stages/toddler/Pages/Physical-Appearance-and-Growth-Your-2-Year-Od.aspx. Last updated August 6, 2013. Accessed April 3, 2015.

16. American Academy of Pediatrics. Physical changes during puberty. Healthy Children web site. http://www.healthychildren.org/English/ages-stages/gradeschool/puberty/Pages/Physical-Development-of-School-Age-Children.aspx. Last updated December 19, 2014. Accessed April 3, 2015.

17. Domino FJ. Teething. In: Domino FJ, Baldor RA, Golding J, Grimes JA, eds. *The 5-Minute Clinical Consult 2015.* 23rd ed. Philadelphia, PA: Wolters Kluwer Health; 2014: 1156–1157.

18. Jarvis C. *Physical Examination and Health Assessment.* 6th ed. St. Louis, MO: Elsevier Saunders; 2012.

19. Felluga D. Modules on Freud: On psychosexual development. Introductory Guide to Critical Theory web site. http://www.purdue.edu/guidetotheory/psychoanalysis/freud.html. Last updated January 31, 2011. Accessed April 3, 2015.

20. Phillips SM, Shulman RJ. Measurements of growth in children. In: Basow DS, ed. *UpToDate*. Waltham, MA: UpToDate; 2015. http://www.uptodate.com/contents/measurement-of-growth-in-children. Last updated February 10, 2014. Accessed April 3, 2015.

21. American Academy of Pediatrics. Corrected age for preemies. Healthy Children web site. http://www.healthychildren.org/English/ages-stages/baby/preemie/pages/Corrected-Age-For-Preemies.aspx. Last updated January 8, 2015. Accessed April 3, 2015.

22. United States Department of Health and Human Services, Centers for Disease Control and Prevention. About BMI for children and teens. http://www.cdc.gov/healthyweight/assessing/bmi/childrens_bmi/about_childrens_bmi.html. Last updated July 11, 2014. Accessed April 3, 2015.

23. Willacy H, Tidy C. Denver Developmental Screening Test. Patient web site. http://www.patient.co.uk/doctor/denver-developmental-screening-test. Reviewed December 3, 2014. Accessed April 3, 2015.

24. Health supervision of the well child. In: Porter RS, Kaplan JL, eds. The Merck Manual Online. http://www.merckmanuals.com/professional/pediatrics/approach_to_the_care_of_normal_infants_and_children/health_supervision_of_the_well_child.html#v1077060. Last reviewed April 2014. Accessed April 3, 2015.

25. Haupt M. 4 Month Well Child visit. University of Chicago Department of Pediatrics web site. http://pediatrics.uchicago.edu/chiefs/ClinicCurriculum/documents/4MonthWellChild.pdf. Accessed April 3, 2015.

26. Norton R, Kobusingye O. Injuries. *N Engl J Med.* 2013; 368(18): 1723–1730. doi: 10.1056/NEJMra1109343.

27. Kelly NR. Prevention of poisoning in children. In: Basow DS, ed. *UpToDate.* Waltham, MA: UpToDate; 2015. http://www.uptodate.com/contents/prevention-of-poisoning-in-children. Last updated December 9, 2014. Accessed April 3, 2015.

28. Gill AC, Wesson DE. Firearm injuries in children: Prevention. In: Basow DS, ed. *UpToDate*. Waltham, MA: UpToDate; 2015. http://www.uptodate.com/contents/firearm-injuries-in-children-prevention. Last updated October 30, 2014. Accessed April 3, 2015.

29. Committee on Injury, Violence, and Poison Prevention, Durbin DR. Child passenger safety. *Pediatrics.* 2011; 127(4): 788–793. doi:10.1542/peds.2011-0213

30. Protecting children in your home. Safe Kids Worldwide web site. http://www.safekids.org/infographic/protecting-children-your-home. Accessed April 3, 2015.

31. Merrick MT, Latzman NE. Child maltreatment: A public health overview and prevention considerations. *Online J Issues Nurs.* 2014; 19(1): 2. doi: 10.3912/OJIN.Vol19No01Man02

32. United States Department of Health and Human Services, Administration for Children and Families, Administration on Children Youth and Families, Children's Bureau. Mandatory reporters of child abuse and neglect. https://www.childwelfare.gov/pubPDFs/manda.pdf#page=1&view=Professionals Required to Report. Published 2014. Accessed April 29, 2015.

33. How are children different? Royal Children's Hospital Melbourne web site. http://www.rch.org.au/paed_trauma/manual/11_How_are_children_different. Accessed April 3, 2015.

34. Brandt BL. Household environmental toxins and neurodevelopment in children [professional paper]. Bozeman, MT: Montana State University; 2012. http://scholarworks.montana.edu/xmlui/bitstream/handle/1/966/BrandtB0512.pdf?sequence=1&isAllowed=y

35. United States Department of Health and Human Services, Centers for Disease Control and Prevention, Agency for Toxic Substances and Disease Registry. Principles of pediatric environmental health: How are newborns, infants, and toddlers exposed to and affected by toxicants? http://www.atsdr.cdc.gov/csem/csem.asp?csem=27&po=9. Issued February 15, 2012. Renewed February 15, 2014. Accessed April 3, 2015.

36. American Academy of Pediatrics. Curriculum for managing infectious diseases in early education and child care settings: Module 1, understanding infectious diseases. Healthy Child Care American web site. http://www.healthychildcare.org/PDF/InfDiseases/Module1.pdf. Published 2010. Accessed April 3, 2015.

37. Thompson GH, Stern LC, Wilber JH, Son-Hing JP. The multiply injured child. In: Mencio GA, Swiontkowski MF, eds. *Green's Skeletal Trauma in Children.* 5th ed. Philadelphia, PA: Elsevier Saunders; 2015: 59–85.

38. Mayo Clinic Staff. Greenstick fractures. Mayo Clinic web site. http://www.mayoclinic.org/diseases-conditions/greenstick-fractures/basics/definition/con-20027302. Reviewed June 18, 2013. Accessed April 3, 2015.

39. Kache S. Pediatric airway and respiratory physiology. Stanford School of Medicine Pediatric Housestaff web site. http://peds.stanford.edu/Rotations/picu/pdfs/10_Peds_Airway.pdf. Accessed April 3, 2015.

40. Pomerantz WJ, Roback MG. Physiology and classification of shock in children. In: Basow DS, ed. *UpToDate*. Waltham, MA: UpToDate; 2015. http://www.uptodate.com/contents/physiology-and-classification-of-shock-in-children?source=search_result&search=shock+children&selectedTitle=4~150#H8. Last updated December 17, 2014. Accessed April 3, 2015.

41. Jevon P. Paediatric advanced life support: A practical guide for nurses. 2nd ed. Chichester, West Sussex: John Wiley & Sons; 2012.

42. Pomerantz WJ, Roback MG. Hypovolemic shock in children: Initial evaluation and management. In: Basow DS, ed. *UpToDate*. Waltham, MA: UpToDate; 2015. http://www.uptodate.com/contents/hypovolemic-shock-in-children-initial-evaluation-and-management?source=see_link#H13. Last updated September 18, 2014. Accessed April 3, 2015.

43. Hypoglycemia and low blood sugar in children. Boston Children's Hospital web site. http://www.childrenshospital.org/health-topics/conditions/hypoglycemia-and-low-blood-sugar. Accessed April 3, 2015.

44. Adolescents and mental health. World Health Organization web site. http://www.who.int/maternal_child_adolescent/topics/adolescence/mental_health/en. Accessed April 3, 2015.

45. Continuing medical education: Frequently asked questions. American Academy of Child & Adolescent Psychiatry web site. http://www.aacap.org/aacap/Families_and_Youth/Resource_Centers/Depression_Resource_Center/FAQ.aspx. Accessed April 3, 2015.

Chapter 2

Immunization Recommendations

QUESTIONS

1. Which of the following vaccines should <u>not</u> be given to patients who are pregnant?

   a. The inactivated polio vaccine

   b. The measles, mumps, rubella vaccine

   c. The influenza vaccine

   d. The tetanus, diptheria, and acellular pertussis vaccine

2. If a newborn's mother is HBsAg-positive, when should the nurse practitioner order the hepatitis B vaccine for the newborn?

   a. Within 12 hours after birth

   b. Prior to home discharge

   c. One week after birth

   d. Not until 1 year of age

3. By the age of 3, a child should have received the third dose of all of the following immunizations <u>except</u>:

   a. Hepatitis B

   b. Diptheria, tetanus, and acellular pertussis

   c. *Haemophilus influenzae*

   d. Varicella

4. The measles, mumps, and rubella vaccine (MMR) may be given simultaneously with tuberculosis testing and the purified protein derivative (PPD) skin test, but it is commonly recommended to postpone the PPD for 4–6 weeks for which reason?

   a. To avoid unwanted protein binding to the MMR vaccine

   b. To avoid adverse effects

   c. To allow the MMR vaccine to form antibodies

   d. To avoid possible false negative on the PPD test

5. You are treating a 24-month-old infant who has completed her PCV13 series. All of the following are possible preexisting conditions that would require administration of one dose of the 23PS formulation <u>except</u>:

   a. Chronic cardiac disease

   b. Hepatitis B

   c. Renal failure

   d. Asplenia

6. Which of the following is <u>not</u> a typical minor adverse reaction to a vaccine?

   a. Low-grade temperature

   b. Local tenderness

   c. Local pallor

   d. Local muscle soreness

7. At least how many months apart should hepatitis A doses of vaccines be administered?

   a. At least 1 month apart

   b. At least 3 months apart

   c. At least 6 months apart

   d. At least 12 months apart

8. Sharon, age 16, has just received her first meningococcal conjugate vaccine. How long should she ideally wait before receiving the booster dose?

   a. Eight weeks

   b. Six months

   c. One year

   d. The patient does not require a booster dose.

9. Jason, age 8 years, is going to South America on vacation with his parents. His parents want to know which vaccinations he needs to keep from getting sick. Assuming he is caught up on all of his other vaccinations, which of the following vaccines would be <u>least</u> necessary for Jason?

   a. Hepatitis A vaccine

   b. Typhoid vaccine

   c. Malaria vaccine

   d. Tetanus, diptheria, acellular pertussis vaccine

10. Jack, a school-aged child, has a 4-year-old brother who has just been diagnosed with acute lymphocytic leukemia. Jack should receive which of the following flu vaccine preparations?

    a. Inhaled influenza vaccine

    b. Quadrivalent inactivated influenza vaccine

    c. Trivalent inactivated influenza vaccine

    d. The child should not receive any influenza vaccine at risk of shedding the virus to the sibling.

RATIONALES

1. b

The measles, mumps, and rubella (MMR) vaccine should not be given to patients who are pregnant or immunosuppressed, as it is a live virus vaccine. It is recommended that women should not become pregnant within 4 weeks after receiving the MMR vaccine, but they can typically be vaccinated after giving birth or while breastfeeding, as the risk to the fetus has passed. The tetanus, diptheria, and acellular pertussis vaccine is usually safe to give to pregnant patients, and the ideal time to vaccinate is between 27 and 36 weeks of gestation. The inactivated poliovirus may be given to pregnant women if clearly needed. The influenza vaccine is commonly recommended for pregnant women to protect both the mother and unborn child.

2. a

Infants who are born to HBsAg-positive mothers should be given the hepatitis B vaccine within 12 hours of being born. Pregnancy is not a contraindication to vaccination, so pregnant mothers can receive the hepatitis B vaccine. However, a newborn born to a hepatitis B carrier would still typically need to receive a vaccination shortly after birth. If the mother tests positive for HBsAg when her status was previously unknown, hepatitis B immune globulin should be given to the infant no later than 1 week of age. The hepatitis A vaccine is commonly given at 1 year of age.

3. d

By the age of 3, a child should have received only one dose of the varicella vaccine, with the subsequent dose administered between the ages of 4 and 6. By 3 years of age, children should have received all three doses of the hepatitis B vaccine, ideally administered at 0, 2, and 6 months of age. The three primary immunizations for diphtheria, tetanus, and acellular pertussis would typically be administered at 2, 4, and 6 months of age, followed by boosters at 15 months and 6 years of age. The *Haemophilus influenzae* vaccine would likewise usually be administered at 2, 4, and 6 months of age, followed by one booster at 12 months.

4. d

The measles, mumps, and rubella (MMR) vaccine may be given simultaneously with tuberculosis testing and the purified protein derivative (PPD) skin test, but it is recommended to postpone the PPD for 4–6 weeks to avoid a possible suppressive response to the PPD, which may potentially yield a false negative response. Unwanted protein binding to MMR and risk of adverse effects are not common contraindications to supplying the vaccine simultaneously. Furthermore, the formation of antibodies from MMR typically has no effect on the efficacy of the PPD test.

5. b

A 24-month-old with hepatitis B who has completed the PCV13 series would not typically need a 23PS vaccination. Chronic cardiac disease, renal failure, and asplenia are all conditions for which the nurse practitioner should consider administering a dose of 23PS, so long as the patient is 24 months of age and has completed the PCV13 series. Other conditions that would typically call for necessary administration of a 23PS dose include splenic dysfunction, HIV, nephrotic syndrome, pulmonary diseases, and diabetes.

6. c

Local pallor is not a typical minor adverse reaction to a vaccine; rather, many vaccines produce localized redness and swelling as common minor side effects. Other typical adverse reactions to vaccines may include local muscle soreness, low-grade temperature, and local tenderness.

7. c

The two doses of the hepatitis A vaccine should ideally be administered at least 6 months apart between 1 and 2 years of age. The first booster dose protects against hepatitis A for 1 year and allows the body to make antibodies against the virus. The subsequent dose, given after 6 months, acts to protect against hepatitis A for 20 years. Giving the second vaccine after 1 or 3 months does not typically allow the body enough time to make antibodies to the virus. Although waiting 12 months for the second vaccination is not recommended because the efficacy of protection from the first vaccine might dwindle, the second vaccination should still be received as soon as possible.

8. d

If the meningococcal conjugate vaccine is given at the age of 16 or older, a booster dose is not considered necessary. However, it is recommended that patients receive the first dose between 11 and 12 years of age. Patients who receive the first vaccination prior to age 16 should require a booster at age 16, at least 8 weeks after the first dose was administered. Although 6 months is the recommended time frame between hepatitis A vaccines, the meningococcal conjugate vaccine requires a different time frame based on the patient's age. The time frame of 1 year would only be relevant if the patient received her first dose of meningococcal conjugate vaccine at age 15, as she would require a booster at age 16.

9. d

Patients who are current on their vaccinations would not typically require a subsequent tetanus, diptheria, and acellular pertussis vaccine, as the vaccine commonly protects for 10 years and is not particularly indicated for foreign travel. Because hepatitis A can be acquired through contaminated food and water, the hepatitis A vaccine is recommended for all travelers. Similarly, the typhoid vaccine is recommended for people travelling to rural areas. The malaria vaccination is recommended to travelers visiting foreign countries that pose a risk of encountering infected mosquitos.

10. c

The sibling should definitely receive a flu vaccine and the trivalent influenza vaccine is the preferred formulation, as the quadrivalent product is commonly recommended after the age of 18. The inhaled influenza vaccine is a live virus and not recommended for families of immunocompromised patients.

DISCUSSION

Hepatitis B Vaccination

Overview

The hepatitis B (HepB) vaccination is given to newborns in a series of three intramuscular (IM) injections that should be completed by 18 months of age.[1] All newborns should receive the first dose prior to hospital discharge. The second and third doses are usually administered 1 month and 6 months after the initial dose. For the initial dose at birth, only a monovalent HepB vaccine should be administered. Either a monovalent or combination vaccine may be used for the second and third doses.[2] Pediatric patients younger than the age of 18 who have not received the vaccine should be vaccinated as soon as possible.[1]

The Centers for Disease Control and Prevention (CDC) recommends that infants born to mothers who are positive for the hepatitis B surface antigen (HBsAg) should receive a HepB vaccine and a 0.5 ml dose of hepatitis B immune globulin (HBIG) within 12 hours of birth. These two injections should be administered at separate sites. The second dose of HepB should then be given at 1–2 months of age, and the last dose should be administered by 6 months of age. An additional HBsAG titre should be drawn at 9–12 months of age, and one additional dose of HepB should be given if the child does not demonstrate immunity.[3]

If the HBsAg status of the mother is unknown, the nurse practitioner (NP) should determine her status, assess the baby's status immediately after birth, and administer HepB within 12 hours of birth. If the mother is positive for the antigen, HBIG should be administered to the newborn by no later than 1 week of age.[3]

Rotavirus Vaccine (Rota)

Overview

The rotavirus vaccine is given as a series of three doses to newborns at 6 and 32 weeks of age. The NP may order the first dose at a minimum 6 weeks of age, and each subsequent dose is given at a minimum of 4-week intervals. The rotavirus vaccination series should be completed by 8 months of age.[4]

Diphtheria/Tetanus/Acellular Pertussis Vaccines (DTaP)

Overview

The DTaP vaccine is given in a series of three primary doses and two boosters. The three primary doses are given at 2 months, 4 months, and 6 months of age. Once this series is completed, the first booster is administered at 15–18 months of age and the second at 4–6 years of age.[5]

Tetanus, Diphtheria, Acellular Pertussis Vaccines (Tdap)

Overview

The Tdap vaccine is administered in a single dose at 11 or 12 years of age. After this dose is given, tetanus-diphtheria (Td) boosters are currently recommended to be given every 10 years.[6]

Children older than 7 years of age who have not received the DTaP series should receive the Tdap vaccine as the first dose of their catch-up series.[7] Due to a resurgence of pertussis, Tdap boosters should also be considered for adults who will be around infants.

Haemophilus Influenzae Type B (Hib) Conjugate Vaccine

Overview

The *Haemophilus influenzae* type b (Hib) conjugate vaccine is given in a series of three primary doses and one booster. The primary doses are administered at 2 months, 4 months, and 6 months of age, and the booster is given at 12–15 months of age. The first dose of the Hib vaccine should not be given before 6 weeks of age, and no dosage of the Hib vaccine is recommended for children at 5 years of age or later.[8]

Pneumococcal Vaccine (PCV13 or PPSV23)

Overview

The pneumococcal vaccine consists of two different types: the 13-valent pneumococcal conjugate vaccine (PCV13) and the 23-valent pneumococcal polysaccharide vaccine (PPSV23).[9]

The PCV13 vaccine (Prevnar) is recommended for children younger than 5 years of age and is given as a series that consists of three primary doses and one booster. The three primary doses of PCV13 should be given at 2 months, 4 months, and

6 months of age, and the booster is given at 12–15 months of age.[10]

The PPSV23 vaccine (Pneumovax) series is recommended for children older than 2 years of age who are at high risk of disease due to immuno-compromising conditions.[11] These conditions may include HIV infection, renal failure, nephrotic syndrome, and diabetes.[10]

Polio Vaccine (IPV)

Overview

The polio vaccine is administered in a series of four doses. The first three are given at 2 months, 4 months, and 6–18 months of age, and a booster is administered at 4–6 years of age.[5] The inactivated polio vaccine is recommended for all four of these scheduled vaccines. The CDC no longer recommends the oral polio vaccine because this formulation is strongly correlated with the onset of paralysis in rare instances.[12]

Influenza Vaccine

Overview

The influenza vaccine should be administered to children 6 months of age and older.[13] In children 6–35 months of age, the recommended annual dose is 0.25 ml IM. The dose increases to 0.50 ml IM for children 3 years of age and older.[11] Children younger than 9 years who have not yet received the influenza vaccine should receive two doses administered 1 month apart. Once children reach 9 years of age, they only need a single dose annually.[13,14]

Inactivated influenza vaccines are offered in either quadrivalent or trivalent formulations.[15] The quadrivalent formulation covers four strains, whereas the trivalent formulation covers three. Additionally, a live attenuated virus can be distributed via FluMist and may serve as an alternative to trivalent vaccines in healthy children older than 2 years.[11]

Measles, Mumps, and Rubella (MMR)

Overview

The MMR vaccine is given in a series of two doses. The first dose should be administered at 12–15 months of age, and the second dose should be administered at 4–6 years of age.[16] Children aged 4–6 years who have not yet received the first dose must wait at least 4 weeks between doses. If a patient is exposed to measles or is travelling to endemic areas, the NP can order the MMR vaccine as early as 6 months of age; however, the primary series must be resumed at the appropriate time.

Varicella

Overview

The varicella vaccine is given in a series of two doses: The first should be administered between 12–15 months of age, and the second should be administered at 4–6 years of age.[17] According to the CDC, these two doses should be a minimum of 3 months apart when administered to children younger than the age of 13.[5] Both doses should be administered after the age of 12 months if no evidence of immunity is available and the parents cannot recall a history of chicken pox. Moreover, it is preferable to separate the varicella vaccine from the MMR vaccine by 1 month, as concomitant administration of the vaccines has been associated with rash and a higher rate of fever.[17]

Hepatitis A Vaccine

Overview

The CDC recommends that two doses of the hepatitis A vaccine should be administered to all children between 1 and 2 years of age.[18] Both of these doses should be given at a minimum of 6 months apart, although these may be separated by up to 18 months.[5]

Meningococcal Vaccine

Overview

The meningococcal vaccine is available as a conjugate vaccine and as a polysaccharide vaccine. The meningococcal conjugate vaccine is recommended for children who are at an increased risk of meningococcal disease and is administered between 2 months and 10 years of age. Booster doses may be given under certain circumstances or conditions that increase the risk of meningococcal disease. For older children and adolescents, the initial dose of the meningococcal polysaccharide vaccine is administered at 11 or 12 years of age with a booster given from age 16 to 18.[19] It is important to adhere to this schedule because incidence of meningococcal disease peaks in patients between the ages of 16 and 21 years.[5] No booster is necessary if an adolescent receives his or her first dose at 16 years of age or later.[19]

Human Papillomavirus Vaccine (HPV)

Overview

HPV is the most common sexually transmitted disease and males and females are both recommended to be vaccinated against HPV.[14] The human papillomavirus (HPV) vaccine is administered in a series of three doses, the first of which is recommended for all adolescents at 11 or 12 years of age. The second dose is then given 1–2 months after the first dose, with the third dose administered 6 months after the initial dose.[5] Adolescents are advised to remain seated for at least 15 minutes after receiving the HPV vaccine, as the vaccine may produce postural hypotension, labile syncope, and vasovagal responses shortly after administration.[11]

Two preparations of the HPV vaccine are commercially available: the HPV quadrivalent vaccine (HPV4), distributed as Gardasil, and the HPV bivalent vaccine (HPV2), which is distributed as Cervarix. Females may be given either HPV2 or HPV4, but males may only be administered HPV4.[5] Both HPV2 and HPV4 protect against oncologic strains of HPV (e.g., types 16 and 18), which cover cancerous lesions of the cervix, anus, penis, and oropharynx, as well as genital warts and recurrent papillomatosis. The HPV4 protects against cancerous lesions and HPV types 6 and 11, which cause the majority of genital warts in both females and males.[20]

References

1. Centers for Disease Control and Prevention. Hepatitis B in short. http://www.cdc.gov/vaccines/vpd-vac/hepb/in-short-adult.htm#who. Last updated August 21, 2012. Accessed April 3, 2015.

2. Centers for Disease Control and Prevention. Hepatitis B vaccination. http://www.cdc.gov/vaccines/vpd-vac/hepb. Last updated February 3, 2014. Accessed April 3, 2015.

3. CDC recommendation for infant vaccination. Hepatitis B Foundation web site. http://www.hepb.org/patients/infant_vaccination_cdc_summary.htm. Accessed April 3, 2015.

4. Centers for Disease Control and Prevention. Rotavirus vaccine – Questions and answers. http://www.cdc.gov/vaccines/vpd-vac/rotavirus/vac-faqs.htm. Last updated September 14, 2012. Accessed April 3, 2015.

5. Centers for Disease Control and Prevention. Recommended immunization schedules for persons age 0 through 18 years. http://www.cdc.gov/vaccines/schedules/hcp/imz/child-adolescent.html. Last updated January 28, 2015. Accessed April 3, 2015.

6. Centers for Disease Control and Prevention. Tdap vaccine: What you need to know. http://www.cdc.gov/vaccines/hcp/vis/vis-statements/tdap.pdf. Published February 24, 2015. Accessed April 3, 2015.

7. DTaP vaccine. A.D.A.M. Medical Encyclopedia. http://www.nlm.nih.gov/medlineplus/druginfo/meds/a682198.html. Last revised May 15, 2014. Accessed April 3, 2015.

8. Haemophilus influenzae type b (Hib) vaccine. A.D.A.M. Medical Encyclopedia. http://www.nlm.nih.gov/medlineplus/druginfo/meds/a607015.html. Last revised April 15, 2014. Accessed April 3, 2015.

9. Centers for Disease Control and Prevention. Pneumococcal vaccination. http://www.cdc.gov/VACCINES/VPD-VAC/pneumo/default.htm#vacc. Last updated February 10, 2015. Accessed April 3, 2015.

10. Healthwise, Inc. Pneumococcal vaccine. WebMD. http://children.webmd.com/vaccines/pneumococcal-vaccine-1?page=2. Reviewed May 26, 2014. Accessed April 3, 2015.

11. Live attenuated influenza vaccine [LAIV] (The nasal spray flu vaccine). Centers for Disease Control and Prevention web site. http://www.cdc.gov/flu/about/qa/nasalspray.htm. Last updated September 9, 2014. Accessed April 3, 2015.

12. A look at each vaccine: Polio vaccine. Children's Hospital of Philadelphia Vaccine Education Center web site. http://www.chop.edu/service/vaccine-education-center/a-look-at-each-vaccine/polio-vaccine.html. Reviewed May 2013. Accessed April 3, 2015.

13. Influenza vaccine, inactivated or recombinant. A.D.A.M. Medical Encyclopedia. http://www.nlm.nih.gov/medlineplus/ency/article/002025.htm. Last reviewed September 15, 2014. Accessed April 3, 2015.

14. Barkley TW Jr. *Pediatric Primary Care Nurse Practitioner Certification Review/Clinical Update Continuing Education Course*. West Hollywood, CA: Barkley and Associates; 2015.

15. Grohskopf LA, Shay DK, Shimabukuro TT, et al. Prevention and control of seasonal influenza with vaccines: recommendations of the Advisory Committee on Immunization Practices — United States, 2013–2014. *MMWR Morb Mortal Wkly Rep*. 2013; 62(RR07): 1–43. http://www.cdc.gov/mmwr/preview/mmwrhtml/rr6207a1.htm.

16. MMR vaccine (measles, mumps, rubella). A.D.A.M. Medical Encyclopedia. http://www.nlm.nih.gov/medlineplus/druginfo/meds/a601176.html. Last reviewed July 18, 2012. Accessed April 3, 2015.

17. Centers for Disease Control and Prevention. Routine varicella vaccination. http://www.cdc.gov/vaccines/vpd-vac/varicella/hcp-routine-vacc.htm. Last updated April 5, 2012. Accessed April 3, 2015.

18. Healthwise, Inc. Hepatitis A and B vaccines. WebMD. http://children.webmd.com/vaccines/hepatitis-a-and-b-vaccines?page=2. Reviewed May 26, 2014. Accessed April 3, 2015.

19. Meningococcal vaccine. Vaccines.gov. http://www.vaccines.gov/diseases/meningitis/#. Accessed April 3, 2015.

20. Centers for Disease Control and Prevention. HPV vaccine - Questions and answers. http://www.cdc.gov/vaccines/vpd-vac/hpv/vac-faqs.htm. Last updated August 6, 2014. Accessed April 3, 2015.

Table 2.1 Recommended immunization schedule for persons 0–18 years, United States, 2015

Vaccine	Birth	1 mo	2 mos	4 mos	6 mos	9 mos	12 mos	15 mos	18 mos	19–23 mos	2–3 yrs	4–6 yrs	7–10 yrs	11–12 yrs	13–15 yrs	16–18 yrs
Hepatitis B	1st dose	2nd dose			3rd dose											
Rotavirus			1st dose	2nd dose												
DTap: < 7 yrs			1st dose	2nd dose	3rd dose			4th dose				5th dose				
Tdap: ≥ 7 yrs														Tdap		
Haemophilus influenzae type b			1st dose	2nd dose	See footnote		3rd or 4th dose									
PCV13			1st dose	2nd dose	3rd dose		4th dose									
PPSV23																
IPV (< 18 yrs)			1st dose	2nd dose	3rd dose							4th dose				
Influenza (IIV; LAIV)					Annual vaccine (IIV only) 1 or 2 doses						Annual vaccine (LAIV or IIV) 1 or 2 doses		Annual vaccine (LAIV or IIV) 1 dose only			
MMR							1st dose					2nd dose				
VAR							1st dose					2nd dose				
Hep A							2 dose series, see footnote									
HPV2: females; HPV4: males and females)														3-dose series		
Meningococcal														1st dose		Booster
Key	Range of recommended ages for all children				Range of recommended ages for catch-up immunization			Range of recommended ages for certain high-risk groups					Range of recommended ages during which catch-up is encouraged and for certain high-risk groups			Not routinely recom-mended

Note. DTap = Diptheria, tetanus, & acellular pertussis; Tdap = Tetanus, diphtheria, & acellular pertussis, PCV13 = Pneumococcal conjugate; PPSV23 = Pneumococcal polysaccharide; IPV = Inactivated polio virus; MMR = Measles, mumps, & rubella, VAR = Varicella; Hep A = Hepatitis A, HPV = Human papillomavirus *Note.* Adapted with permission from *Recommended immunization schedule for persons 0–18 years, United States, 2015*, The Centers for Disease Control and Prevention. http://www.cdc.gov/vaccines/schedules/downloads/child/0-18yrs-schedule.pdf. Published 2015. Accessed April 2015.

Chapter 3

Genetic Evaluation

QUESTIONS

1. Which of these couples in the early stages of their pregnancy would least require a genetic screening for mutations in the HEXA gene?

    a. An Inuit mother and a Louisiana Cajun father

    b. An African-American mother and a Druze father

    c. An Ashkenazi Jewish mother and a Scots-Irish father

    d. A Pinoy mother and a French Canadian father

2. Seizures and dementia can manifest in infants and young pediatric patients as a typical result of which of the following hereditary disorders?

    a. Klinefelter's syndrome

    b. Tay-Sachs disease

    c. Turner's syndrome

    d. Marfan syndrome

3. Alex, an 11-year-old male, comes to your clinic for a physical examination. During the examination, you notice that his spine is severely curved in the lumbar and thoracic areas. Although the diagnosis is concurrent, you also know that this finding is most consistent with which of the following genetic conditions?

    a. Marfan syndrome

    b. Down syndrome

    c. Turner's syndrome

    d. DiGeorge syndrome

4. Which of these factors is not a typical indication to recommend a prenatal evaluation for genetic disorders?

    a. The mother has experienced two stillbirths.

    b. The father has a brother with Down syndrome.

    c. The father worked with pesticides 3 years ago.

    d. The mother is of African descent.

5. Which of these genetic disorders is not associated with cardiac defects?

    a. DiGeorge syndrome

    b. Marfan syndrome

    c. Turner's syndrome

    d. Tay-Sachs disease

6. Which of these factors is most likely to increase the risk of Down syndrome in infants?

   a. Advanced maternal age

   b. Intrauterine infection during the second trimester

   c. Alcoholism during pregnancy

   d. Smoking during pregnancy

7. Which of the following is true regarding Turner syndrome?

   a. It presents as a result of mutations in the HEXA gene.

   b. It is the most common sex-chromosome anomaly found in females.

   c. It typically presents with tall stature and kyphoscoliosis.

   d. It typically presents with increased risk of infection due to thymus aplasia.

8. Which of these conditions is least likely to be inherited through genetics or other parental factors?

   a. Down syndrome

   b. Marfan syndrome

   c. Klinefelter's syndrome

   d. Tay-Sachs disease

9. Which of these genetic disorders is most likely to lead to blindness in later life?

   a. Turner's syndrome

   b. DiGeorge syndrome

   c. Kleinfelter's syndrome

   d. Marfan syndrome

10. You are counseling one of your pregnant patients on the prevalence of genetic disorders. If the baby has no predisposition for a specific genetic disorder, his chance of being born with a major malformation is most likely:

   a. Approximately 2%

   b. Approximately 5%

   c. Approximately 8%

   d. Approximately 10%

RATIONALES

1. b

The mutations in the HEXA gene that result in Tay-Sachs disease are not particularly common in either African-American or Druze populations. Tay-Sachs disease is closely linked to Ashkenazi Jewish populations; however, the mutations that produce the condition are also common in French Canadian and Louisiana Cajun populations.

2. b

Tay-Sachs disease is a progressive disorder that destroys nerve cells in the brain and spinal cord, commonly producing symptoms such as dementia in pediatric patients diagnosed with the disease and eventually leading to death. Some cases of Klinefelter's syndrome may lead to seizures due to hypocalcemia; however, dementia is not typically associated with the condition, and patients with Klinefelter's are more likely to present with learning disabilities and personality impairment. Turner's syndrome and Marfan syndrome are not degenerative disorders affecting neurological development; however, some patients with Turner's syndrome may develop learning disabilities. Marfan syndrome is not typically known to produce dementia.

3. a

Kyphoscoliosis, a combination of both kyphosis and scoliosis, is a common phenotypic presentation of Marfan syndrome. Children with Down syndrome or DiGeorge syndrome may develop scoliosis, but rarely present with kyphoscoliosis. Turner syndrome may likewise present with scoliosis; however, this condition only presents in females as the result of a missing X chromosome.

4. c

Exposure to toxic chemicals is a common indicator for genetic evaluation if the fetus itself is exposed; as it was the father, not the fetus, who experienced prior exposure to toxic chemicals, this scenario does not strongly indicate the need for genetic evaluation. A history of miscarriages and stillbirths, as well as a family history of mental retardation, are common indicators for genetic evaluation. Depending on circumstances, ethnic background may be an indicator as well, as the gene responsible for sickle cell anemia is more likely to present in individuals with African or African-American ancestry.

5. d

Tay-Sachs disease is an irreversible condition associated with neurological degeneration, not cardiac defects. DiGeorge syndrome often results in congenital heart defects such as aortic arch anomalies, resulting in significant morbidity and mortality in pediatric patients. Patients with Marfan syndrome may present with aortic regurgitation and mitral valve prolapse at birth, and coarctation of the aorta is a common congenital heart defect in patients with Turner's syndrome.

6. a

Advanced maternal age is a strong risk factor for Down syndrome. As the disorder typically occurs as a result of trisomy that develops at conception, intrauterine infection during the second trimester is not viewed as a risk factor. Some studies suggest a link between alcohol intake and smoking during pregnancy and Down syndrome; results, however, are inconclusive.

7. b

Turner's syndrome, also known as XO karyotype, is the most common sex-chromosome anomaly found in females occurring as a result of a missing or altered X chromosome. Tay-Sachs disease, a genetic disorder particular to the Ashkenazic Jewish population and other ethnic groups, is not a sex-chromosome anomaly. Although Turner's syndrome may present with scoliosis, tall stature and kyphoscoliosis are more common indicators of Marfan's syndrome. DiGeorge syndrome often manifests with cardiac malformations, thymus aplasia, and an associated increased susceptibility to infection; Turner's syndrome, on the other hand, is more likely to produce increased risk of autoimmune disorders later in life.

8. c

Klinefelter's syndrome is not an inherited condition, since one of its mainstay characteristics is infertility; rather, it is commonly attributed to the failure of chromosomal separation during meiosis. Although maternal age may be a factor for the onset of the condition, Klinefelter's is not inherited via the genetic pool. Down syndrome may typically be attributed to parental age or presence of the genetic translocation for Down syndrome. Marfan syndrome is an inherited condition caused by mutations in the FBN1 gene. Tay-Sachs disease primarily presents among populations with common mutations in the HEXA gene, which primarily appear in Ashkenazi Jews, but have been seen in Louisiana Cajuns and Quebecois French-Canadians.

9. d

Patients with Marfan syndrome often exhibit ectopia lentis and have an increased chance of experiencing retinal detachment and glaucoma, which can lead to blindness. Patients with Turner's syndrome are more likely to experience strabismus, cataracts, and red-green color blindness. DiGeorge syndrome may produce strabismus and amblyopia but does not significantly increase the risk of blindness. Although patients with Klinefelter's syndrome have presented with myopia and bilaterial retinal detachment, structural eye abnormalities are not a common feature of the condition.

10. a

Approximately 2% of all live births are affected by a major genetic malformation. About 40%–45% of these accountable genetic disorders are usually diagnosed during the neonatal period and 80% are commonly diagnosed before the child is 6 months old.

DISCUSSION

Genetic Evaluation

Overview

Genetic disorders are basically uncommon, with major malformations occurring in approximately 2% of all live births.[1,2] Genetic disorders include single gene disorders, chromosomal abnormalities, and multifactorial disorders.[3] Single gene disorders occur after a mutation in the DNA sequence of a single gene. This mutation can occur within the sperm or egg, or can be passed on to a child from either parent. Single gene disorders can be autosomal (e.g., sickle cell disease) or X-linked (e.g., fragile X syndrome).[3]

Chromosomal abnormalities occur when the normal 23 pairs of chromosomes are altered to be more or less than 23 pairs. Conditions that derive from this kind of abnormality include such problems as Down syndrome and Turner's syndrome.[3] Multifactorial disorders involve variations in multiple genes and environmental factors.[3] Alzheimer's disease and hypothyroidism are two multifactorial disorders.

Only 40%–45% of all genetic disorders are diagnosed in the neonatal period, but about 80% are identified before the age of 6 months.[1]

Presentation

A genetic evaluation should be conducted if certain risk factors are present. Some indications include advanced parental age, which is classified as about 35 years or older,[4] and a maternal history of miscarriages or stillbirths.[5] Genetic testing is warranted if the mother has abnormal tests during pregnancy, has been exposed to teratogenic substances (e.g., x-rays, chemicals, drugs), has had difficulty with conception, or has experienced a genetic condition with a previous pregnancy.[6] Finally, many conditions in a patient's family history may necessitate a genetic evaluation, such as a history of birth defects, mental retardation, growth retardation, neurologic conditions, or familial conditions.[7]

Routine newborn screening tests vary from state to state; however, all states screen for phenylketonuria, congenital hypothyroidism, and galactosemia, in addition to other metabolic or genetic-associated disorders. Parents in specific ethnic groups that are at higher risk for certain genetically-acquired conditions (e.g., sickle cell anemia, 1 per 600 people of African descent; Tay-Sachs, 1 per 3,500 Ashkenazi Jews) may choose to be evaluated for carrier status.[8,9]

When evaluating a child for genetically-acquired conditions, a child's phenotype and genotype should be considered. Phenotypic indications for genetic evaluation include: dysmorphic features, developmental delay, below average intelligence, short stature, failure to thrive, progressive deterioration of health status, and seizures.[3]

A genogram is a genetic family history used to assess a child's genotype. Family members' histories of miscarriages, stillbirths, and other abnormalities should also be obtained. If the child's pedigree is concerning, a prenatal screening and diagnosis should be conducted for subsequent pregnancies.[4,10]

Trisomy 21 (Down Syndrome)

Overview

A variety of chromosomal abnormalities, collectively known as "syndromes," may develop spontaneously or as a result of either parent's genetic influence. Trisomy 21, or Down syndrome, occurs if a third chromosome 21 is present. The condition occurs in approximately 1:691 births.[11] The incidence of Down syndrome is greater when the maternal parent is of advanced age; however, recent studies have found advanced paternal age is also a contributing factor.[12] Down syndrome can be diagnosed prenatally via blood and fetal cell sampling or morphologically after birth.[13] Although a high percentage of patients with Down syndrome die within the first year of life, recent health care advancements have increased the median life expectancy to approximately 49 years.[13]

Presentation

Children with Down syndrome often display delayed growth and development. The degree of retardation may range from mild to severe. Facial features characteristic of Down syndrome include a flat facial profile or abnormal head shape, a flattened nasal bridge, a protruding tongue, inner epicanthal folds, and slanted palpebral fissures. Other physical manifestations may include short broad hands with a single palmar crease, short broad fingers, and hypotonia. Down syndrome infants may also have small ears, a short neck, tiny white spots on the iris, and unstable joints.[6]

Those affected are more likely to have epilepsy, congenital heart disease, endocrine abnormalities, esophageal and duodenal atresia, and hearing and vision impairment. Children with Down syndrome are also at increased risk of leukemia and early dementia.[13,14]

XXY Syndrome (Klinefelter's Syndrome)

Overview

Klinefelter's syndrome, the most common sex-linked chromosomal abnormality in males, is characterized by an extra X chromosome.[15] Although the mortality rate of those with Klinefelter's syndrome is over half, those that do survive do not have a significantly increased rate of mortality compared to healthy individuals.[16]

Presentation

Patients are typically born with no apparent abnormalities. The condition is often diagnosed later in life when the patient experiences infertility.[3] Klinefelter's syndrome is the most common cause of hypogonadism, gynecomastia, and infertility in men.[17]

Phenotypic manifestations of Klinefelter's syndrome include osteoporosis, subnormal libido, and reduction in gross and fine motor skills. Individuals may also have behavioral or mental health problems, poor muscle tone, tremors, and an increased incidence of vascular, endocrine, and autoimmune diseases.[16]

XO Karyotype (Turner's Syndrome)

Overview

Turner's syndrome, or XO karyotype, is the most common sex-chromosome anomaly in females. This syndrome occurs in about 1 in every 2,000 live births. Fetuses with the XO karyotype account for about 10% of all miscarriages.[1,18] Approximately 95% of all embryos affected by Turner's syndrome do not survive to term.[1,19] Although there is limited conclusive data, it is suggested that the life expectancy of an individual is shortened by about ten years.[18]

Presentation

Although karyotype testing may diagnose the condition in early childhood, Turner's syndrome is usually diagnosed around puberty when there is a lack of common signs of sexual maturation.[18] A patient with Turner's syndrome may present with a webbed neck, low hairline, scoliosis, and a "shield"-shaped chest with widely spaced nipples. Other presentations may include learning disabilities, lack of secondary sexual characteristics, and strabismus. Congenital heart disease and urinary tract anomalies are also prevalent concerns in patients with Turner's syndrome.[20,18]

Marfan Syndrome

Overview

Marfan syndrome is an inherited connective tissue disorder in which there is a mutation on the gene that produces the protein fibrillin-1. This results in an increase of the transforming growth factor beta protein, which subsequently causes complications within the connective tissue.[21] These complications affect the skeletal, cardiac, and ophthalmic body systems.[22] Due to these complications, most commonly cardiovascular, Marfan syndrome results in a slightly lower life expectancy than that of a person without Marfan syndrome.[22] Marfan syndrome occurs in approximately 1:5,000 births.[21]

Presentation

The phenotypic presentation of Marfan syndrome may include tall stature, long and thin extremities and fingers, pectus carinatum or excavatum, hyperextension of joints, genu recurvatum, and kyphoscoliosis. Manifestations specific to the head may include a long narrow face and a high-arched, narrow palate.[21] Pediatric patients with Marfan's syndrome may also exhibit cardiovascular issues, such as aortic regurgitation and mitral valve prolapse.[23] Ophthalmic complications may include ectopia lentis and iridodonesis.[21,24,25] The most severe complications may include aortic dissection resulting in sudden death, as well as blindness from lens complications.[21]

Tay-Sachs Disease

Overview

Tay-Sachs disease is a condition occurring from the absence of the enzyme hexosaminidase-A.[26] The disease is mostly found in the Ashkenazic Jewish population and occurs in approximately 1:2,500 live births.[27] Approximately 1 in every 27 Ashkenazic Jews in the United States is a carrier. Other populations that have an increased incidence of the condition include French Canadians and Louisiana Cajuns.[26] Patients with Tay-Sachs disease present normally at birth, but they begin to deteriorate typically between 3 and 6 months of age.[26]

Presentation

Around three to six months of age, those with Tay-Sachs begin to regress while fatty enzymes begin to build up in the brain.[26] Patients may experience decreased muscle tone, listlessness, blindness, deafness, seizures, and dementia. Regression to a vegetative state typically occurs, with death usually occurring around the age of 5.[26]

DiGeorge (Velocardiofacial) Syndrome

Overview

DiGeorge (velocardiofacial) syndrome is a congenital defect involving the parathyroid glands, thymus, and the conotruncal region of the heart[28] that affects 1 out of every 2,000–4,000 individuals in the United States.[29] Although infants with DiGeorge syndrome have an increased risk of mortality, those that live past infancy may live a similar lifespan to that of an individual without DiGeorge syndrome.[29]

Presentation

DiGeorge syndrome often presents with phenotypic manifestations, such as increased susceptibility to infection due to thymic aplasia. Abnormal facies are common as well, such as lateral displacement of inner canthi, short palpebral fissures, short philtrum, micrognathia, and ear anomalies.[29] Pediatric patients with DiGeorge syndrome are often born with congenital heart defects, such as aortic arch anomalies, resulting in significant neonatal morbidity and mortality.[30] DiGeorge syndrome may cause cognitive and behavioral psychiatric problems, such as attention-deficit/hyperactivity disorder or anxiety.[29] Additionally, pediatric patients may be afflicted with hypoparathyroidism and hypocalcaemia, which can cause seizures in infancy.[31,32]

References

1. Barkley TW Jr. Genetic evaluations. In: Barkley TW Jr, ed. *Pediatric Primary Care Nurse Practitioner Certification Review.* West Hollywood, CA: Barkley and Associates; 2015: 24–28.

2. Centers for Disease Control and Prevention, National Center on Birth Defects and Developmental Disabilities. Birth defects: Data and Statistics. http://www.cdc.gov/ncbddd/birthdefects/data.html. Last updated October 20, 2014. Accessed April 3, 2015.

3. Centers for Disease Control and Prevention, National Center on Birth Defects and Developmental Disabilities. Family health history and genetics: Genetics basics. http://www.cdc.gov/ncbddd/genetics/basics.html. Last updated March 3, 2015. Accessed April 3, 2015.

4. Genetic Alliance & The New York-Mid-Atlantic Consortium for Genetic and Newborn Screening Services. Indications for a genetic referral. In *Understanding Genetics: A New York, Mid-Atlantic Guide for Patients and Health Professionals.* Washington, DC: Genetic Alliance; 2009: 29–32. http://www.ncbi.nlm.nih.gov/books/NBK115554/

5. Fretts RC. Stillbirth: diagnosis and management. In: Basow DS, ed. *UpToDate.* Waltham, MA: UpToDate; 2015. http://www.uptodate.com/contents/diagnosis-and-management-of-stillbirth. Last updated June 13, 2014. Accessed April 3, 2015.

6. Centers for Disease Control and Prevention, National Center on Birth Defects and Developmental Disabilities. Family health history and genetics: Genetic counseling. http://www.cdc.gov/ncbddd/genetics/genetic_counseling.html. Last updated March 3, 2015. Accessed April 3, 2015.

7. Interpreting family history. National Coalition for Health Professional Education in Genetics Web site. http://www.nchpeg.org/index.php?option=com_content&view=article&id=170&Itemid=64. Accessed April 3, 2015.

8. Wiener DL. Inborn errors of metabolism. In: Kemp S, ed. Medscape. http://emedicine.medscape.com/article/804757-overview. Updated February 18, 2015. Accessed April 3, 2015.

9. U.S. Department of Health and Human Services, Health Resources, and Services Administration, Discretionary Advisory Committee on Heritable Disorders in Newborns and Children. Newborn screening: Towards a uniform screening panel and system. http://www.hrsa.gov/advisorycommittees/mchbadvisory/heritabledisorders. Chartered April 24, 2013. Accessed April 3, 2015.

10. U.S. Department of Health and Human Services, National Institutes of Health (NIH), U.S. National Library of Medicine, Lester Hill National Center for Biomedical Communications. Handbook: Help me understand genetics. http://ghr.nlm.nih.gov/handbook.pdf. Published March 30, 2015. Accessed April 3, 2015.

11. Down syndrome facts. National Down Syndrome Society Web site. http://www.ndss.org/Down-Syndrome/Down-Syndrome-Facts. Accessed April 3, 2015.

12. Centers for Disease Control and Prevention, National Center on Birth Defects and Developmental Disabilities. Facts about Down syndrome. http://www.cdc.gov/ncbddd/birthdefects/DownSyndrome.html. Last updated October 20, 2014. Accessed April 3, 2015.

13. Chen H, Down syndrome. In: Descartes M, ed. Medscape. http://emedicine.medscape.com/article/943216-overview#showall. Updated August 18, 2014. Accessed April 3, 2015.

14. U.S. Department of Health and Human Services, NIH, Eunice Kennedy Shriver National Institute of Child Health and Human Development. What conditions or disorders are commonly associated with Down syndrome? http://www.nichd.nih.gov/health/topics/down/conditioninfo/Pages/associated.aspx. Last updated April 9, 2014. Accessed April 3, 2015.

15. Frühmesser A, Kotzot D. Chromosomal variants in Klinefelter syndrome. *Sex Dev.* 2011; 5(3): 109–123. doi: 10.1159/000327324

16. Chen H. Klinefelter syndrome clinical presentation. In: Rohena LO, ed. Medscape. http://emedicine.medscape.com/article/945649-clinical#showall. Updated August 20, 2014. Accessed April 3, 2015.

17. Larner AJ. *Neuropsychological Neurology: The Neurocognitive Impairments of Neurological Disorders.* 2nd ed. Cambridge, UK: Cambridge University Press; 2013: 110–144.

18. Overview. Turner Syndrome Society of the United States Web site. http://www.turnersyndrome.org/#!overview/ctzx. Accessed April 3, 2015.

19. Davenport ML, Ross J, Backeljauw PF. Turner syndrome. In: Radovick S, MacGillivray MH, eds. *Pediatric Endocrinology: A Practical Clinical Guide.* 2nd ed. Heidelberg, Germany: Springer; 2013; 109–136.

20. U.S. Department of Health and Human Services, NIH, U. S. National Library of Medicine, Lester Hill National Center for Biomedical Communications. Genetics home reference: Conditions: Turner syndrome. http://ghr.nlm.nih.gov/condition/turner-syndrome. Reviewed January 2012. Published March 30, 2015. Accessed April 3, 2015.

21. What is Marfan syndrome? The Marfan Foundation Web site. http://www.marfan.org/about/Marfan. Accessed April 3, 2015.

22. U.S. Department of Health and Human Services, NIH, National Heart, Lung, and Blood Institute (NHLBI). What is Marfan syndrome? http://www.nhlbi.nih.gov/health/health-topics/topics/mar. Updated October 1, 2010. Accessed April 3, 2015.

23. U.S. Department of Health and Human Services, NIH, NHLBI. What are the signs and symptoms of Marfan syndrome? http://www.nhlbi.nih.gov/health/health-topics/topics/mar/signs.html. Updated October 1, 2010. Accessed April 3, 2015.

24. Eifrig CW. Ectopic lentis clinical presentation. In: Roy H Sr, ed. Medscape. http://emedicine.medscape.com/article/1211159-clinical. Updated March 10, 2015. Accessed April 3, 2015.

25. Hoang QV, Leong JA, Gallego-Pinazo R. Myopia: Ocular and systemic disease. In: Spaide RF, Ohno-Matsui K, Yannuzzi LA. *Pathologic Myopia*. New York, NY: Springer; 2014: 333–344.

26. U.S. Department of Health and Human Services, NIH, National Human Genome Research Institute. Learning about Tay-Sachs disease. http://www.genome.gov/10001220. Last reviewed March 17, 2011. Accessed April 3, 2015.

27. Tegay DH. GM2 gangliosidoses: Introduction and epidemiology. In: Rohena LO, ed. Medscape. http://emedicine.medscape.com/article/951943-overview. Updated December 11, 2014. Accessed April 3, 2015.

28. Horenstein MS, Ardinger R Jr, Ardinger H. Velocardiofacial syndrome. In: Weber HS, ed. Medscape. http://emedicine.medscape.com/article/892655-overview. Updated February 13, 2014. Accessed April 3, 2015.

29. Bawle EV. DiGeorge Syndrome. In: Jyonouchi H, ed. Medscape. http://emedicine.medscape.com/article/886526-overview. Updated March 12, 2014. Accessed April 3, 2015.

30. Chin AJ. Interrupted aortic arch. In: Neish SR, ed. Medscape. http://emedicine.medscape.com/article/896979-overview#showall. Updated August 29, 2013. Accessed April 3, 2015.

31. Immune Deficiency Foundation. DiGeorge syndrome. In: Blaese RM, Stiehm ER, Bonilla FA, Younger ME, eds. *Patient and Family Handbook for Primary Immunodeficiency Diseases*. 5th ed. Towson, MD: Immune Deficiency Foundation; 2013: 72–76. http://primaryimmune.org/idf-publications/patient-family-handbook/

32. Pitukcheewanont P. Pediatric hypoparathyroidism. In: Kemp S, ed. Medscape. http://emedicine.medscape.com/article/922204-overview#showall. Updated March 6, 2014. Accessed April 3, 2015.

Chapter 4

Prenatal Assessment/ Screening

QUESTIONS

1. You are examining a newborn in the nursery. As part of your examination, you stimulate the Moro reflex. How would you do this, and what reaction would you look for in the patient?

   a. Turn his head to one side and watch for contralateral upper extremity to extend.

   b. Release your support of the newborn's head to observe nervous system response.

   c. Stroke the infant's lower foot to observe an upward curling of his big toe.

   d. Hold the baby aloft to see if he extends his arms towards the ground.

2. During a physical examination, a newborn is found to have length, width, and head circumference all at less than the 10th percentile for her age. All of the following factors should likely be considered as potential sources for her condition <u>except</u>:

   a. Residing at high altitudes

   b. Bacterial intrauterine infection

   c. Inborn errors of metabolism

   d. Congenital or chromosomal abnormalities

3. Which of the following skin variations that occurs in newborns would be of most concern?

   a. Milia

   b. Hemangioma

   c. Erythema toxicum

   d. Port wine stain

4. While examining a newborn infant, which of the following would be most indicative of a neuromuscular problem?

   a. Arms and legs flexed over abdomen

   b. Inability to track with eyes

   c. No response to clapping of hands

   d. Three café au lait spots on back

5. In the correct method for assessing an infant for developmental hip dysplasia, the nurse practitioner would have the baby on his back with knees flexed and:

   a. Abduct knees, listening for click as femoral head slips into acetabulum

   b. Adduct knees, listening for click as femoral head slips into acetabulum

   c. Abduct knees, feeling femoral head enter acetabulum

   d. Adduct knees, feeling femoral head slip into acetabulum

6. Which of these abdominal findings would be of most concern in newborns?

   a. Umbilical hernia

   b. Diastasis recti

   c. Flat abdomen

   d. Abdomen rising with inspiration, falling with expiration

7. Which of the following findings in a newborn would be <u>least</u> likely to indicate an abnormality?

   a. Heart murmurs

   b. White forelocks

   c. Wide fontanels

   d. Four junctional nevi clustered on trunk

8. You are examining the newborn child of a recovering alcoholic. During the interview, she mentions she was still drinking early into her pregnancy and did not know she was pregnant for some time. You examine the newborn's mouth. Which of the following findings would most strongly indicate fetal alcohol syndrome?

   a. Shrunken, contracted mouth

   b. Enlarged tongue

   c. Triangular upper lip

   d. Whitish-yellow cysts on gums

9. You are performing an eye exam on a newborn child. When you perform the red reflex test, a black spot presents instead. Which of these conditions would this finding typically indicate?

   a. Optic nerve hypoplasia

   b. Retinoblastoma

   c. Heterochromia

   d. Absence of a clear retinal pathway

10. According to the normal stage of primitive reflex development, which of the following reflexes is expected to <u>not</u> disappear by about 12 months of age?

    a. The head turning towards anything that strokes the cheek or mouth

    b. The arms spreading or contracting in response to loss of balance

    c. Sucking in response to objects touching the roof of the mouth

    d. Toes fanning out in response to stroking of the sole

RATIONALES

1. b

The Moro reflex is best tested by releasing the newborn's head in order to observe the nervous system's response to surprise; most infants will respond by abducting or adducting their arms in an attempt to regain balance. An impaired or absent response may indicate motor or neurologic disorders. Turning the head to one side with ipsilateral arm extension is the fencing reflex. Stroking the infant's lower foot tests the Babinski reflex, which, barring pathology, commonly vanishes by 2 years of age. Holding the infant aloft and rotating him or her forward to test the response to a simulated fall is part of the parachute test and should not typically stimulate the startle reflex.

2. a

Symmetric intrauterine growth retardation (IUGR) presents with length, weight, and head circumference at less than the 10th percentile, whereas asymmetric IUGR presents with weight under the 10th percentile but length and head circumference within normal range; residing at high altitudes is more likely to produce asymmetric IUGR, due to decreased oxygen available to the fetus, than symmetric IUGR. Bacterial intrauterine infection, inborn errors of metabolism, and congenital or chromosomal abnormalities are known factors that may contribute to symmetric IUGR.

3. d

Port wine stains are vascular birthmarks consisting of superficial and deep dilated capillaries that cause permanent reddish to purplish discoloration of the skin and may signify neurologic concerns. Milia are pinpoint white papules on the face that spontaneously disappear within 3–4 weeks of life. A hemangioma is characterized by raised, soft, red lumps on the skin and is not usually a concern. Erythema toxicum is a benign newborn rash.

4. c

A newborn should respond to a startle with a loud sound; failure to elicit this response could indicate hearing damage or other neuromuscular challenges. The normal posture of a newborn is flexion of extremities over trunk. Newborns may look at an object or face, but are not commonly expected to track. Café au lait spots are often counted and measured, and could be indicative of a problem if larger than 5 or 6 mm in size.

5. a

Ortolani's click, commonly used to assess for developmental hip dysplasia, is performed by abducting the knees, then listening and feeling for the femoral head to re-enter the acetabulum. Barlow's maneuver, which also assesses for developmental hip dysplasia, is done by adducting the knees and feeling the femoral head pop out of, not into, the acetabulum.

6. c

A flat contour to the abdomen is abnormal in infants and may indicate malnutrition or intrauterine growth retardation. Reduction in nutrients to the fetus can cause a decrease in intra-abdominal fat. This can be caused by poor blood flow, decreased transplacental concentration of amino acids, or impairment of the ability of the placenta to transfer nutrients. Slight distension is normal and the nurse practitioner should see a slight protuberance in a healthy infant. A rounded, symmetrical contour to the abdomen that rises with inspiration is normal in infants; an asymmetrical abdomen may indicate an abdominal mass. An umbilical hernia may present in the infant, but this condition is fairly harmless and often resolves itself by 1 year of age. Likewise, diastasis recti may present in newborns, but this condition typically resolves on its own accord.

Erythema toxicum
- benign newborn rash

7. a

Heart murmurs may present in 85%–90% of all newborns; despite this high percentage, structural heart disease typically only presents in 8–10 live births out of 1000. White forelocks may indicate Waardenburg syndrome, whereas wide fontanels may indicate hydrocephalus, Down syndrome, or hypothyroidism. Although junctional nevi may be present in newborns, groupings of the spots may signal a precursor tuberous sclerosis or generalized neurofibromatosis.

8. c

A triangular upper lip with fish-like mouth, or the fish mouth deformity, is commonly observed in neonates and pediatric patients born with fetal alcohol syndrome. Microstomia, on the other hand, presents as a shrunken, contracted mouth and is usually observed in trisomy 18 and trisomy 21. Macroglossia, or enlarged tongue, may be due to hypothyroidism or mucopolysaccharidoses. Epstein pearls present as whitish-yellow cysts on the gums and roof of the mouth; these pearls are common in newborns and are not considered an abnormal sign because they typically disappear within 1–2 weeks of birth.

9. d

The red reflex replaced by a black spot commonly indicates that there is no clear pathway from the lens to the retina and is a crucial finding for congenital cataracts, corneal scar, or ocular hemorrhage. Optic nerve hypoplasia, on the other hand, is a midline defect of the central nervous system and may present with colobomas. Heterochromia simply refers to a difference in coloration of the iris and usually does not indicate an underlying condition. Further, retinoblastoma and congenital cataracts may be indicated by the red reflex being replaced by a whitish color, not a black spot.

10. d

The Babinski reflex, or fanning of the toes upon stroking of the sole, is expected to disappear after 12 months or when the infant starts walking, but may last for up to 2 years; if it persists past this point, it may indicate a nervous system disorder. The turning of the head towards anything that strokes the cheek is a sign of the rooting reflex, whereas sucking on anything that touches the roof of the mouth demonstrates the sucking reflex; both these reflexes are expected to disappear at 3–4 months of age. The Moro reflex, indicated by stretching or contracting the arms upon perceiving a loss of balance, is also expected to disappear during this window.

DISCUSSION

The Newborn Assessment: History

Prenatal History

A newborn assessment should begin with a prenatal history. The prenatal history should consist of a review of the pregnancy, past pregnancies, and mother's and father's medical and genetic histories.[1] When reviewing the pregnancy, the nurse practitioner (NP) should determine if the mother used any foreign substances.[2,3] Any health problems the mother experienced during pregnancy (e.g., placenta previa, abruptio placentae, gestational diabetes, hypertension) should also be documented. The NP should review the results of any prenatal screening tests performed and determine if there are any abnormal findings that warrant further evaluation.

A review of past pregnancies should include a history of congenital anomalies, still births, and genetic conditions. When reviewing the mother's medical and genetic history, maternal illnesses prior to and during pregnancy should be discussed.[4] Any maternal medications should also be discussed, and medications should be reviewed for intrauterine effects or the potential for excretion in breast milk.[1] The father's medical and genetic history should also be included in the prenatal history.

Perinatal History

The perinatal history should include a record of events surrounding labor, the newborn's weight and length, and the Apgar score. A review of the events of labor should include the duration of labor, the duration of rupture of membranes, and the use of analgesia or anesthesia.[1] The type of delivery and whether the labor was spontaneous or induced should also be included in the report. Any complications (e.g., prolonged labor, meconium staining or aspiration, or use of forceps or vacuum) should be noted.[3] Resuscitative measures used on the newborn should be included in the history as well.

Apgar scores, which assess the clinical status of infants immediately after delivery, should be recorded at 1 minute and 5 minutes after birth. The Apgar score contains five areas of assessment for a total of 10 points, as displayed in table 4.1.

Each component of the test receives a score of 0, 1, or 2. If the newborn scores below 7 at 5 minutes, the test should be repeated every 5 minutes for 20 minutes or until the newborn scores above 7 in two consecutive tests.[3,5,6]

The birth weight and length of the newborn should also be recorded. Low birth weight (LBW) is characterized as less than 2,500 grams, very low birth weight (VLBW) is less than 1,500 grams, and extremely low birth weight (ELBW) is less than 1,000 grams.[7,8,5]

Table 4.1 APGAR Sign

	2	1	0
Appearance (skin coloration)	Pink color all over (hands and feet are pink)	Pink color (but hands and feet are bluish)	Bluish-gray or pale all over
Pulse	Normal (above 100 beats per minute)	Below 100 beats per minute	Absent (no pulse)
Grimace (responsiveness or "reflex irritability")	Pulls away, sneezes, or coughs with stimulation	Facial movement only (grimace) with stimulation	Absent (no response to stimulation)
Activity (muscle tone)	Active, spontaneous movement	Arms and legs flexed with little movement	No movement, "floppy" tone
Respirations	Normal rate and effort (30–60 breaths per minute), good cry	Slow or irregular breathing, weak cry	Absent (no breathing)

Used with permission from Barkley TW Jr. Prenatal/newborn assessment and newborn screening. In: Barkley TW Jr, ed. *Pediatric Primary Care Nurse Practitioner Certification Review/Clinical Update Continuing Education Course.* West Hollywood, CA: Barkley and Associates; 2015: 30.

Postnatal History

The NP should review any maternal problems, such as bleeding, anesthesia reactions, breastfeeding complications, and depression.[3,9] The NP should also review any infant problems, such as ABO/Rh blood type incompatibilities, hyperbilirubinemia, hip dysplasia, murmurs, or talipes equinovarus congenita (i.e., club feet).[10,11,12,13]

The Newborn Assessment: Physical Examination

Measurements

The newborn's weight, length, and head circumference should be plotted on standard growth curves. The average length of a newborn is 51 cm, the average weight is 3.6 kg for males and 3.5 kg for females, and the average head circumference is 35 cm.[1] The newborn's length should be measured by using a measurement board or standard tape measure and measuring from the crown to the heel. Newborns should be unclothed and quiet while being weighed to ensure an accurate reading.[6]

Gestational Age

Gestational age is frequently assessed using the New Ballard Score. The New Ballard Score can estimate the gestational age of full term and extremely premature newborns alike, but the score tends to overestimate the gestational age of extremely premature newborns. To increase accuracy, the assessment should be conducted within 12 hours of birth.[6]

The New Ballard Score maturational assessment consists of six neuromuscular and six physical characteristics.[14] The six portions of the neuromuscular section are posture, square window, arm recoil, popliteal angle, scarf sign, and heel–to-ear. The NP should assess the newborn's posture at rest, noting the position of arms and legs. Square window refers to the newborn's wrist flexibility. The NP should estimate the angle measurement between the palm of the newborn's hand and forearm. Arm recoil is the measurement of the angle of recoil following brief extension of the upper extremity. The popliteal angle assesses the maturation of the passive flexor tone around the knee point. The scarf sign tests the passive tone of flexors around the shoulder girdle. The heel to ear maneuver tests for passive flexion or resistance to extension of posterior hip flexor muscles.[15]

The six portions of the physical section are skin, lanugo, plantar surface, breast, ear, and genitals. The maturation level of fetal skin, the amount of lanugo covering the body, and the amount of major foot creases are noted. Palpating the breast tissue beneath the skin and holding it between the thumb and forefinger helps to estimate the amount of tissue. The ear examination consists of assessing the cartilage thickness and folding forward the pinna. If the pinna does not recoil, the eyelid development should be assessed. In males, the descent of testes and amount of rugae is assessed. In females, the prominence of clitoris and labia minora is noted.[15]

Each of the 12 sections is scored based on the degree of development. Gestational age is determined based upon the sum of these scores. Low scores indicate immaturity, whereas high scores indicate a mature or post-mature infant.[3,14]

Newborns born at 37–41 weeks gestation are considered at term and have the best health outcomes. Newborns born prior to 37 weeks gestation are premature, and newborns born after 42 weeks are post-term.[16,17,18]

Newborns whose weight is within the 10th and 90th percentiles for their gestational age are considered appropriate for gestational age (AGA).[19] Infants large for gestational age (LGA) are born with a weight above the 90th percentile for gestational age.[20,21] Genetic risk factors for LGA include genetic syndromes (e.g., Beckwith-Wiedemann syndrome, Simpson-Golabi-Behmel syndrome) and race and ethnicity (e.g.,

Caucasian, American Indian, Samoan). Maternal risk factors include maternal diabetes and maternal obesity.[22]

Infants small for gestational age (SGA) are born with a weight below the 10th percentile for their gestational age.[20,21] Some SGA infants may also have experienced intrauterine growth restriction (IUGR), which is diminished growth velocity in the fetus. IUGR can be caused by maternal, placental, or neonatal factors. Maternal factors include severe maternal starvation, medical disorders, substance abuse, and intrauterine infection.[22,23] Placental factors include placental injuries and structural anomalies.[22] Neonatal factors include inborn errors of metabolism, genetic syndromes, and karyotypic abnormalities.[3,22]

Fifty-five percent of all SGA newborns have asymmetric IUGR. Asymmetric IUGR newborns typically have a head circumference and length within normal limits and weight below the 10th percentile.[22,24,25,26] Asymmetric IUGR is often caused by a reduction in fetal nutrients.[22] Other causes include chronic hypertension, pre-eclampsia, renal or cyanotic heart disease, hemoglobinopathies, abruptio placentae, multiple gestation, or high altitude.[3] Symmetric IUGR is characterized by a reduction in both body and head growth. Symmetric IUGR is usually caused by intrinsic factors, such as congenital infections or chromosomal abnormalities.[6]

Vital Signs

Vital signs should be recorded every 30–60 minutes during the first 4–6 hours, and then every 8–12 hours. A normal temperature ranges from 36.1– 37 °C (97–98.6 °F). A normal respiratory rate falls between 30 and 60 breaths per minute. The newborn's heart rate should be between 120 and 160 beats per minute (bpm).[1,27,28] Newborns suspected of cardiovascular or renal abnormalities should also have their blood pressure monitored. A reading less than 112/74 mmHg is normal.[3]

Skin

Within 2–3 days, a newborn's skin usually becomes dry and flaky. The skin turns red when the newborn cries. When cold, the extremities typically turn bluish with a mottled tint.[29]

Skin abnormalities that may indicate an underlying disorder include abnormal pigmentation, macular stains, and hemangiomas.[1] Congenital nevi often begin as flat, evenly pigmented patches but later may become uneven and speckled. There is a small risk that congenital nevi will develop into melanoma.[30] Macular stains are blanchable, pink-red patches. Macular stains may be associated with extracutaneous disorders, such as spinal dysraphism or Beckwith-Wiedemann syndrome.[31] Hemangiomas (i.e., strawberry marks) are vascular neoplasms that typically present as red or crimson macules. Although most hemangiomas are benign and disappear by age 5, some, depending on placement, may interfere with vital functions. Large cutaneous or visceral hemangiomas, in particular, may result in high-output cardiac failure and structural abnormalities.[32]

Some common, benign skin findings in newborns are milia, erythema toxicum, Mongolian spots, and miliaria. Milia (i.e., milk spots) are white papules frequently found on the nose and cheeks. Milia tend to disappear within 3–4 weeks.[1,29,33] Erythema toxicum are white papules on an erythematous base commonly found on the face and trunk. Erythema toxicum usually resolves within 2 weeks.[1,29,33] Mongolian spots, more common in African-American and Asian newborns, are blue-black macules with indefinite borders. Mongolian spots are usually located on the buttocks and gradually disappear within the first year of life.[1,6] Miliaria are thin-walled vesicles with a nonerythematous and nonpigmented base caused by blockage of sweat glands. The rash usually resolves when the newborn is removed from the warm, humid environment.[6]

Port wine stains and café au lait spots are usually benign. Port wine stains are low flow capillary malformations. Port wine stains are initially pink in color with sharply delineated borders. Over time, the pink color progresses to dark red or purple. Port wine stains may sometimes be associated with structural anomalies (e.g., Sturge-Weber syndrome).[1,6,31] Café au lait spots are light brown macules with well-defined borders. Six or more café au lait spots may indicate neurofibromatosis.[6]

Neurological Exam

A neurological exam consists of a general assessment and an assessment of motor function, cranial nerves, reflexes, senses, and behavior. A general assessment examines the newborn's vital signs, levels of alertness, and skin, head, and spine. A neurological exam is best conducted when the newborn is quiet and awake because portions of the exam, such as motor function, are difficult to assess when the newborn is asleep. Altered levels of alertness (e.g., mild stupor, moderate stupor, deep stupor, coma) are seen in infants with cortical dysfunction.[34]

In a healthy newborn, muscle function should be symmetric, smooth, and spontaneous. Sustained tremulousness beyond the fourth day may indicate cortical dysfunction.[34] When at rest, a term newborn should present with hips abducted and partially flexed with knees flexed, arms abducted, elbows flexed, and fists clenched.[35]

All 12 cranial nerves can be assessed, but the olfactory nerve very rarely needs to be assessed in newborns. The optic nerve is assessed by examining the fundi. A term infant should be able to turn toward soft lights. The oculomotor, trochlear, and abducens nerves can be assessed by observing spontaneous eye movements. To assess the trigeminal nerve, observe the newborn's response to tactile stimuli. The facial nerve can be assessed by noting whether the newborn closes both eyelids during vigorous crying. The vestibulo cochlear nerve can be assessed by examining the newborn for a startle or blink response to sudden loud noises. When the glossopharyngeal or vagus nerves are impaired, the newborn will have difficulty swallowing. Impairment of the hypoglossal nerve is indicated by the tongue resting to one side.[34,35]

The reflex portion of the exam should include an assessment of superficial and developmental reflexes. The abdominal reflex can be assessed by gently stroking each of the four quadrants in an axial to peripheral direction. This should result in contraction of the abdominal wall.[34] The anal wink reflex can be exhibited by gently stroking the perianal region. The perianal muscle should contract. The lack of a contraction may indicate a spinal cord lesion.[34] Developmental (i.e., primitive) reflexes are generally present at birth and resolve with maturation. The developmental reflexes are presented in table 4.2.[35,36]

The sensory examination is rarely performed because it is challenging to determine an infant's response to sensory stimuli. The rooting reflex, however, can be used to detect perioral tactile sensation.[34,35]

Two key elements of the behavioral evaluation are consolability and habituation. Healthy newborns can be consoled within about fifteen seconds. Infants with brain injury typically are more difficult to console. Habituation measures the newborn's ability to diminish response to repetitive stimuli. A lack of habituation is associated with cortical dysfunction and prenatal substance abuse exposure.[34]

Head/Neck

An inspection of the newborn's head should include an examination of size, shape, and symmetry.[1,6] Bony abnormalities, such as frontal bossing, should be noted and may indicate a hormonal or skeletal disorder.[37,38] Microcephaly, a head circumference smaller than two standard deviations,

Table 4.2 Primitive Reflexes in Newborn Neurological Development

Reflex	Appears	Disappears
Rooting	Newborn	3–4 months
Sucking	Newborn	3–4 months
Moro	Newborn	3–4 months
Grasp (palmar, plantar)	Newborn	3–6 months; 4 months
Pacing/stepping	Newborn	1–2 months
Tonic neck	Newborn	3 months
Babinski	Newborn	12 months or when walking

Used with permission from Barkley TW Jr. Prenatal/newborn assessment and newborn screening. In: Barkley TW Jr, ed. *Pediatric Primary Care Nurse Practitioner Certification Review/Clinical Update Continuing Education Course*. West Hollywood, CA: Barkley and Associates; 2015: 32.

and macrocephaly, a head circumference larger than two standard deviations, may be detected at the newborn screening but would require further examination over the coming weeks.[3,39,40,41]

The newborn's hair should be uniform in color and distribution.[1] White forelocks may indicate deafness.[1,42,43] Multiple hair whorls may indicate Down syndrome. The scalp should also be examined for defects, unusual lesions, or protuberances.

The head should be palpated to detect fontanelles, which should be flat and soft.[6] In normal newborns, the anterior fontanelle is diamond shaped and persists until about 18 months. The posterior fontanelle is triangle-shaped, and closes by 2–3 months. The posterior fontanelle is not always palpable at birth, however. Tense or bulging fontanelles may indicate intracranial pressure. Sunken fontanelles may indicate dehydration. Fontanelles that are smaller than expected are a potential indicator for premature fusion of skull bones and should be investigated. Wide fontanelles may indicate underlying conditions, such as IUGR, hydrocephalus, Down syndrome, or hypothyroidism.[44,45] Sutures should also be palpated. An asymmetric skull after birth is normal, but may indicate craniosynostosis if it remains after 2 or 3 days.[1]

Caput succedaneum, edema that crosses the midline, should resolve within a few days.[1,46] Cephalohematoma, blood under the periosteum that does not cross the midline, requires closer examination, however.[1,47,48]

The face should be examined for shape, symmetry, and bruises or dysmorphic features.[1] Facial palsies, such as loss of nasolabial fold, partial closing of the eye, or the appearance of a "drooping" mouth, typically resolve within a few weeks.[34] Asymmetric crying facies are the congenital absence or hypoplasia of the depressor angularis muscle. Asymmetric crying facies are benign and become less noticeable as the child gets older. The condition may be associated with a cardiovascular anomaly.[34]

The position, spacing, and symmetry of the newborn's eyes should be noted.[1] Abnormally wide interpupillary distance may indicate trisomy 13 or Apert syndrome. Asymmetry due to epicanthal folds usually suggests a genetic syndrome, such as trisomy 21. Sclera should be white and clear.[1] Blue sclera may indicate osteogenesis imperfecta.[49] Pupils should be round and equal in diameter. The pupils should constrict in response to the light from an ophthalmoscope.[6] An infant may present with colobomas, which are an embryonic fissure defect. Mild forms of colobomas may only affect the iris.[50] In more severe cases, the choroid and optic nerve may be involved; these severe cases may also indicate central nervous system midline defects, such as optic nerve hypoplasia.[51] The newborn should have a normal red reflex.[52,53] Dark spots or a white reflex justify a referral to an ophthalmologist.[6]

The position of the ears should be similar bilaterally.[6] The size and appearance should also be inspected.[1] The ears should be examined for branchial cleft cysts, sinuses, and skin tags. Any external ear abnormalities increase the risk of abnormalities in the middle and inner ear.[1]

The shape and patency of the nose should be examined. The birth process may cause the nose to be abnormally shaped, but this should correct itself within a few days. The patency of each naris should be checked because newborns are predominantly nose breathers.[6]

The mouth should be symmetric and in proportion to the chin and tongue. Mucous membranes should be pink and moist. Oral secretions should be thin and clear. The NP should also check for any clefts.[1,6]

The newborn examination should reveal a relatively short neck that is symmetric with the head. The newborn should have full range of motion.[6] Any excess skin, such as webbing, may indicate a genetic disorder, such as Turner syndrome.[1] The NP should palpate the clavicle. Tenderness or swelling may indicate a fracture.[1]

Pulmonary/Chest

A full-term newborn's chest circumference should be about two centimeters smaller than the head circumference.[6] A small or malformed thorax may indicate pulmonary hypoplasia or a neuromuscular disorder. The newborn's chest should be symmetrical. An asymmetrical chest may be from an absent pectoralis muscle or abscess. Pectus excavatum (i.e., funnel chest) and pectus carinatum (i.e., pigeon breast) should also be noted.[1,54,55]

The newborn's breast size and nipples should be noted. The breast size can be used in determining the gestational age because a newborn's breast tissue may hypertrophy as a result of maternal hormones.[1,6] Supernumerary nipples are a common finding, especially among African-American newborns.[1,34] A newborn's breast may secrete a milky fluid (i.e., witch's milk) for several weeks, but this will resolve on its own.[6]

The majority of newborn lung examinations do not require the use of a stethoscope. At rest, the newborn should exhibit unlabored breathing without grunting, nasal flaring, or intercostal retractions. Auscultation may reveal rales or decreased breath sounds, which may indicate disease (e.g., pulmonary edema, neonatal pneumonia).[56]

Cardiovascular

A cardiovascular examination of a newborn includes an examination of rate, rhythm, quality of heart sounds, murmurs, and femoral pulses. In the first few days of life, the point of maximal impulse is located at the fourth intercostal space at or to the left of the midclavicular line. The NP should auscultate at the second and fourth intercostal spaces, cardiac apex, and axilla.[6] The normal heart rate for a newborn is 120–160 bpm but may dip to 85–90 bpm while the newborn is sleeping.[1,6]

Asymptomatic rhythms are relatively common in preterm infants. Sinus bradycardia and tachycardia are the two most common benign dysrhythmias. Premature atrial or ventricular contractions are also common. An electrocardiogram is needed to properly identify the condition.[6]

Heart sounds should be auscultated to evaluate the quality. The split second heart sound, which should be expected, indicates the presence of two semilunar valves. Any gallops detected would require further evaluation. Ejection clicks, which also require further evaluation, may indicate pulmonary or aortic valve stenosis or a bicuspid aortic valve.[56]

About 85% of all newborns have murmurs.[57,58] Many cases of slight murmurs cease once the ductus arteriosus closes, but innocent murmurs may present in infants, children, and adolescents. However, murmurs still require examination to rule out the possibility of congenital heart defects (CHDs).[59] Pulse oximetry is often performed at birth to determine the possibility of CHD in the newborn.[60]

The femoral pulses should be palpated when the infant is quiet. Diminished femoral pulses may indicate coarctation of the aorta.[1] Blood pressure of the upper and lower extremities should be measured if there is still doubt about detecting the femoral pulses at the time of discharge.[34] Increased femoral pulses may occur with patent ductus arteriosus.[1]

Blood pressure should be assessed at birth as well. Hypotension should be recognized and treated in order to avoid complications such as intraventricular hemorrhage. Hypertension should also be noted and may indicate several abnormalities, but frequently presents with bronchopulmonary dysplasia.[61]

Abdomen

The NP should examine the newborn's abdomen while the newborn is quiet because it will make palpation easier. The abdomen should be slightly protuberant. Distention may indicate intestinal obstruction, organomegaly, or ascites.[1] Palpation should reveal a liver that is soft with a smooth edge.[1,6] The NP may also be able to locate the tip of the spleen.[6] The kidneys should be smooth and firm to the touch.[6] Enlarged kidneys may indicate hydronephrosis or cystic renal disease.[1] Any other masses that the NP detects would be considered abnormal.[1]

The umbilical cord should have two arteries and one vein. It should be bluish-white in color, shiny, and moist.[6] An erythema or odorous discharge may indicate omphalitis.[1] The average diameter of the umbilical cord in a normal term infant is 1.5 cm; poor nutritional status may result in a small cord.[1,62] Umbilical hernias may present in newborns and young children but are generally benign and resolve spontaneously.[34,63]

Genitourinary

The newborn should be inspected immediately after birth to identify the gender.[1] Female newborns should have their labia minora and labia majora examined.[56] A pre-term newborn will present with a prominent labia minora and clitoris.[1] A term newborn, however, will present with a prominent labia majora. The labia majora may be reddened and swollen. Clear and white vaginal discharge, sometimes tinged with blood, may occur within the first few days.[56,64] The hymen should also be inspected. An imperforate hymen should prompt a referral to a pediatric gynecologist.[56]

The penis and scrotum should be examined in male newborns. The penis should be stretched to assess the length.[1] Phimosis is normal in newborns.[6] The degree of hypospadias, if apparent, should be noted. Circumcision should be postponed if hypospadias is present.[56] The scrotum should be palpated for testes. The testes should be firm, smooth, and comparatively equal in size.[6] Blue testes visible through the scrotal skin is a sign of torsion.[56] Undescended testes are not a cause for concern unless the testes have not descended by 6 months of age.[56]

In both males and females, the anus should be checked for patency, position, and size.[56]

Musculoskeletal

The spine should be examined for curvature, patency, and presence of structural abnormalities. The spine should be straight and flexible with no visible defects.[6] Both sides of the back should be symmetrical.[6] The NP should palpate along the spine to check for any abnormal growths. Soft tissue masses covered with normal skin may be lipomas or myelomeningocele.[1] Sacral dimpling is not a cause for concern unless the dimples are larger than 0.5 cm or located more than 2.5 cm from the anal verge.[56] If this is the case, the newborn should be screened for a neural tube defect.[1] The lower back should also be examined for tufts of hair or skin tags, which may indicate spina bifida.[65]

The hands and feet should be inspected for syndactyly and polydactyly.[1] Newborns should also be examined for palmar creases. A single palmar crease may suggest trisomy 21. Newborns with talipes equinovarus genita (i.e., clubfoot) require orthopedic intervention as soon as possible.[56] Limbs should be proportional and equal in length and exhibit full range of motion.[6]

Every newborn should be observed for developmental dysplasia of the hips (DDH).[56] The Barlow maneuver and Ortolani maneuver are two common maneuvers for assessing newborns for DDH. The Barlow maneuver causes posterior dislocation of an unstable hip.[12,43,56] The Ortolani maneuver makes a click sound with reduction of dislocation.[12,43,56] Newborns with suspected DDH should be referred to an orthopedic surgeon.[66]

The Newborn Assessment: Selected Screening Tests

Screening Principles

The goal of newborn screening is to detect life-threatening disorders while the disorders are asymptomatic.[67] Screening can detect inborn errors of metabolism, endocrine disorders, hemoglobinopathies, immunodeficiencies, cystic fibrosis, and CHDs. Not all diseases that can be screened will become part of a mass screening program. When determining which conditions to screen for, several principles are considered: if a lack of treatment for the disease can result in significant morbidity or death, if effective treatment is readily accessible, if early treatment leads to better outcomes, if the test has a low false-negative rate, and if the test is simple and inexpensive. Results should be received in a timely manner, and a definitive follow-up test should be available.[67,68]

Mandatory Screening Program

The Recommended Uniform Screening Panel created by the Secretary's Advisory Committee on Heritable Disorders in Newborns and Children includes 32 core conditions and 26 secondary conditions.[69] Each state has its own mandated screening program.[70] Some conditions that every state screens for are phenylketonuria (PKU), galactosemia, sickle cell disease, and congenital hypothyroidism.[3,60]

Considerations for Newborn Screening

Overview

Screening typically occurs while the newborn is still in the hospital. The blood spot specimen is collected as close to discharge as possible so abnormal compounds have time to accumulate. If the specimen is collected while the newborn is younger than 24 hours old, a repeat test should be conducted. If the test is positive, a confirmatory test should be performed as soon as possible. Hearing loss and critical CHD should also be screened for prior to discharge.[67]

Screened Considerations

A newborn's hearing can be screened by observing the infant's response to loud noises and voices, also known as the startle reflex. Hearing screening can also be conducted via the brain stem auditory evoked response test (BSAER). The BSAER measures the auditory brainstem response to click stimuli. Delayed or absent waves may indicate neurologic or cochlear deficit.[71] If hearing loss is indicated, treatment should begin by 6 months of age.

Critical CHDs can be screened through pulse oximetry screening, an effective, noninvasive, and inexpensive test. The seven critical CHDs are hypoplastic left heart syndrome, pulmonary atresia, tetralogy of Fallot, total anomalous pulmonary venous return, transposition of the great arteries, tricuspid atresia, and truncus arteriosus. Critical CHDs must be diagnosed and treated shortly after birth to prevent death or disability.[72]

Inborn errors of metabolism, such as PKU and galactosemia, are screened using dried blood spots from a heel prick. PKU occurs in 1 out of every 10,000–25,000 infants and may produce developmental delay, seizures, aggression, autism, and hyperactivity. When galactosemia is present, liver dysfunction and coagulopathies will often manifest. Galactosemia occurs in 1 out of every 60,000–80,000 infants; 25% of all infants who carry the condition unrecognized run the risk of developing sepsis.[3]

Dried blood spots are also used to screen for hemoglobinopathies, including sickle cell disease and thalassemia. Certain hemoglobinopathies are more common in certain populations, with sickle cell disease occurring in 1 out of every 400 African-American infants. Hemoglobinopathies commonly result in anemia.[3]

Cystic fibrosis can also be screened using a dried blood spot. Most newborns who have a positive screen do not have cystic fibrosis, however. Therefore, a confirmatory sweat test is required.[3,73]

References

1. McKee-Garrett TM. Assessment of the newborn infant. In: Basow DS, ed. *UpToDate*. Waltham, MA: UpToDate; 2015. http://www.uptodate.com/contents/assessment-of-the-newborn-infant?-source=search_result&search=assess-ment+of+the+newborn+infant&selected-Title=1~150. Last updated February 19, 2015. Accessed May 6, 2015.

2. Prouillac C, Lecoeur S. The role of the placenta in fetal exposure to xenobiotics: importance of membrane transporters and human models for transfer studies. *Drug Metab Dispos.* 2010; 38(10): 1623–1635. doi: 10.1124/dmd.110.033571

3. Barkley TW Jr. Prenatal/newborn assessment and newborn screening. In: Barkley TW Jr, ed. *Pediatric Primary Care Nurse Practitioner Certification Review/Clinical Update Continuing Education Course*. West Hollywood, CA: Barkley and Associates; 2015: 29–37.

4. Sackey JA. The preconception office visit. In: Basow DS, ed. *UpToDate*. Waltham, MA: UpToDate; 2015. http://www.uptodate.com/contents/the-preconception-office-visit. Last updated March 19, 2015. Accessed April 3, 2015.

5. Wheeler BJ. Health promotion of the newborn and family. In: Hockenberry MJ, Wilson D, eds. *Wong's Essentials of Pediatric Nursing.* 9th ed. St. Louis, MO: Elsevier Mosby; 2012: 185–227.

6. Cavaliere TA, Sansoucie DA. Assessment of the newborn and infant. In: Kenner C, Wright Lott J, eds. *Comprehensive Neonatal Nursing Care.* 5th ed. New York, NY: Springer Publishing Company; 2014: 71–112.

7. Ogawa M, Matsuda Y, Kanda E, et al. Survival rate of extremely low birth weight infants and its risk factors: Case-control study in Japan. *ISRN Obstet Gynecol.* 2013; 2013: 873563. doi: 10.1155/2013/873563.

8. Subramanian KNS, Seo SC, Barton AM, Montazami S. Extremely low birth weight infant. In: Rosenkrantz T, ed. Medscape. http://emedicine.medscape.com/article/979717-overview#showall. Updated December 17, 2014. Accessed April 3, 2015.

9. Pregnancy complications. Centers for Disease Control and Prevention Web site. http://www.cdc.gov/reproductivehealth/maternalinfanthealth/pregcomplications.htm. Last updated January 22, 2014. Accessed April 3, 2015.

10. Krauspe R, Weimann-Stahlschmidt K, Westhoff B. The current state of treatment for clubfoot in Europe. In: Bentley G, ed. *European Instructional Lectures, Vol. 11.* Copenhagen, Denmark: Springer; 2011: 47–66.

11. Wong RJ, Bhutani VK. Patient information: Jaundice in newborn infants (Beyond the Basics). In: Basow DS, ed. *UpToDate.* Waltham, MA: UpToDate; 2015. http://www.uptodate.com/contents/jaundice-in-newborn-infants-beyond-the-basics. Last updated February 28, 2014. Accessed April 3, 2015.

12. Infant and child hip dysplasia: Infant signs and symptoms. International Hip Dysplasia Institute Web site. http://hipdysplasia.org/developmental-dysplasia-of-the-hip/infant-signs-and-symptoms. Accessed April 3, 2015.

13. U.S. Department of Health and Human Services, National Institutes of Health (NIH), National Heart, Lung, and Blood Institute. How is a heart murmur diagnosed? http://www.nhlbi.nih.gov/health/health-topics/topics/heartmurmur/diagnosis.html. Updated September 20, 2012. Accessed April 3, 2015.

14. Smith VC. The high-risk newborn: Anticipation, evaluation, management, and outcome. In: Cloherty JP, Eichenwald EC, Hansen AR, Stark AR, eds. *Manual of Neonatal Care.* 7th ed. Philadelphia, PA: Lippincott, Williams, & Wilkins; 2012: 74–90.

15. New Ballard Score Maturational Assessment of Gestational Age. The New Ballard Score Web site. http://www.ballardscore.com/. Accessed May 6, 2015.

16. Lissauer T. Physical examination of the newborn. In: Martin RJ, Fanaroff AA, Walsh MC, eds. *Neonatal-Perinatal Medicine: Diseases of the Fetus and Infant.* 9th ed. St. Louis, MO: Elsevier Mosby; 2011: 485–500.

17. Premature infant. A.D.A.M. Medical Encyclopedia. http://www.nlm.nih.gov/medlineplus/ency/article/001562.htm. Updated November 14, 2011. Accessed April 3, 2015.

18. Donahue SMA, Kleinman KP, Gillman MW, Oken E. (2010).Trends in birth weight and gestational length among singleton term births in the United States. *Obstet Gynecol.* 2010; 115(2 Pt 1): 357–384. doi: 10.1097/AOG.0b013e3181cbd5f5

19. Appropriate for gestational age (AGA). A.D.A.M. Medical Encyclopedia. http://www.nlm.nih.gov/medlineplus/ency/article/002225.htm. Updated December 4, 2013. Accessed April 3, 2015.

20. Resnik R, Creasy RK. Intrauterine growth restriction. In: Creasy RK, Resnik R, Iams JD, Lockwood CJ, Moore T, Greene MF, eds. *Creasy and Resnik's Maternal-Fetal Medicine: Principles and Practice.* 7th ed. Philadelphia, PA: Elsevier Saunders; 2013: 743–755.

21. Small for gestational age. A.D.A.M. Encyclopedia. http://www.nlm.nih.gov/medlineplus/ency/article/002302.htm. Updated August 11, 2013. Accessed April 6, 2015.

22. Mandy GT. Small for gestational age infant. In: Basow DS, ed. *UpToDate.* Waltham, MA: UpToDate; 2015. http://www.uptodate.com/contents/small-for-gestational-age-infant. Last updated January 20, 2015. Accessed April 6, 2015.

23. Mandy GT. Large for gestational age newborn. In: Basow DS, ed. *UpToDate.* Waltham, MA: UpToDate; 2015. http://www.uptodate.com/contents/large-for-gestational-age-newborn?source=search_result&search=large+for+gestational+age&selectedTitle=1~45. Last updated September 3, 2014. Accessed May 6, 2015.

24. Carlo WA. Prematurity and intrauterine growth restriction. In: Kliegman RM, Stanton BF, Schor NF, St. Geme JW III, Behrman RE, eds. *Nelson Textbook of Pediatrics.* 19th ed. Philadelphia, PA: Saunders Elsevier; 2011: 532–535.

25. Soliman AT, ElAwwa A. Catch-up growth: Role of GH-IGF-I axis and thyroxine. In: Preedy VR, ed. *Handbook of Growth and Growth Monitoring in Health and Disease, Vol. 1.* New York, NY: Springer Science and Business Media; 2011: 935–962.

26. Brown JE, Isaacs JS, Krinke UB, et al. *Nutrition Through the Life Cycle.* 5th ed. Stamford, CT: Cengage Learning; 2013: 87–137.

27. American Academy of Pediatrics, American College of Obstetricians and Gynecologists. Care of the newborn. In: Riley LE, Stark AR, eds. *Guidelines for Perinatal Care.* 7th ed. Elk Grove Village, IL: American Academy of Pediatrics; 2012: 265.

28. Lo MD, Mazor SS. Neonatal resuscitation. In: Marx JA, Hockberger RS, Walls RM, et al., eds. *Rosen's Emergency Medicine: Concepts and Clinical Practice.* 8th ed. Philadelphia, PA: Elsevier Saunders; 2013: 112–118.

29. Skin characteristics in newborns. A.D.A.M. Medical Encyclopedia. http://www.nlm.nih.gov/medlineplus/ency/article/002301.htm. Updated December 4, 2013. Accessed April 6, 2015.

30. Schaffer JV, Bolognia JL. Congenital melanocytic nevi. In: Basow DS, ed. *UpToDate.* Waltham, MA: UpToDate; 2015. http://www.uptodate.com/contents/congenital-melanocytic-nevi?source=search_result&search=-congenital+melanocytic+nevus&selectedTitle=1~11. Last updated October 14, 2014. Accessed May 6, 2015.

31. Pielop JA. Vascular lesions in the newborn. In: Basow DS, ed. *UpToDate.* Waltham, MA: UpToDate; 2015. http://www.uptodate.com/contents/vascular-lesions-in-the-newborn?source=search_result&search=vascular+lesions+in+the+newborn&selectedTitle=1~150. Last updated May 4, 2015. Accessed May 6, 2015.

32. Antaya RJ. Infantile hemangioma. In: James WD, ed. Medscape. http://emedicine.medscape.com/article/1083849-overview#showall. Updated March 31, 2014. Accessed April 6, 2015.

33. Lewis ML. A comprehensive newborn examination: Part II. Skin, trunk, extremities, neurologic. *Am Fam Physician.* 2014; 90(5): 297–302. http://www.aafp.org/afp/2014/0901/p297.html

34. Kotagal S. Neurologic examination of the newborn. In: Basow DS, ed. *UpToDate.* Waltham, MA: UpToDate; 2015. http://www.uptodate.com/contents/neurologic-examination-of-the-newborn?source=search_result&search=neurologic+examination+of+the+newborn&selectedTitle=1~150. Last updated May 28, 2014. Accessed May 6, 2015.

35. Khan OA, Garcia-Sosa R, Hageman JR, Msall M, Kelley KR. Core concepts: Neonatal neurological examination. *Neoreviews,* 2014; 15(8): e316–e324. http://pediatrics.uchicago.edu/Research/Publications/Khan.Hageman%20NeonatalNeuroExam%20NeoReviews%2008.2014.pdf

36. Infant reflexes. A.D.A.M. Medical Encyclopedia. http://www.nlm.nih.gov/medlineplus/ency/article/003292.htm. Updated December 4, 2013. Accessed April 6, 2015.

37. What causes frontal bossing? Healthline Web site. http://www.healthline.com/symptom/frontal-bossing. Accessed May 6, 2015.

38. Dibas B, Srivastava T. Vitamin D in health and bone disease. In: Vijayakumar M, Nammalwar BR, eds. *Principles and Practices of Pediatric Nephrology.* 2nd ed. New Delhi, India: Jaybee Brothers Medical Publishers; 2013: 785–794.

39. Ul Hassan A. *Platinum Notes USMLE Step-2: The Complete Preparatory Guide.* New Delhi, India: Jaypee Brothers Medical Publishers; 2013: 304–306.

40. Kinsman SL, Johnston MV. Congenital anomalies of the central nervous system. In: Kliegman RM, Stanton BF, St. Geme JW III, Schor NF, Behrman RE, eds. *Nelson Textbook of Pediatrics.* 19th ed. Philadelphia, PA: Elsevier Saunders; 2011: 2007.

41. Increased head circumference. A.D.A.M. Medical Encyclopedia. http://www.nlm.nih.gov/medlineplus/ency/article/003305.htm. Updated May 10, 2013. Accessed April 7, 2015.

42. U.S. Department of Health and Human Services, NIH, U.S. National Library of Medicine, Lister Hill National Center for Biomedical Communications, Genetics Home Reference. Waardenburg syndrome. http://ghr.nlm.nih.gov/condition/waardenburg-syndrome/show/print. Reviewed October 2012. Published April 6, 2015. Accessed April 8, 2015.

43. Benjamin K, Furdon SA. Physical assessment. In: Verklan MT, Walden M, eds. *Core Curriculum for Neonatal Intensive Care Nursing.* 5th ed. St. Louis, MO: Elsevier Saunders; 2014: 110–145.

44. Gallagher ER, Hing AV, Cunningham ML. Evaluating fontanels in the newborn skull. *Contemp Pediatr.* 2013, November 1. http://contemporarypediatrics.modernmedicine.com/contemporary-pediatrics/content/tags/cerebrospinal-fluid-dynamics/evaluating-fontanels-newborn-skull?page=full

45. Carlo WA. Physical examination of the newborn infant. In: Kliegman RM, Stanton BF, Schor NF, St. Geme JW III, Behrman RE, eds. *Nelson Textbook of Pediatrics.* 19th ed. Philadelphia, PA: Saunders Elsevier; 2011: 541–544.

46. Newborn head molding. A.D.A.M. Medical Encyclopedia. http://www.nlm.nih.gov/medlineplus/ency/article/002270.htm. Updated December 4, 2013. Accessed April 6, 2015.

47. Cephalohematoma. Stanford School of Medicine: Newborn Nursery at LPCH Web site. http://newborns.stanford.edu/PhotoGallery/Cephalohematoma1.html. Accessed April 7, 2015.

48. Doerr S. Newborn jaundice (neonatal jaundice). In: Mersch J, ed. MedicineNet. http://www.medicinenet.com/newborn_jaundice_neonatal_jaundice/page3.htm. Reviewed March 24, 2014. Accessed April 7, 2015.

49. Ramachandran M, Achan P, Jones DHA, Panchbhavi VK. Osteogenesis imperfecta. In: Gellman H, ed. Medscape. http://emedicine.medscape.com/article/1256726-overview#showall. Updated November 24, 2014. Accessed April 8, 2015.

50. Olitsky SE, Hug D, Plummer LS, Stass-Isern M. Abnormalities of pupil and iris. In: Kliegman RM, Stanton BF, Schor NF, St. Geme JW III, Behrman RE, eds. *Nelson Textbook of Pediatrics.* 19th ed. Philadelphia, PA: Elsevier Saunders; 2011: 2154–2156.

51. Warner-Rogers J. Clinical neuropsychological assessment of children. In: Goldstein LH, McNeil JE, eds. *Clinical Neuropsychology: A Practical Guide to Assessment and Management for Clinicians.* 2nd ed. Chichester, West Sussex, UK: Wiley-Blackwell; 2013: 317–346.

52. Blosser CG, Woo TM. Eye disorders. In: Burns CE, Dunn AM, Brady MA, Starr NB, Blosser CG, eds. *Pediatric Primary Care.* 5th ed. Philadelphia, PA: Elsevier Saunders; 2012: 622–651.

53. Tuli SY, Giordano BP, Kelly M, Fillipps D, Tuli SS. Newborn with an absent red reflex. *J Pediatr Health Care.* 2013; 27(1): 51–55. doi: 10.1016/j.pedhc.2011.10.010

54. Lesnick BL, Davis SD. Infant pulmonary function testing: Overview of technology and practical considerations – new current procedural terminology codes effective 2010. *Chest.* 2010; 139(5): 1197–1202. doi:10.1378/chest.10-1423

55. Wanger J. *Pulmonary Function Testing: A Practical Approach.* 3rd ed. Sudbury, MA: Jones & Bartlett Learning; 2012: 263–280.

56. Johnson L, Cochran WD. Assessment of the newborn history and physical examination of the newborn. In: Cloherty JP, Eichenwald EC, Hansen AR, Stark AR, eds. *Manual of Neonatal Care.* 7th ed. Philadelphia, PA: Lippincott, Williams, & Wilkins; 2012: 91–102.

57. Blundell A, Harrison R. *OSCEs at a Glance.* 2nd ed. Hoboken, N.J.: John Wiley & Sons; 2013: 304–306.

58. Parikh AS, Mitchell AL. Congenital anomalies. In: Martin RJ, Fanaroff AA, Walsh MC, eds. *Fanaroff and Martin's Neonatal-Perinatal Medicine: Diseases of the Fetus and Infant.* 10th ed. St. Louis, MO: Elsevier Saunders; 2014: 577–596.

59. Frank JE, Jacobe KM. Evaluation and management of heart murmurs in children. *Am Fam Physician.* 2011; 84(7): 793–800. http://www.aafp.org/afp/2011/1001/p793.html

60. Pulse oximetry screening for critical congenital heart defects. Centers for Disease Control and Prevention Web site. http://www.cdc.gov/Features/CongenitalHeartDefects. Last reviewed August 29, 2014. Accessed April 8, 2015.

61. Department of Health and Human Services, State Government of Victoria, Australia. Blood pressure – neonates. http://www.health.vic.gov.au/neonatalhandbook/procedures/blood-pressure.htm. Accessed April 8, 2015.

62. Palazzi DL, Brandt ML. Care of the umbilicus and management of umbilical disorders. In: Basow DS, ed. *UpToDate*. UptoDate: Waltham, MA; 2015. http://www.uptodate.com/contents/care-of-the-umbilicus-and-management-of-umbilical-disorders?source=search_result&search=care+of+the+umbilicus+and&selectedTitle=1~150. Last updated February 20, 2015. Accessed May 6, 2015.

63. Drutz JE. The pediatric physical examination: Chest and abdomen. In: Basow DS, ed. *UpToDate*. UptoDate: Waltham, MA; 2015. http://www.uptodate.com/contents/the-pediatric-physical-examination-chest-and-abdomen. Last updated October 14, 2013. Accessed April 8, 2015.

64. Bowden VR, Greenberg CS. *Children and Their Families: The Continuum of Care.* 2nd ed. Philadelphia, PA: Wolters Kluwer Health/Lippincott Williams & Wilkins; 2010: 860–935.

65. Mayo Clinic Staff. Sacral dimple: complications. Mayo Clinic Web site. http://www.mayoclinic.org/diseases-conditions/sacral-dimple/basics/complications/con-20025266. Reviewed October 24, 2012. Accessed April 9, 2015.

66. Rosenfeld SB. Developmental dysplasia of the hip: Clinical features and diagnosis. In: Basow DS, ed. *UpToDate*. UptoDate: Waltham, MA; 2015. http://www.uptodate.com/contents/developmental-dysplasia-of-the-hip-clinical-features-and-diagnosis?source=search_result&search=developmental+dysplasia+of+the+hip&selectedTitle=1~33. Last updated April 14, 2015. Accessed May 6, 2015.

67. Kemper AR. Newborn screening. In: Basow DS, ed. *UpToDate*. UptoDate: Waltham, MA; 2015. http://www.uptodate.com/contents/newborn-screening?source=search_result&search=newborn+screening&selectedTitle=1~146. Last updated July 14, 2014. Accessed May 6, 2015.

68. Anderson R, Rothwell E, Botkin JR. Newborn screening: Ethical, legal, and social implications. In: Pepper GA, Wysocki KJ, eds. *Annual Review of Nursing Research, Vol. 29: Genetics.* New York, NY: Springer Publishing Company; 2012: 113–132.

69. The Recommended Uniform Screening Panel. Baby's First Test Web site. http://babysfirsttest.org/newborn-screening/the-recommended-uniform-screening-panel. Accessed may 6, 2015.

70. Lewis JA. Human genetics and genomics: Impact on neonatal care. In: Kenner C, Wright Lott J, eds. *Comprehensive Neonatal Nursing Care.* 5th ed. New York, NY: Springer Publishing Company; 2014: 829–848.

71. Adcock LM, Freysdottir D. Screening the newborn for hearing loss. In: Basow DS, ed. *UpToDate*. UptoDate: Waltham, MA; 2015. http://www.uptodate.com/contents/screening-the-newborn-for-hearing-loss?source=search_result&search=screening+the+newborn+for+hearing+loss&selectedTitle=1~150. Last updated April 20, 2015. Accessed May 6, 2015.

72. Riley C, Spencer B, Prater LS. Normal term newborn. In: Kenner C, Wright Lott J, eds. *Comprehensive Neonatal Nursing Care.* 5th ed. New York, NY: Springer Publishing Company; 2014: 113–132.

73. What are the chances my baby has CF? Cystic Fibrosis Foundation Web site. http://www.cff.org/AboutCF/Testing/Newborn-Screening/UnderstandingtheResults/. Last updated January 27, 2014. Accessed May 6, 2015.

Chapter 5

Infant Health and Issues

QUESTIONS

1. You are conducting a Well Child Check on a 5-month-old boy, as per the Bright Futures guidelines. At this point in time, which of the following would <u>least</u> qualify as a concerning finding?

   a. Undescended testes

   b. Galactorrhea

   c. Head lag when pulled to sitting position

   d. Failure to hold head up when lying on stomach

2. A mother brings her 3-month-old male child to your office with complaints of sudden difficulty feeding the child, as well as an inability to console his screaming. Although the child shows a response to her efforts, his crying and agitation have not decreased. The mother also notes that she noticed a bump on his head, which she assumed was from him hitting his head during one of his screaming fits. Which of the following would be the best initial course of action?

   a. Lumbar puncture

   b. Administration of ceftriaxone

   c. Immediate admission to hospital

   d. Blood count and culture

3. A mother brings her 7-month-old infant daughter to your office because, over the past week, she's felt the daughter's lymph nodes in the neck "getting harder." Upon physical examination, you notice that the lymph nodes feel small, round, and slightly hardened. Which of the following is the most likely cause?

   a. Pyelonephritis

   b. Lymphoma

   c. Respiratory infection

   d. Leukemia

4. According to the psychosocial development model, at which age would an infant be <u>least</u> likely to cry when she is handed to her new babysitter?

   a. Four months

   b. Six months

   c. Eight months

   d. Ten months

5. Which of the following standardized tests may be performed by parents with no formal training?

   a. Denver Developmental Screening Test II

   b. Ages and Stages Questionnaire

   c. Bayley Scales of Infant Development

   d. Newborn Behavioral Assessment Scale

6. A 9-month-old infant presents to the clinic fussy, with decreased appetite and a fever of 102.3 °F. Upon examining the patient, you find it difficult to find a localized site of infection. Which of the following is the most likely condition?

   a. Otitis media

   b. Group B streptococcal infection

   c. Occult bacteremia

   d. Urinary tract infection

7. Which of the following findings would most strongly indicate that a febrile infant is moderately ill?

   a. The infant has a temperature of 101.8 °F but smiles often.

   b. The infant is fussy but calms quickly when offered support.

   c. The infant appears listless and does not feed well.

   d. The infant has a temperature of 103 °F but appears alert and active.

8. During the examination of a 3-month-old patient, you place the infant in the supine position with the hips flexed 90° and abducted. You then grab the patient's legs by the thigh and gently adduct the leg while applying downward, lateral pressure. What is the name of the supplementary exam that is commonly performed in conjunction with the exam you are performing on your patient?

   a. Klisic

   b. Barlow

   c. Ortolani's

   d. Galeazzi

9. What is the name of the condition in which the foreskin is not retractable over the tip of the penis?

   a. Epispadias

   b. Chordee

   c. Hypospadias

   d. Phimosis

10. You are consulting a mother who is worried about her 8-month-old male infant. She states that he has a fever, and she wants to give him ibuprofen. You recommend giving him 90 mg of ibuprofen every 6 hours. Based on the above treatment guidelines, what is the most likely weight of this infant?

    a. 7.5 kg

    b. 8.18 kg

    c. 9 kg

    d. 10 kg

RATIONALES

1. c

Although infants should mostly maintain head control by 4 months of age, it is still normal for an infant to reach this developmental milestone anywhere between 4 and 6 months of age. The inability to raise the head when lying on the stomach, galactorrhea, and undescended testes are all considered to be developmental warning signs starting at 3 months of age.

2. c

The signs that the child is displaying—persistent screaming with no evidence of fever and a soft, bulging fontanel—are indicative of intracranial pressure in the infant, which warrants immediate hospital admission. A bulging fontanel typically occurs when fluid builds up in the brain, causing increased intracranial pressure. A lumbar puncture would be appropriate if the aim was to measure the intracranial pressure. Administering ceftriaxone would be warranted in cases of bacterial infection, which is often indicated by a temperature change in the infant. Performing a blood count test and obtaining cultures are often used to detect bacteremia in infants.

3. c

The most likely cause is a respiratory infection because the infant is presenting with shotty lymph nodes, which often indicate a past infection. Although pyelonephritis is an infection, it is less likely than a respiratory infection to cause shotty lymph nodes in the neck. Lymphoma would be more strongly indicated by enlarged lymph nodes, as opposed to shotty lymph nodes. Leukemia would be characterized by generalized lymphadenopathy, not localized to one area.

4. a

An infant would be least likely to cry when introduced to a stranger at around 4 months, as stranger anxiety typically develops at around 6 months. Thus, the 6-month-old, the 8-month-old, and the 9-month-old are more likely than the 4-month-old to have developed a fear of strangers, and would be more likely to cry when introduced to a new babysitter.

5. b

The Ages and Stages Questionnaire is a standardized test that may be utilized by parents or care takers and does not require a professional. The Denver Developmental Screening Test II and the Bayley Scales of Infant Development test typically require the employment of professionals. The Newborn Behavioral Assessment Scale may be performed by Brazelton-certified individuals.

6. d

A diagnosis of urinary tract infection (UTI) should be considered if a local site of infection cannot be found in a febrile infant. Typically, an unexplained fever is the most characteristic symptom in an infant with a UTI. Pneumonia and otitis media are also associated with causing fever in infants, but both conditions would likely present with other findings as well, such as tachypnea or respiratory distress in pneumonia and irritability and vertigo in otitis media. Gastroenteritis in infants would also cause other symptoms and would not be the most likely diagnosis.

7. a

Moderately ill infants typically display irritable or fussy behavior and have a fever temperature below 102 °F, yet are easy to console, may smile, and continue to feed normally. Infants that present with a temperature above 100.4 °F but smile, feed normally, and appear alert and active are typically classified as mildly ill. Severely ill infants normally present with a temperature higher than 104 °F; these infants often appear listless, may not feed at all or feed poorly, and are typically recommended for hospital admission.

8. c

The scenario describes the Barlow test, which is used to assess for developmental dysplasia of the hip (DDH); the Ortolani test is typically performed with the Barlow test and is also used to assess for developmental dysplasia of the hip. These two tests evaluate hip stability and are the favored diagnostic exams for patients 3 months of age and younger. The Klisic and Galeazzi signs are often performed on patients older than 3 months of age to assess for decreased hip abduction and unequal thigh length.

9. d

Phimosis presents with foreskin that is not retractable over the tip of the penis. This condition is considered common in infant patients and is often resolved by 3 years of age. Hypospadias results in the opening of the urethra manifesting on the underside, rather than the tip, of the penis; epispadias similarly affects the urethra, causing it to open on the top or side of the penis. Chordee refers to curvature of the penis at the junction of head and shaft.

10. c

The suggested ibuprofen regimen for managing a fever in infants older than 6 months is
10 mg/kg every 6 hours; thus, a 90-mg dose of ibuprofen would be recommended for an infant weighing 9 kg. A recommended dose of 90 mg for an infant who weighs 7.5 kg would suggest that the dose is 12 mg/kg, which is not the case. If the suggested dose were 11 mg/kg, the nurse practitioner would recommend 90 mg for an infant who weighs approximately 8.18 kg. These dosing regimens would be appropriate for acetaminophen, however, because the recommended dose is 10–15 mg/kg. For a 10 kg patient taking 90 mg of ibuprofen, the recommended dosing ratio would have to be 9 mg/kg.

DISCUSSION

Child Health Supervision

Overview

The American Academy of Pediatrics' (AAP) *Bright Futures: Guidelines of Health Supervision of Infants, Children, and Adolescents* acts as a primary guide for supervision of child health and promotes optimal health development in children through preventive care.[1] To accomplish this goal, supervision of infant health includes screenings at regularly scheduled intervals, known as Well Child Checks (WCCs), starting at 1 month of age.[2] In addition to measuring the child's growth and development, WCCs help detect and treat diseases early and prevent diseases through routine vaccinations, education, and anticipatory guidance.[3]

Definition

In child health supervision, the newborn period begins at birth and lasts up to the first month of life; infancy, on the other hand, is the period after birth through 11 months of age. Early childhood spans ages 1–4 years. Middle childhood spans from 5 to 10 years of age, and adolescence occurs thereafter until 21 years of age.[4]

Focus

Physical

Infant WCCs should include an assessment of the child's growth and development. The physical examination should include a measurement of weight, height, and head circumference.[5] Additionally, the child's gross and fine motor development should be assessed, as should social interaction.[6]

Cognitive

The nurse practitioner (NP) should assess the cognitive and sensorimotor development of children. The NP can make these assessments through direct observations, a thorough history, and observations from parents, teachers, and child care providers.[4]

Psychosocial

Psychosocial development of infants is marked by development of trust.[7] The infant's social development and parent-child interactions should also be assessed.[3]

Well Child Checks

Overview

WCCs should begin 1 month post-birth, followed by visits at 2, 4, 6, 9, and 12 months of age.[2,8] If the infant is discharged from the hospital prior to 48 hours, his or her first visit should be within 48 hours of discharge.[8] Many providers also choose to check weight gain and feeding at a 2 week visit.

Stage Appropriate Screening

WCCs use both subjective and objective data to assess a child's health. The WCC may include a physical exam; laboratory tests; health and developmental history; immunizations; lead, hearing, vision, and dental screenings; and health education.[9] Additionally, developmental screening can be assessed by the Ages and Stages Questionnaire (ASQ), which is the parents' assessment of their child's language, social, motor, and problem solving skills. The Denver Developmental Screening Test, second edition (Denver II), can also be implemented to detect developmental delays or children at risk of development problems.[10] Management plans for the infant are determined by the results of screening.

The Physical Examination: Necessary Elements

Overview

A complete physical examination is recommended for all children and should be performed at regular intervals.[11] The examination should measure the infant's height and weight; head circumference should also be measured until the child is 3 years of age.[11] These measurements are recorded on approved growth charts for the specific child. The NP should also assess the infant's vital signs, including temperature, blood pressure, respiratory rate, and heart rates.[11]

Head control is expected in infants by 4 months of age, and no lag is expected when the infant is pulled to sitting at 6 months. A lag may indicate a neurodevelopmental concern such as palsy.[12] The infant's fontanels should also be assessed. The posterior fontanel usually closes within the first few months, and the anterior fontanel typically closes around 15–18 months. Early or late closure of fontanels may signal significant anomalies, such as hyperthyroidism, trisomy disorders, or microcephaly.[13] The nose should be assessed for nasal flaring, which may indicate difficulty breathing, or a flattened bridge, which may indicate an underlying congenital disorder such as fetal alcohol syndrome.[14] The NP should also examine the child's skin for lesions, rashes, or other abnormalities.[11,15]

A nose, mouth, and throat exam can help detect infections and common childhood abnormalities.[16] These abnormalities may be caused by too little or too much fluoride, sleeping with a bottle, or an unusual tooth eruption sequence. Fissures at the patient's lip corners may indicate vitamin deficiencies, and asymmetrically enlarged tonsils may suggest infection, as well as immunologic or anatomic anomalies.[17]

Voice abnormalities in infants may indicate underlying disorders. For instance, a shrill or high-pitched cry may indicate increased intracranial pressure.[18] In addition to assessing the infant's voice, the NP should perform a chest and lung exam, assessing for normal heart sounds and breathing. Mild pectus carinatum (pigeon chest) and pectus excavatum (sunken chest) are common findings in children, and gynecomastia and galactorrhea may present up to 3 months of age; if these presentations persist or exacerbate, however, the patient may have a genetic disorder.[5,17] An abdominal exam should likewise be performed. In most infants, the abdomen is prominent and the liver edge is palpable 1–2 cm below the right costal margin.[17] Diastasis recti, a disorder marked by the separation of the rectus abdominis muscle, is a common abnormal abdominal finding in infants; this condition typically resolves on its own and does not necessitate intervention.[12]

The genitals should be examined in infants of both genders. When dealing with female patients, the NP should assess for signs of labial adhesions and ensure that the vaginal opening is fully visible. When dealing with male patients, the NP should assess for abnormalities of the penis and testes. The testes typically descend by the age of 3 months, and many male infants present with a large scrotum. When examining the penis, the NP should assess for genitourinary abnormalities such as phimosis, where the foreskin is unable to fully retract, or hypospadias, where the urethra appears on the underside of the penis.[12,17]

Developmental dysplasia of the hip (DDH), a dislocation of the hip, is typically present at birth but may develop within the first year of life. DDH may be indicated by findings such as asymmetry of skin fold thickness and unequal leg length. DDH can be detected by the Ortolani maneuver, in which a palpable "clunk" is present upon reduction of the hip.[19,20] DDH can also be detected by the Galeazzi sign, which manifests an inequality in the height of the pediatric patient's knees while the patient lies down with his or her feet drawn in towards the buttocks.[21]

In normal infants, lymph nodes are not typically palpable.[22] Infants may present with enlargements in the inguinal and cervical nodes, which are normal variants that typically only last a short period of time.[12] Shotty nodes may indicate past infection in the infant, but do not typically indicate active infection unless they are warm, tender, and enlarged.[22] Palpable supraclavicular lymph nodes or nodes larger than 3 mm should warrant urgent referral for possible malignancy.[22]

Standardized Tests

According to the AAP, children should be screened for developmental disabilities during WCCs at 9 months, 18 months, and 24 or 30 months of age.[23] Several standardized tests may be used to assess the development of infants, including the Denver II, the Bayley Scales of Infant Development, the Bayley Infant Neurodevelopmental Screener, and the ASQ, among others.[17] The Newborn Behavioral Assessment Scale includes 27 behavioral responses and 20 reflex items to assess higher cortical function, including consolability and habituation.[24] The Modified Checklist for Autism in Toddlers should also be used in pediatric screening protocols.[12]

Reflexes and Motor Skills

The presence and strength of an infant's reflexes, such as the Moro reflex and tonic neck reflex, is important in assessing the infant's nervous system development and function. If an infant's reflex persists after the age at which the reflex normally disappears, this may be a sign of neurodevelopmental abnormalities.[12]

Cognitive Development

When evaluating the cognitive development of an infant, the NP should assess the infant's response to environment and voice. Visual acuity is measured by the blink reflex and pupil constriction. Hearing screening, using tests such as otoacoustic emissions and auditory brainstem response, is indicated for all infants.[25]

Sensorimotor development, as defined by Jean Piaget, should also be assessed. By these standards, infants should be able to adapt their reflexes to their environment and engage in simple problem-solving.[26]

Psychosocial Development

There is a range of temperaments in infants; some may adapt easily to situations and people, but others may have a more difficult time adapting and may react more intensely.[12] Infants typically develop a fear of strangers and a fear of separation from their parents at approximately 7–9 months of age.[12] Attachment is defined as an affective bond that develops over the course of the first year of life and will differentiate into other emotions later. Although breastfeeding promotes maternal sensitivity and attachment development, breastfeeding is not necessary for, and does not always result in, secure attachment. Insecure attachment results in infants with detachment issues, such as avoidance, anxiety, and disorganization.[4,17]

Nutrition/Feeding

There are many benefits to breastfeeding, as breast milk has the optimal combination of nutrients for the growth and development of infants.[8,27] In addition to breast milk, infants should also receive supplements to ensure an adequate intake of vitamin D.[28] According to the AAP, children should be breastfed exclusively until 6 months of age, at which time solid foods should begin to be introduced. Breastfeeding should continue until approximately 12 months of age. After 12 months of age, infants should be transitioned to whole milk with a limit of 24 ounces per day to avoid micro-gastrointestinal bleeding with resultant iron deficiency anemia. Excessive milk intake can also lead to poor nutrition from lack of food intake due to satiety from milk.[4,12] Weaning may be delayed if breastfeeding is mutually desired by both the mother and infant.[28]

Dental Health

The NP should assess the infant for tooth decay due to use of a baby bottle. Before the patient's teeth erupt, the infant's mouth should be cleaned by wiping with a soft cloth; this process will help to minimize the risk of tooth decay once primary dentition begins. Once the teeth erupt, the parents should be encouraged to clean their child's mouth twice daily with a soft brush. The infant's fluoride intake should also be monitored; if supplements are necessary, administration should begin at 6 months of age.[29] The AAP recommends that infants have their first dental visit by the time they reach 1 year of age.[30]

Sleep

Infants between the ages of 2 months and 1 year should sleep 16–18 hours per day, including two to three naps daily.[31] It is strongly recommended that parents or caregivers avoid sleeping with infants because bed-sharing can increase the risk of sudden infant death syndrome (SIDS).[8,32]

SIDS can also be prevented by putting infants to sleep on their back, using a firm sleep surface, keeping soft objects out of the crib, offering a pacifier at naptime and bedtime, and breastfeeding.[33]

Injury Prevention: Special Consideration for Infants

Knowledge of developmental phases, awareness of external occurrences that may cause the infant harm, and constant supervision of the infant are ways to facilitate injury prevention. Because infants do not yet understand consequences, they are at an increased risk of unintentional injury, such as falls, burns, poisoning, choking, and drowning. Constant supervision and educating the infant (e.g., teaching the importance of approaching authority figures and staying away from strangers) are also ways to safeguard against potential harm.[8]

Developmental Warning Signs (see table 5.1)

Visual delays, such as retinopathy, infant cataracts, and strabismus, are developmental warning signs in infants.[4,12] Other developmental warning signs include an infant's failure to raise his or her head when lying on his or her stomach by 3 months of age, and the failure to manually play with toys by 6 months of age.

Fever in the Very Young Infant

Infants generally have higher temperatures than older children and adults because they have a greater surface-area-to-body-weight ratio and a higher metabolic rate.[34] An infant is considered to have a fever when the infant's rectal temperature is greater than 100.4 °F (38 °C). In newborns, however, fevers can be indicated by lower than normal temperatures because newborns are unable to regulate their body temperatures when they are very ill.

Fever in Early Infancy (the first 2 months of life)

Although almost any infection can cause fevers in infants, fevers in this population are usually indicative of an upper respiratory illness or other type of viral infection. The degree of the fever does not always directly correlate with the severity of the illness.[35] Group B *Streptococcus* and Gram-negative enteric organisms are common causes of fevers in the first month of age, whereas *Streptococcus pneumoniae* and *Haemophilus influenzae* are more likely causes of fevers in the second month of age.[17]

Assess the Degree of Illness: Responses are Behavioral

Infants who are mildly ill often act relatively normal, appearing alert and active, feeding well, and smiling. Moderately ill infants, on the other hand, may be fussy or irritable. They may, however, eat normally, be consolable, and smile. Severely ill infants with temperatures of 104 °F (40 °C) or higher typically appear listless, cannot be consoled, and either feed poorly or do not feed at all. Hospital admission is recommended if the infant's fever is above 100.4 °F.[17] Diagnostic studies depend on the infant's age: Neonates should receive a full sepsis evaluation, whereas infants older than 28 days should undergo studies to determine the source of the fever. These studies may include lumbar punctures, urine and stool cultures, or complete blood counts, depending on the presentation. Additionally, radiographic studies may be indicated if the patient presents with signs of respiratory illness, such as coughing, wheezing, or coryza.[36] When no local site of infection can be clearly identified, the NP should consider the diagnosis of a urinary tract infection, pneumonia, or another type of infection.[17]

Management

Over-the-counter medications, such as acetaminophen, are recommended to

Table 5.1	Developmental Warning Signs During the Infant Stage
2 months	Doesn't respond to loud sounds
	Doesn't watch things as they move
	Doesn't smile at people
	Doesn't bring hands to mouth
	Can't hold head up when pushing up from stomach
4 months	Doesn't watch things as they move
	Doesn't smile at people
	Can't hold head steady
	Doesn't coo or make sounds
	Doesn't bring things to mouth
	Doesn't push down with legs when feet are on hard surface
	Has trouble moving one or both eyes in all directions
6 months	Doesn't try to get things in reach
	Doesn't show affection to caregivers
	Doesn't respond to sounds
	Has difficulty putting things in mouth
	Doesn't make vowel sounds
	Doesn't roll over in either direction
	Doesn't laugh/make squealing sounds
	Seems stiff with tight muscles
	Seems floppy like a rag doll
9 months	Doesn't bear weight on legs with support
	Doesn't sit with help
	Doesn't babble
	Doesn't play games back and forth
	Doesn't respond to name
	Doesn't seem to recognize familiar people
	Doesn't look where you point
	Doesn't transfer toys from one hand to the other
1 year	Doesn't crawl
	Can't stand when supported
	Doesn't search for things that she sees you hide
	Doesn't say single words
	Doesn't learn gestures (waving, shaking head)
	Doesn't point to things
	Loses skills he/she once had
18 months	Doesn't point to things to show others
	Can't walk
	Doesn't know what familiar things are used for
	Doesn't copy others
	Doesn't gain new words
	Doesn't have a vocabulary of 6 words or more
	Doesn't notice/care when caretaker leaves/returns
	Loses skills he/she once had

Note. Adapted with permission from Developmental milestones. CDC. http://www.cdc.gov/ncbddd/actearly/milestones/index.html. Published 2014. Accessed April 2015.

manage fevers in infants as long as the source of fever is located and treated.[35] Ibuprofen should only be used in infants younger than 6 months of age when they are not responding to acetaminophen and they are being closely monitored in the hospital or undergoing a septic workup.[37] Alternating medications is not recommended because medication errors are common as a result of dosage and timing inaccuracies. Moreover, there is no evidence that a patient's temperature is better controlled by alternating medications.[8,35]

References

1. Hagan JF, Shaw JS, Duncan PM, eds. *Bright Futures: Guidelines for Health Supervision of Infants, Children, and Adolescents.* 3rd ed. Elk Grove Village, IL: American Academy of Pediatrics; 2008.

2. Well-child visits. MedlinePlus Web site. http://www.nlm.nih.gov/medlineplus/ency/article/001928.htm. Updated January 27, 2013. Accessed April 8, 2015.

3. Consolini DM. Health supervision of the well child. In: Porter RS, Kaplan JL, eds. The Merck Manual Online. http://www.merckmanuals.com/professional/pediatrics/health_supervision_of_the_well_child/health_supervision_of_the_well_child.html?qt=colson%20held%20and%20chapman&alt=sh. Updated April 2014. Accessed April 13, 2015.

4. Kliegman RM, Stanton BF, St. Geme JW III, Schor NF, Behrman RE. *Nelson Textbook of Pediatrics.* 19th ed. Philadelphia, PA: Elsevier Saunders; 2011.

5. Drutz JE. The pediatric physical examination: Chest and abdomen. In: Basow DS, ed. *UpToDate.* Waltham, MA: UpToDate; 2015. http://www.uptodate.com/contents/the-pediatric-physical-examination-chest-and-abdomen?source=search_result&search=pediatric+physical+examination&selectedTitle=3~150. Updated October 14, 2013. Accessed April 13, 2015.

6. Boyse K. Developmental milestones. University of Michigan Health System Web site. http://www.med.umich.edu/yourchild/topics/devmile.htm. Updated August 2013. Accessed April 13, 2015.

7. Crocetti E, Meeus WHJ, Ritchie RA, Meca A, Schwartz SJ. Adolescent identity: Is this the key to unraveling associations between family relationships and problem behaviors? In: Scheier LM, Hansen WB, eds. *Parenting and Teen Drug Use: The Most Recent Finding from Research, Prevention, and Treatment.* New York, NY: Oxford University Press; 2014: 92–109.

8. Recommendations for preventive pediatric health care. American Academy of Pediatrics Web site. http://www.aap.org/en-us/professional-resources/practice-support/Periodicity/Periodicity%20Schedule_FINAL.pdf. Published 2014. Accessed April 14, 2015.

9. Well child exams. Lake Cumberland District Health Department Web site. http://www.lcdhd.org/children/well_child_exams. Accessed April 14, 2015.

10. Ringwalt S. Developmental screening and assessment instruments with an emphasis on social and emotional development for young children ages birth through five. National Early Childhood Technical Assistance Center Web site. http://www.nectac.org/~pdfs/pubs/screening.pdf. Published May 2008. Accessed April 14, 2015.

11. Drutz JE. The pediatric physical examination: General principles and standard measurements. In: Basow DS, ed. *UpToDate.* Waltham, MA: UpToDate; 2015. http://www.uptodate.com/contents/the-pediatric-physical-examination-general-principles-and-standard-measurements. Updated March 2015. Accessed April 14, 2015.

12. Burns CE, Dunn AM, Brady MA, Starr NB, Blosser CG. *Pediatric Primary Care.* 5th ed. Philadelphia, PA: Elsevier Saunders; 2013.

13. Gallagher ER, Hing AV, Cunningham ML. Evaluating fontanels in the newborn skull. *Contemp Peds.* 2013; 30(11): 12. http://contemporarypediatrics.modernmedicine.com/contemporary-pediatrics/content/tags/cerebrospinal-fluid-dynamics/evaluating-fontanels-newborn-skull?page=full

14. Fuller RA. Newborn assessment. In: Sawyer SS, ed. *Pediatric Physical Examination & Health Assessment.* Sudbury, MA: Jones & Bartlett Learning; 2012: 103–142.

15. PEDS: Basic pediatric clerkship. University of Washington Department of Pediatrics Web site. https://www.washington.edu/medicine/pediatrics/docs/students/PEDS%20Clerkship%20Manual_Website_0614.pdf. Last updated May 2014. Accessed April 14, 2015.

16. Allen PJ. Nose, mouth, and throat. In: Duderstadt K, ed. *Pediatric Physical Examination: An Illustrated Handbook.* 2nd ed. St. Louis, MO: Elsevier Mosby; 2014: 178–197.

17. Barkley TW Jr. Infant health and issues. In *Pediatric Primary Care Nurse Practitioner: Certification Review/Clinical Update Continuing Education Course.* West Hollywood, CA: Barkley & Associates; 2015: 38–44.

18. Increased intracranial pressure. Nationwide Children's Hospital Web site. www.nationwidechildrens.org/Document/Get/40003. Updated January 2015. Accessed April 14, 2015.

19. Schwend RM, Shaw BA, Segal LS. Evaluation and treatment of developmental hip dysplasia in the newborn and infant. *Pediatr Clin North Am.* 2014; 61(6): 1095–1107. doi: 10.1016/j.pcl.2014.08.008

20. Tamai J, McCarthy JJ. Developmental dysplasia of the hip. In: Jaffe WL, ed. Medscape. http://emedicine.medscape.com/article/1248135-overview#showall. Updated March 31, 2014. Accessed April 14, 2015.

21. Storer SK, Skaggs DL. Developmental dysplasia of the hip. *Am Fam Physician.* 2006; 74(8): 1310–1316. http://www.aafp.org/afp/2006/1015/p1310.html

22. Drutz JE. The pediatric physical examination: Back, extremities, nervous system, skin, and lymph nodes. In: Basow DS, ed. *UpToDate.* Waltham, MA: UpToDate; 2015. http://www.uptodate.com/contents/the-pediatric-physical-examination-back-extremities-nervous-system-skin-and-lymph-nodes?source=-search_result&search=pediatric+physical+examination&selectedTitle=5~150. Updated March 2015. Accessed April 14, 2015.

23. U.S. Department of Health and Human Services, Centers for Disease Control and Prevention. Developmental monitoring and screening. http://www.cdc.gov/ncbddd/childdevelopment/screening.html. Updated February 12, 2015. Accessed April 14, 2015.

24. Kotagal S. Neurological examination of the newborn. In: Basow DS, ed. *UpToDate.* Waltham, MA: UpToDate; 2015. http://www.uptodate.com/contents/neurologic-examination-of-the-newborn?source=search_result&search=neurological+examination+of+the+newborn&selectedTitle=1~150. Updated May 28, 2014. Accessed April 14, 2015.

25. Delaney AM. Newborn hearing screening. In: Meyers AD, ed. Medscape.. http://emedicine.medscape.com/article/836646-overview#showall. Updated September 11, 2014. Accessed April 14, 2015.

26. Cherry K. Sensorimotor stage of cognitive development. About Education Web site. http://psychology.about.com/od/piagetstheory/p/sensorimotor.htm. Accessed April 14, 2015.

27. Infant feeding and nutrition module. Oregon Health Authority Web site. https://public.health.oregon.gov/HealthyPeopleFamilies/wic/Documents/modules/infant-feeding-and-nutrition-staff.pdf. Updated April 2014. Accessed April 14, 2015.

28. American Academy of Pediatrics. Breastfeeding and the use of human milk. *Pediatrics.* 2012; 129(3): 600–603. doi: 10.1542/peds.2011-3553

29. Nowak AJ, Warren JJ. (2015). Preventive dental care and counseling for infants and young children. In: Basow DS, ed. *UpToDate*. Waltham, MA: UpToDate; 2015. http://www.uptodate.com/contents/preventive-dental-care-and-counseling-for-infants-and-young-children?source=search_result&search=Preventive+dental+care+and+counseling+for+infants+and+young+children&selectedTitle=1~150. Updated February 13, 2015. Accessed April 14, 2015.

30. Your child's age 1 dental visit. Simple Steps Web site. http://www.simplestepsdental.com/SS/ihtSSPrint/r.WSIHW000/st.31840/t.31887/pr.3/c.354252.html. Updated July 3, 2012. Accessed April 14, 2015.

31. U.S. Department of Health and Human Services, Centers for Disease Control and Prevention. How much sleep do I need? http://www.cdc.gov/sleep/about_sleep/how_much_sleep.htm. Updated July 1, 2013. Accessed April 14, 2015.

32. UNICEF UK Baby Friendly Initiative statement on bed sharing research. UNICEF Web site. http://www.unicef.org.uk/BabyFriendly/News-and-Research/News/UNICEF-UK-Baby-Friendly-Initiative-statement-on-new-bed-sharing-research. Published May 21, 2014. Accessed April 14, 2015.

33. American Academy of Pediatrics. SIDS and other sleep-related infant deaths: Expansion of recommendations for a safe infant sleeping environment. *Pediatrics*. 2011; 128(5): e1341–e1367. doi: 10.1542/peds.2011-2285

34. Ward MA. Fever in infants and children: Pathophysiology and management. In: Basow DS, ed. *UpToDate*. Waltham, MA: UpToDate; 2015. http://www.uptodate.com/contents/fever-in-infants-and-children-pathophysiology-and-management?source=search_result&search=Pathophysiology+and+management+of+fever+in+infants+and+children&selectedTitle=1~150. Updated December 15, 2014. Accessed April 14, 2015.

35. Sullivan JE, Farrar HC, Section on Clinical Pharmacology and Therapeutics, Committee on Drugs. Fever and antipyretic use in children. *Pediatrics*. 2011; 127(3): 580–587. doi: 10.1542/peds.2010-3852

36. Gould JM, Aronoff SC. Fever in the infant and toddler workup. In: Steele RW, ed. Medscape. http://emedicine.medscape.com/article/1834870-workup#showall. Updated January 30, 2014. Accessed April 14, 2015.

37. Hockenberry MJ, Wilson D. *Wong's Essentials of Pediatric Nursing*. 9th ed. St. Louis, MO: Elsevier; 2013.

Chapter 6

Toddler/Preschool Health and Issues

QUESTIONS

1. Johnny, age 3, is brought into the clinic by his parents, who state that he has been unable to perform certain skills that he used to be able to perform. They also say that his ability to use language has started to deteriorate, and he does not want to play with the other children at school. Which of the following conditions would be the most likely diagnoses?

   a. Autistic disorder

   b. Asperger's syndrome

   c. Rett's disorder

   d. Childhood disintegrative disorder

2. By what age would a lack of awareness of cars and animals be first considered a developmental delay?

   a. At 1 year

   b. At 2 years

   c. At 3 years

   d. At 4 years

3. Dan and Kara bring their toddler son, Ian, to your office because they are worried about his feeding habits. They explain that they still have to feed him because he is unable to use utensils—even a spoon—on his own. As the practitioner, you know that at what earliest age would Ian have to be for this issue to be a developmental concern?

   a. Twelve months old

   b. Fifteen months old

   c. Seventeen months old

   d. Twenty months old

4. Two 2 year olds are playing in a sandbox. They are both scooping and pouring sand, occasionally glancing over at each other but not interacting. How would the nurse practitioner best characterize this type of play?

   a. This behavior is abnormal, as by now they should want to play together.

   b. This behavior demonstrates parallel play, which is common in this age group.

   c. These children are participating in associative play, which is not expected in this age group.

   d. This is active play and is typical in this age group.

5. What is the average age by which toddlers achieve daytime control of bowel and bladder movements?

   a. By 18 months of age

   b. By 2 years of age

   c. By 2.5 years of age

   d. By 3 years of age

6. A 3-year-old male patient presents for a well-child checkup. While interviewing his parents, you learn that the patient's family comes from a working-class neighborhood in downtown Los Angeles. All of the following laboratory exams are especially indicated at this age <u>except</u>:

   a. Hemoglobin and hematocrit

   b. Vitamin D level

   c. Cholesterol

   d. Lead level

7. At what age does taking a blood pressure reading usually become a part of a child's physical examination?

   a. At 2 years

   b. At 3 years

   c. At 4 years

   d. At 5 years

8. Which of the following values most likely indicates the normal visual acuity of a 5-year-old child?

   a. Vision is 20/80

   b. Vision is 20/50

   c. Vision is 20/30

   d. Vision is 20/20

9. A concerned father says that his daughter recently turned 5 years old, and he has noticed she is beginning to stutter. The nurse practitioner tells the father that his daughter's condition is probably normal, but you will be watching with him to see if it persists or if she avoids speaking. As the nurse practitioner, you know that it is usually acceptable to wait before referring the son for his stuttering until how long?

   a. Three months

   b. Six months

   c. Nine months

   d. Twelve months

10. Leonard, a 4-year-old toddler, is brought to your office by his parents who have some concerns regarding his development. Which of the following factors should Leonard's parents be most concerned about?

    a. He has only eaten mashed potatoes for the previous 4 weeks.

    b. He has had a stutter for the previous 4 months.

    c. He struggles with nighttime bowel and bladder control.

    d. He has never acquired the motor skill of skipping.

RATIONALES

1. d

Based on the age of the patient and the recent decline in multiple areas of functioning, the most likely condition is childhood disintegrative disorder. This condition generally presents with a regression after at least 2 years of normal development. Autistic disorder, on the other hand, typically presents with impaired social interaction or language delay within the patient's first year. Asperger's syndrome does not typically result in language delays and would likely present with repetitive behaviors or interests. Lastly, Rett's disorder typically manifests after the first 5 months of the patient's life and results in neurodegenerative development. This condition has predominately been diagnosed in females; thus, it would not likely present in a male patient.

2. b

It would be considered a developmental warning sign for a toddler to not notice animals or cars by the age of 2 years. At the age of 1 year, an infant is not yet expected to notice animals or cars. A child not being aware of his or her external environment could be considered a developmental warning sign at 3 years of age. Not listening or not speaking in sentences would be a developmental warning sign at 4 years.

3. d

The inability to use a spoon would not be considered a warning sign for developmental delay until 18 months of age or after; so, of the choices, 20 months would be the earliest age at which this would be considered a warning sign for Ian. Children are typically still using their hands to eat food at 12 months of age. A spoon could be introduced as early as 15 months of age, and the ability to use the spoon is often acquired by 17 months.

4. b

Two year olds most frequently exhibit parallel or onlooker play. Parallel play is characterized by children mimicking each other's behavior without actively engaging with one another. Preschoolers exhibit associative, dramatic, and interactive play.

5. b

Although toddlers may be physiologically and psychologically ready for toilet training at 18 months of age, they are, on average, able to control daytime bowel and bladder movements by 2 years of age. Since toilet training does not start at a specific age, some children may be ready to begin toilet training at 2.5 years; this age does not, however, represent the median age at which the child achieves daytime control. By 3 years of age, toddlers should be able to control nighttime bowel and bladder control, which usually lags behind daytime control by 1 year.

6. b

Children in inner city and impoverished environments are expected to be tested for anemia; thus, hemoglobin/hematocrit, lead poisoning (which is common in this population) and cholesterol (if greater than the 95th percentile) tests are usually warranted. Vitamin D is frequently measured but there are no requirements for this test at this age.

7. b

Blood pressure (BP) readings usually become part of a child's physical examination at 3 years of age. Although BP readings may be conducted before the age of 3 years, results are often difficult to isolate; as such, these readings are usually only considered in cases when the child shows signs of underlying renal or cardiovascular disease. BP readings should already be part of a child's physical examination by 4 or 5 years of age.

8. c

Normal visual acuity for a 5-year-old child is usually 20/30. A 5-year-old with a visual acuity of 20/80 or 20/50 is lower than the average visual acuity for this age and, in such cases, the child should be referred to an optometrist or ophthalmologist. Likewise, 20/20 vision is not expected at this stage of development.

9. b

The nurse practitioner should advise the father to bring in his daughter for an evaluation if her stuttering persists for more than 6 months or if she avoids speaking. Because stuttering normally resolves within anywhere from a few weeks to 6 months, bringing a child in for evaluation after 3 months does not allow enough time for the condition to resolve spontaneously. However, if the stuttering persists, waiting up to 9 months or longer may be detrimental to language development as therapy practices should be implemented prior to that point.

10. c

The fact that Leonard still struggles with nighttime bowel and bladder control gives most substantial grounds for concern. On average, daytime bowel and bladder control is acquired by 2 years of age, and nighttime control is acquired within the following year. Toilet training is often completed by 4 years of age. Food jags are common behaviors in toddlers. This behavior is taken on by toddlers to assert their independence, and may be relieved by continuing to offer new foods, and encouraging kids to at least taste them. Stutters that present before 6 years of age are not of concern unless the stuttering persists for longer than 6 months or leads to the child avoiding speaking. Lastly, skipping is a motor skill that is generally acquired by age 5, so the fact that Leonard has never skipped is of little concern at this point in his life.

DISCUSSION

Definition

The toddler age is defined as 1 to 3 years of age, whereas the preschool age is considered to last from ages 4 to 5 years.[1]

Focus

Physical

The physical development of toddlers is assessed by measurements of the child's body. These measurements consist of the toddler's length, height, weight, and head circumference, which are taken at each checkup until the toddler is 2 years of age.[1,2]

Cognitive

According to Jean Piaget's theory of cognitive development, the preoperational thinking stage lasts from 2 to 7 years of age.[3] During this stage, children are typically egocentric in their thoughts and communications. One characteristic of childhood egocentrism is the concept of animism, in which the child believes that inanimate objects are alive and have feelings.[4] Moreover, children typically begin to engage in pretend play during the preoperational stage.[3] Around age 4 years, children enter the intuitive thinking substage, which lasts until approximately age 7 years. In this substage, children often learn by asking questions and display centration in their thinking.[5]

Psychosocial

Erik Erikson's theory of psychosocial development categorizes toddlers as entering the autonomy vs. shame and doubt stage, whereas preschoolers enter the initiative vs. guilt stage. During the autonomy vs. shame and doubt stage, toddlers commonly develop a greater sense of personal control which, in turn, promotes confidence.[6] The initiative vs. guilt stage, on the other hand, is usually marked by the child asserting power and control over the world via directing social interactions such as play.[6]

Well Child Checks

Overview

Well Child Checks (WCCs) measure a toddler's health by gathering subjective and objective data. A physical examination commonly measures anthropometrics, including the child's height, weight, and head circumference.[2]

Numerous tools are used in developmental screening, such as the Ages and Stages Questionnaire produced by the American Academy of Pediatrics (AAP) and the Denver Developmental Screening Test, second edition (Denver II). These tools are often used for developmental screening of children 6 years of age and under. Children should receive blood pressure assessments annually, starting at 3 years of age.[7] The AAP also recommends that additional screening for anemia should occur between 1 and 5 years of age.[8] To meet these recommendations, children may be screened for anemia via hematocrit testing. Furthermore, for children who live in high-risk areas such as large, urban cities, the Centers for Disease Control and Prevention (CDC)[9] recommend lead screening with questionnaires. Preschoolers should be screened for tuberculosis with a purified protein derivative test between the ages of 4 and 6 years if they are at risk for the disease. Finally, children should undergo cholesterol screenings at around 10 years of age to assess for cardiovascular risk factors.[10]

Management of toddlers should include the continuation and completion of the primary series of immunizations. The toddler's illnesses should be managed with appropriate supportive care or medications, and the nurse practitioner (NP) should also give health promotion strategies with anticipatory guidance. Moreover, the AAP recommends that the child's first dental screening should ideally occur after the first tooth eruption and no later than age 1.[11]

According to the recommended schedule for WCCs, toddlers should be screened at 12, 15, and 18 months of age. Beginning at 2 years of age, children should be screened annually.[12]

The Interview

Overview

When interviewing a toddler, the NP should be mindful that toddlers are often striving for autonomy. Tantrums are common in toddlers, and major fears emerge during this age as well. The NP should allow children to touch equipment, give choices when possible, and continue progression from a non-invasive exam to an invasive exam. Additionally, the child should be undressed for as little of the exam as possible in order to keep discomfort to a minimum.[1,13]

The Physical Examination: Necessary Elements

Overview

Measurement of the standard growth parameters is essential for assessing a child's normal development.[14] In a physical examination, a toddler's weight and length (i.e., height) should be measured at each visit up to 2 years of age, at which point these measurements should then be taken annually. Body mass index measures the proportion between the child's weight and height, and is the best clinical standard for defining obesity in children older than age 2 years.[15] Furthermore, head circumference is measured during each visit up to 2 years of age. The anterior fontanel usually closes between 12 and 18 months of age; delayed closure may indicate an underlying condition, such as hypothyroidism or Down syndrome.[1,13] Chest circumference, on the other hand, is usually measured in the examination of a newborn, but is not a typical part of subsequent routine examinations for toddlers.[14] A child's chest and head are typically equal until the age of 2 years, after which the chest size usually becomes larger than the head.[16]

In addition to these measurements, the toddler's vital signs should also be measured, including temperature, respiratory and heart rates, and blood pressure.[14] Typical dental development consists of the appearance of primary teeth at 6 months of age and permanent teeth at 6 years of age.[1,13] An eye exam should be performed at each WCC to assess for conditions, such as strabismus, which often appear shortly after birth.[1,13] In an ear examination, the child's tympanic membrane may appear red as a result of crying. Children should be assessed for neck masses. Shotty nodes are normal findings, as are nodes with 1–2 cm enlargement; both typically present post-infection.[17,18] Moreover, children should be assessed for periorbital edema, which is the presenting symptom in nearly all children with nephrotic syndrome.[19]

The NP should conduct a mouth and throat exam to assess for abnormalities. Dental abnormalities, such as cavities, may occur due to lack of fluoride; less commonly, too much fluoride can cause changes in the child's enamel.[20] Fissures at the lip corners may indicate a vitamin deficiency, and mouth breathing may be indicative of allergic rhinitis.[13] Furthermore, a nasal voice may be indicative of enlarged adenoids or tonsils, whereas a raspy voice may be indicative of laryngitis.[21]

Cardiac disorders may be indicated by increased respiratory rate at rest or during sleep, as well as eyelid or orbital edemas. If the child is squatting during play or sleeping in a knee-to-chest position, this may also indicate cardiac disorders.[22] The NP should perform a chest exam, and the point of maximal impulse (PMI) can usually be found near the fourth intercostal space in the midclavicular line; a displaced PMI may indicate a cardiac disorder.[23] Additionally, a lung exam should be performed to assess the pediatric patient's respiratory rate, diaphragm movement, and breath sounds.[24]

Prominent abdomens are often normal in toddlers, and palpation of the abdomen may be helpful in assessing whether or not the prominent abdomen is caused by an underlying complication.[25] A liver edge is palpable 1–2 cm beneath the right costal margin in most children. Labial adhesions are common in prepubertal females, and males may present with undescended testes or phimosis, a condition where the foreskin is too tight to be pulled back from the head of the penis.[26,27] Genu varum (bowed legs) and genu valgum (knock-knees) are both normal musculoskeletal variants in young children.[22] Genu varum, however, often resolves by age 2 years and warrants an orthopedic referral if it persists any longer; genu valgum typically resolves itself by age 7 years.[18] A turned-in foot may indicate femoral anteversion or tibial torsion.[18]

Developmental Monitoring

Motor Skills

The CDC outlines developmental milestones that indicate whether a toddler is developing normally.[28] At 2 years of age, the child should be able to walk up and down steps, run, kick a ball, and build a tower of four or more blocks. At 3 years of age, the child should be able to ride a tricycle and copy a circle. At age 4 years, children typically begin to hop and show the ability to draw a person with at least two body parts. Lastly, at 5 years of age, the child should be able to skip, as well as copy squares and other types of shapes.

Cognitive Development

According to Jean Piaget's theories of cognitive development, the preoperational period lasts from 2 to 7 years of age. During this stage, children display a tendency to understand their environment only through their own point of view, a tendency known as egocentrism. Moreover, children in this stage of development tend to demonstrate animism, which is the belief that inanimate objects are capable of feeling and thinking.[3]

Piaget's preoperational stage can be further divided into the preconceptual substage, which lasts from 2 to 4 years of age, and the intuitive substage, which lasts from 4 to 7 years of age. The preconceptual substage is characterized by the child's inability to understand the properties of classes used to identify objects. During the intuitive stage, on the other hand, children typically develop a more complete understanding of concepts.[29]

Visual acuity is often the best measurement to help determine if a child's vision is developing normally; visual acuity testing should be performed on all children older than 3 years of age. A toddler's visual acuity is about 20/30 and often continues to improve with age.[30] Furthermore, toddlers commonly begin to orient themselves with sound and language development at 2 years of age.[1] The recommended hearing test for children 3 years of age and older is play audiometry, which is similar to pure tone audiometry, except that the child performs specific play actions when he or she hears tones.[31]

By age 2 years, language development typically progresses to the point where the child has at least a 50-word vocabulary, talks constantly, and can follow simple instructions.[1,13,28] The child's vocabulary usually expands to include up to 900 words by 3 years of age, 1,500–1,600 words by 4 years of age, and more than 2,000 words by 5 years of age.[32] Moreover, at age 4 years, the child can understand phrases and simple analogies; by age 5 years, children use sentences regularly and know at least four colors. A tip in remembering meaningful word usage in sentences is recalling that children typically use two words in conjunction by 2 years of age, three words in conjunction by 3 years of age, four words in conjunction by 4 years of age, and five words in conjunction by 5 years of age.[18]

Psychosocial Development

According to Erik Erikson's stages of psychosocial development, the toddler years are characterized by the autonomy vs. shame and doubt stage, which lasts from 2 to 3 years of age. The autonomy versus shame and doubt stage is characterized by the child's development of a sense of independence by gaining personal control.[33] In order to curb aggression and encourage impulse control during this stage, discipline should be introduced. Furthermore, play is a major psychosocial medium during the autonomy vs. shame and doubt stage; toddlers often engage in onlooker and parallel play, and preschoolers often engage in associative, cooperative, dramatic, and physical play.[1,13]

Standardized Testing

Overview

The Bayley Scales of Infant and Toddler Development, third edition (BAYLEY-III), are the gold standard for recognizing and diagnosing developmental delays in infants and toddlers up to 42 months of age. The BAYLEY-III test measures a child's development with separate cognitive, language, motor, social-emotional, and adaptive functioning scales.[34] As mentioned earlier, the Denver II test may be used to screen a child's development up to 6 years of age. Additionally, the Ages and Stages Questionnaire is used to screen children from 4 months to 5 years of age.[35] The Modified Checklist for Autism in Toddlers is also used during this time, and is used to screen children and assess the risk of autism spectrum disorder.[13]

Nutrition/Feeding

As soon as parents begin introducing cow's milk, the bottle should be weaned to reduce the risk of tooth decay.[36] A sippy cup can even begin to be used around 10 months of age to reduce the time needed to wean from the bottle. The use of utensils should also be encouraged, and most toddlers are able to use forks and spoons by 18 months of age.[13] Concerning the toddler's diet, it is important to not force eating, to avoid simple sugar snacks and drinks, and to remember that food jags are common.[18]

Dental Health

According to the AAP, children should receive their first dental exam by 1 year of age.[37] Additionally, brushing is recommended for toddlers twice a day, including before bed.[38]

Sleep

Toddlers require 10–12 hours of sleep per night in addition to a daily afternoon nap.[39] During the toddler age, rituals and consistency at bedtime are necessary.[18] Nightmares, when they occur, generally start between 3 and 6 years of age; children at this age may also experience night terrors, which are episodes of extreme panic.[40] Most children outgrow night terrors as they grow older.[18]

Toilet Training

Toilet training does not start at a specific age, but depends on the toddler's physical and emotional readiness.[41] Usually, children are physiologically and psychologically ready for toilet training between 1.5 and 2.5 years of age. Daytime control of elimination is typically attained by 2 years of age. However, nighttime control often lags behind by approximately one year. Day and night control is typically achieved around 3–4 years of age.[13] Toilet training should not be started during stressful times, and children should be rewarded for all good efforts; a child should never be punished for incontinence.[41,42]

Developmental Warning Signs (see table 6.1)

Stuttering

Overview

Stuttering is defined as abnormal speech patterns marked by the presence of repetitions and pauses in speech, known as dysfluencies.[43] The precise cause of stuttering is unknown, but stuttering in young children is generally believed to

Table 6.1	Developmental Warning Signs During the Toddler Stage
2 years	Doesn't use 2 word phrases
	Doesn't know what to do with common things (i.e., brush, phone, fork)
	Doesn't copy actions and words
	Doesn't follow simple instruction
	Doesn't walk steadily
	Loses skills he/she once had
3 years	Falls down a lot or has trouble with stairs
	Drools or has very unclear speech
	Can't work simple toys (such as peg boards, simple puzzles, turning handle)
	Doesn't speak in sentences
	Doesn't understand simple instructions
	Doesn't play pretend or make believe
	Doesn't want to play with other children or with toys
	Doesn't make eye contact
	Loses skills he/she once had
4 years	Can't jump in place
	Has trouble scribbling
	Shows no interest in interactive games or make believe
	Ignores other children or doesn't respond to people outside of family
	Resists dressing, sleeping, using toilet
	Can't retell favorite story
	Doesn't follow 3 part commands
	Doesn't understand "same" and "different"
	Doesn't use "me" and "you" correctly
	Speaks unclearly
	Loses skills he/she once had
5 years	Doesn't show a wide range of emotions
	Shows extreme behavior
	Usually withdrawn, inactive
	Easily distracted
	Doesn't respond to people or responds superficially
	Can't tell what's real or make believe
	Doesn't play a variety of games
	Can't give first and last name
	Doesn't use plurals or tenses properly
	Doesn't talk about daily activities or experiences
	Doesn't draw pictures
	Can't brush teeth, wash and dry hands, or get undressed without help
	Loses skills he/she once had

Note. Adapted with permission from Developmental milestones. CDC. http://www.cdc.gov/ncbddd/actearly/milestones/index.html. Published 2014. Accessed April 2015.

be the result of developmental causes.[44] Stuttering is more common among males and has a high familial incidence.[45] The condition typically lasts anywhere from several weeks to 6 months but usually resolves without specialized care. Parents often need considerable reassurance that this is not uncommon and usually resolves spontaneously.[13]

Differential Diagnosis

Stuttering is diagnosed clinically by a speech language pathologist, who assesses factors such as the child's case history, stuttering behaviors, and speech and language abilities.[44] Furthermore, hearing and visual impairment should also be considered in the differential diagnosis.[18]

Management

The NP should recognize the initial presentation of stuttering and encourage the child's parents to be patient; however, health professionals recommend that children be referred if the stutter lasts longer than 6 months, if they are older than 6 years of age and stutter, or if they avoid speaking.[18,44] Stuttering may be treated with methods such as electronic devices, controlled fluency, and cognitive behavior therapy.[44,46]

Pervasive Development Disorders (PDD)

Overview

According to the fifth edition of the Diagnostic and Statistical Manual of Mental Disorders (DSM-5), pervasive development disorders (PDDs), also known as autism spectrum disorders, are a collection of disorders distinguished by impaired social interactions and altered reactions to environmental stimuli.[47] Individuals may avoid eye contact or not understand social cues. Repetitive movements and self-abusive behavior is also typical. Autism is the most common pervasive development disorder.[48] Autism is characterized by a marked impaired or abnormal social development, especially in terms of interaction; signs and symptoms may appear as early as infancy.[49] Moreover, autistic children often have a narrowly focused repertoire of interests and activities, and may exhibit language delay.

Unlike autism, Asperger's syndrome (AS) does not commonly present with any clinically significant delays in language acquisition; however, AS overlaps with high-functioning autism in its often severe and sustained impairments in social interaction.[50] Children with AS may exhibit obsessive compulsive tendencies, and may also develop narrow, repetitious patterns of interests, behavior, and activities.[51]

Rett's disorder (RTT) is a neurologic disorder that causes developmental reversals and occurs exclusively in females.[52] RTT is characterized by a clear and specific pattern of neurodegenerative developmental regression after a 5-month period of normal functioning and growth. After this period of normal development, there is commonly a lack of gain in developmental milestones, as well as loss of skills previously mastered, such as speech and hand skills. Typically, the first stage of the onset of RTT is a developmental arrest in which signs and symptoms, such as hypertonicity, become evident.[53] Delayed head growth is also a common finding and is often the first sign that a child has RTT. Stereotypic hand movements present in almost all patients with RTT, and scoliosis is common and typically increases with age.[54] Additional signs and symptoms may include central nervous system irritability, withdrawal symptoms, and seizures.

Childhood disintegrative disorder (CDD) begins with about two years of normal development, followed by significant regression in multiple areas of functioning. Although the cause of CDD is unknown, the condition may be caused by infections or neurological disorders due to brain insult in utero. Unlike RTT, CDD is overall more common in males, but is more severe in females.[18,55]

Presentation

Although signs and symptoms of PDDs vary depending on the specific disorder, the onset of developmental delay by the age of 3 years is common and is part of the diagnostic criteria.[1,13] Furthermore, the DSM-5 requires six total behaviors from three categories for a PDD diagnosis. These three categories are motor, language, and communication and social.[47] Classic autistic disorder usually appears during the child's first year and almost always manifests by 3 years of age.[56] Autism is characterized by speech and language delays; however, language often develops normally in children with Asperger's syndrome.[57] Autistic children with advanced speech may use speech abnormally and inappropriately. This is known as echolalia, characterized by repeating another person's words mechanically and meaninglessly.[58]

Management

Referral and early screening is of the utmost importance in the management of PDDs.[1,13] The NP may assess the child's behavior with diagnostics, such as the Autism Behavior Checklist, as well as first-stage screening tools, such as the Checklist for Autism in Toddlers and the Modified Checklist for Autism in Toddlers.[59] Treatment of PDDs is individualized, and children should be referred for community resources and family support.

References

1. Kliegman RM, Stanton BF, St. Geme JW III, Schor NF, Behrman RE, eds. *Nelson Textbook of Pediatrics*. Philadelphia, PA: Elsevier Saunders; 2011.

2. Growth charts: Taking your toddler's measurements. Baby Center web site. http://www. babycenter.com/0_growth-charts-taking-your-toddlers-measurements_10870.bc. Accessed April 10, 2015.

3. McLeod S. Preoperational stage. Simply Psychology web site. http://www. simplypsychology.org/ preoperational.html. Published 2010. Accessed April 10, 2015.

4. Piaget's stages of cognitive development. In a Nutshell web site. http://www. telacommunications.com/ nutshell/stages. htm. Accessed April 10, 2015.

5. Oswalt A. Early childhood cognitive development: Intuitive thought. Gulf Bend Center web site. http:// www.gulfbend.org/poc/view_doc. php?type=doc&id=12759&cn=462. Accessed April 10, 2015.

6. Heffner CL. Chapter 3: Section 3: Erikson's stages of psychosocial development. AllPsych web site. http://allpsych.com/ psychology101/social_development/#. VSfxCPnF_kU. Accessed April 10, 2015.

7. Riley M, Bluhm B. High blood pressure in children and adolescents. *Am Fam Physician*. 2010; 85(7): 693–700.

8. Dave H, Wayne AS. Childhood hematologic diseases. In: Rodgers GP, Young NS, eds. *The Bethesda Handbook of Clinical Hematology*. 3rd ed. Philadelphia, PA: Wolters Kluwer Health/Lippincott Williams & Wilkins; 2013: 121–136.

9. United States Department of Health and Human Services, Centers for Disease Control and Prevention. What do parents need to know to protect their children? http://www.cdc.gov/nceh/lead/acclpp/blood_lead_levels.htm. Last reviewed October 30, 2012. Last updated June 19, 2014. Accessed April 10, 2015.

10. Physicians recommend all children, ages 9-11, be screened for cholesterol. American Academy of Pediatrics web site. http://www. aap.org/en-us/about-the-aap/aap-press-room/ pages/Physicians-Recommend-all-Children,-Ages-9-11,-Be-Screened-for-Cholesterol.aspx. Published November 14, 2011. Accessed April 10, 2015.

11. Krol DM. Policy statement: Maintaining and improving the oral health of young children. *Pediatrics*. 2014; 134(6): 1224–1229. doi: 10.1542/peds.2014-2984

12. Well-child visits. A.D.A.M. Medical Encyclopedia. http://www.nlm.nih.gov/medlineplus/ency/article/001928.htm. Updated January 27, 2013. Accessed April 10, 2015.

13. Burns CE, Dunn AM, Brady MA, Starr NB, Blosser CG, eds. *Pediatric Primary Care*. 5th ed. Philadelphia, PA: Elsevier Saunders; 2013.

14. Drutz JE. The pediatric physical examination: General principles and standard measurements. In: Basow DS, ed. *UpToDate*. Waltham, MA: UpToDate; 2015. http://www.uptodate.com/contents/the-pediatric-physical-examination-general-principles-and-standard-measurements. Last updated August 13, 2013. Accessed April 10, 2015.

15. Phillips SM, Shulman RJ. Measurement of growth in children. In: Basow DS, ed. *UpToDate*. Waltham, MA: UpToDate; 2015. http://www.uptodate.com/contents/measurement-of-growth-in-children. Last updated February 10, 2014. Accessed April 10, 2015.

16. Increased head circumference. A.D.A.M. Medical Encyclopedia. http://www.nlm.nih.gov/medlineplus/ency/article/003305.htm. Updated May 10, 2013. Accessed April 10, 2015.

17. Drutz JE. The pediatric physical examination: HEENT. In: Basow DS, ed. *UpToDate*. Waltham, MA: UpToDate; 2015. http://www.uptodate.com/contents/the-pediatric-physical-examination-heent. Last updated September 25, 2014. Accessed April 10, 2015.

18. Barkley TW Jr. *Pediatric Primary Care Nurse Practitioner Certification Review/Clinical Update Continuing Education Course*. West Hollywood, CA: Barkley and Associates; 2015.

19. Lane JC. Pediatric nephrotic syndrome clinical presentation. In: Langman CB, ed. Medscape. http://emedicine.medscape.com/article/982920-clinical#showall. Updated October 27, 2014. Accessed April 10, 2015.

20. Fluoride in diet. A.D.A.M. Medical Encyclopedia. http://www.nlm.nih.gov/medlineplus/ency/article/002420.htm. Updated June 14, 2013. Accessed April 10, 2015.

21. Robin S. Laryngitis in toddlers. Global Post web site. http://everydaylife.globalpost.com/laryngitis-toddlers-9754.html. Accessed April 10, 2015.

22. Reuter-Rice K, Bolick B. *Pediatric Acute Care: A Guide for Interprofessional Practice*. Burlington, MA: Jones & Bartlett Learning; 2012.

23. Allen HD, Driscoll DJ, Shaddy RE, Feltes TF, eds. *Moss and Adams' Heart Disease in Infants, Children, and Adolescents: Including the Fetus and Young Adult*. 8th ed. Philadelphia, PA: Wolters Kluwer Health/Lippincott, Williams, & Wilkins; 2012.

24. Draper R. Paediatric examination. Patient web site. http://www.patient.co.uk/doctor/Paediatric-Examination.htm. Last reviewed June 13, 2014. Accessed April 10, 2015.

25. Hutson JM, Beasley SW. *The Surgical Examination of Children*. Berlin, Germany: Springer Science & Business Media; 2012.

26. Nepple KG, Cooper CS, Alagiri M. Labial adhesions. In: Zuckerman AL, ed. Medscape. http://emedicine.medscape.com/article/953412-overview#a0101. Updated July 14, 2014. Accessed April 11, 2015.

27. Phimosis and paraphimosis in children. Boston's Children Hospital web site. http://www.childrenshospital.org/health-topics/conditions/phimosis-and-paraphimosis. Accessed April 11, 2015.

28. United States Department of Health and Human Services, Centers for Disease Control and Prevention. Developmental milestones. http://www.cdc.gov/ncbddd/actearly/milestones. Last updated March 27, 2014. Accessed April 13, 2015.

29. The stages of cognitive development. Jean Piaget web site. http://piaget.weebly.com/stages-of-cognitive-development.html. Accessed April 13, 2015.

30. Coats DK. Visual development and vision assessment in infants and children. In: Basow DS, ed. *UpToDate*. Waltham, MA: UpToDate; 2015. http://www.uptodate.com/contents/visual-development-and-vision-assessment-in-infants-and-children. Last updated December 9, 2014. Accessed April 13, 2015.

31. Hearing assessments for young children. Australian Hearing web site. http://www.hearing.com.au/hearing-assessments-young-children. Published December 28, 2013. Accessed April 13, 2015.

32. Zundel I. Speech and language development from birth to age five. EduGuide web site. http://www.eduguide.org/article/speech-and-language-development-from-birth-to-age-five. Accessed April 13, 2015.

33. Erikson's stages of development. Learning Theories web site. http://www.learning-theories.com/eriksons-stages-of-development.html. Accessed April 13, 2015.

34. Weiss LG, Oakland T, Aylward GP, eds. *Bayley-III Clinical Use and Interpretation*. San Diego, CA: Academic Press; 2010.

35, LaRosa A. Developmental and behavioral screening tests in primary care. In: Basow DS, ed. *UpToDate*. Waltham, MA: UpToDate; 2015. http://www.uptodate.com/contents/developmental-and-behavioral-screening-tests-in-primary-care. Last updated September 2, 2014. Accessed April 13, 2015.

36. Weaning from the bottle. American Academy of Pediatrics web site. http://www.aap.org/en-us/about-the-aap/aap-press-room/aap-press-room-media-center/Pages/Weaning-from-the-Bottle.aspx. Accessed April 13, 2015.

37. Your child's age 1 dental visit. Palm Valley Pediatric Dentistry web site. http://www.palmvalleypediatricdentistry.com/index.php/about-us/item/76-your-child-s-age-1-dental-visit. Accessed April 13, 2015.

38. Caring for your toddler's teeth. Baby Centre web site. http://www.babycentre.co.uk/a539851/caring-for-your-toddlers-teeth. Last reviewed July 2012. Accessed April 13, 2015.

39. Toddler sleep: What to expect. Raising Children Network web site. http://raisingchildren.net.au/articles/toddlers_sleep_nutshell.html. Last updated February 15, 2012. Accessed April 13, 2015.

40. Cleveland Clinic Staff. Nightmares. Cleveland Clinic web site. http://my.clevelandclinic.org/disorders/sleep_disorders/hic_nightmares.aspx. Last reviewed May 17, 2013. Accessed April 13, 2015.

41. Wilson D. Health promotion of the toddler and family. In: Hockenberry MJ, Wilson D, eds. *Wong's Nursing Care of Infants and Children*. 9th ed. St. Louis, MO: Elsevier Mosby; 2011: 553–584.

42. Zweiback M. Rewards and potty training. Baby Center web site. http://www.babycenter.com/0_rewards-and-potty-training_65029.bc?page=1. Accessed April 13, 2015.

43. Stuttering. American Speech-Language-Hearing Association web site. http://www.asha.org/public/speech/disorders/stuttering.htm. Accessed April 13, 2015.

44. United States Department of Health and Human Services, National Institutes of Health (NIH), National Institute on Deafness and Other Communication Disorders. Stuttering. http://www.nidcd.nih.gov/health/voice/pages/stutter.aspx. Updated March 2010. Accessed April 13, 2015.

45. Carter J, Musher K. Etiology of speech and language disorders in children. In: Basow DS, ed. *UpToDate*. Waltham, MA: UpToDate; 2015. http://www.uptodate.com/contents/etiology-of-speech-and-language-disorders-in-children. Last updated April 1, 2015. Accessed April 13, 2015.

46. Mayo Clinic Staff. Stuttering. Mayo Clinic web site. http://www.mayoclinic.org/diseases-conditions/stuttering/basics/definition/CON-20032854. Updated August 20, 2014. Accessed April 13, 2015.

47. American Psychiatric Association. *Diagnostic and statistical manual of mental disorders: DSM-5.* Washington, D.C: American Psychiatric Association; 2013.

48. American Psychiatric Association. Autism spectrum disorder. American Psychiatric Association web site. http://www.dsm5.org/Documents/Autism%20Spectrum%20Disorder%20Fact%20Sheet.pdf. Published 2013. Accessed April 13, 2015.

49. United States Department of Health and Human Services, NIH, National Institute of Neurologic Disorders and Stroke (NINDS). Autism fact sheet. http://www.ninds.nih.gov/disorders/autism/detail_autism.htm. Last updated November 6, 2014. Accessed April 13, 2015.

50. Brasic JR. Asperger syndrome. In: Pataki C, ed. Medscape. http://emedicine.medscape.com/article/912296-overview. Updated March 26, 2014. Accessed April 13, 2015.

51. United States Department of Health and Human Services, NIH, NINDS. Asperger syndrome fact sheet. http://www.ninds.nih.gov/disorders/asperger/detail_asperger.htm. Last updated November 6, 2014. Accessed April 13, 2015.

52. Rett syndrome. Penn State Hershey web site. http://pennstatehershey.adam.com/content.aspx?productId=117&pid=1&gid=001536. Reviewed November 12, 2012. Accessed April 13, 2015.

53. Bernstein BE, Glaze DG. Rett syndrome. In: Pataki C, ed. Medscape. http://emedicine.medscape.com/article/916377-overview. Updated January 5, 2015. Accessed April 13, 2015.

54. Schultz RJ, Glaze DG. Rett syndrome. In: Basow DS, ed. *UpToDate*. Waltham, MA: UpToDate; 2015. http://www.uptodate.com/contents/rett-syndrome. Last updated October 22, 2013. Accessed April 13, 2015.

55. Childhood disintegrative disorder. Autism Program at Yale web site. http://medicine.yale.edu/childstudy/autism/information/cdd.aspx. Accessed April 13, 2015.

56. Autism spectrum disorders (ASD). In: Porter RS, Kaplan JL, eds. The Merck Manual Online. http://www.merckmanuals.com/professional/pediatrics/learning_and_developmental_disorders/autism_spectrum_disorders_asd.html. Last reviewed March 2013. Accessed April 13, 2015.

57. Chiu S, Hagerman RJ. Pervasive developmental disorder. In: Pataki C, ed. Medscape. http:// emedicine.medscape.com/article/914683-overview. Updated December 12, 2013. Accessed April 13, 2015.

58. Heffner GJ. Echolalia – repetitive speech. Synapse web site. http://www.autism-help.org/communication-echolalia-autism.htm. Accessed April 13, 2015.

59. Bridgemohan C. Autism spectrum disorder: Screening tools. In: Basow DS, ed. *UpToDate*. Waltham, MA: UpToDate; 2015. http://www.uptodate.com/contents/autism-spectrum-disorder-screening-tools. Last updated April 9, 2014. Accessed April 13, 2015.

Chapter 7

School Age Health and Issues

QUESTIONS

1. Jack, age 12, is diagnosed with attention deficit hyperactivity disorder (ADHD). Which of the following is most strongly recommended regarding Jack's medication regimen?

   a. There should be a drug holiday at nighttime during the week.

   b. There should be a drug holiday on the weekends.

   c. There should be a drug holiday during holiday breaks from school.

   d. There should be no drug holiday in the course of treatment.

2. Jerome, an 11-year-old, wakes up every morning at 6 a.m. At what time should he go to bed in order to get the minimum recommended amount of sleep for his age?

   a. 8 p.m.

   b. 9 p.m.

   c. 10 p.m.

   d. 11 p.m.

3. A 7-year-old child arrives at your practice with a radial fracture and bruising around the lower arm. When asked how he received the fracture, the child says he fell while riding his bike earlier that day. Suspecting abuse, you decide to undertake a more thorough examination. All of the following signs would increase your concern of child abuse <u>except</u>:

   a. The child appears shy with a limited vocabulary.

   b. Closer examination of the lower arm reveals thin, finger-like bruises.

   c. You learn that the child exhibits poor academic performance.

   d. You note that the child has 'fallen off his bike' before and presented with a slight concussion.

4. According to Erik Erikson, the industry vs. inferiority stage occurs during school age. Which of the following would Piaget expect for appropriate cognitive development during this stage?

   a. Being active, energetic, and curious

   b. Magical thinking

   c. Understanding the concept of space

   d. Seeking rewards and approval

5. Which of the following is <u>not</u> a developmental warning sign in younger school age children?

   a. Lack of social interaction

   b. Not paying attention in class

   c. Worrying about the opinions of peers

   d. Dropping in test score performance

6. Between what ages should typical pediatric patients first receive a purified protein derivative test for tuberculosis?

   a. Two to 4 years

   b. Four to 6 years

   c. Six to 8 years

   d. Eight to 10 years

7. Which of the following is thought to be a predisposing psychosocial factor for attention deficit hyperactivity disorder?

   a. Family history of alcoholism

   b. Near-death experience from perinatal asphyxia

   c. Depression

   d. Current lack of friends

8. A parent wants to know when the best time is to give the medication being prescribed for attention deficit hyperactivity disorder. Your instructions are based on your knowledge that the earliest onset of action after the ingestion of methylphenidate in children is usually:

   a. 15 minutes

   b. 30 minutes

   c. 45 minutes

   d. 90 minutes

9. What are the last permanent teeth to fully erupt during development?

   a. Bicuspids

   b. Molars

   c. Incisors

   d. Canines

10. All of the following are school age fears the nurse practitioner should expect when interviewing a child <u>except</u>:

    a. Pain

    b. Death

    c. Isolation

    d. Loss of control

RATIONALES

1. d

It is recommended that children do not take drug holidays from their attention deficit hyperactivity disorder (ADHD) medication. Although some parents and practitioners of patients with ADHD encourage drug holidays on nights, weekends, and school breaks, this is typically based on the belief that continuous medication use will lead to dependency or significant adverse effects, for which there is no evidence.

2. c

School age children are recommended to get at least 8 hours of sleep, with a maximum of 11 hours of sleep per night; therefore, a child who wakes up at 6 a.m. should go to sleep at 10 p.m. to receive the minimum recommended amount of sleep. If he goes to bed at 8 p.m. or 9 p.m., the child would receive 10 and 9 hours of sleep, respectively; while designating the recommended amount of sleep, these answer choices do not refer to the minimum recommended amount of sleep. On the other hand, going to bed at 11 p.m. would only give him 7 hours of sleep, which would be the proper amount of sleep for an adult because adults require 7–8 hours of sleep; this amount of sleep, however, is not sufficient for a school age child.

3. c

Although notable changes in school performance and attendance may indicate possible child abuse, poor academic performance in itself is not sufficient to justify the suspicion of child abuse. Along with the vague and incompatible history ascribed to the injury, all of the other signs strongly indicate abuse. A limited vocabulary and a lack of self-esteem may indicate developmental delays, which may be a result of child abuse. Fractures and bruises in various stages of healing may indicate a delay in seeking care. Soft tissue markings in the shape of a hand, object, or weapon, as well as cigarette burns, may indicate non-accidental trauma or a human source of injury.

4. c

Piaget felt that concrete operational thinking—including understanding the concept of space—marked cognitive development during school age years. Erik Erikson's industry versus inferiority stage, which occurs during school age, is marked by a child becoming active, energetic, and curious. Magical thinking is a preschool trait and should not be dominant during this stage. Although children generally seek rewards and approval, this is not a specific tenet of Piaget's concrete operational thinking stage.

5. c

Putting increased emphasis on the opinions of peers is not a warning sign in school age children; rather, it shows normal psychosocial development because the child is now interested in his or her peers and capable of behaving in a peer environment. Developmental warning signs in younger school age children include poor adjustment to school (e.g., not paying attention in class), failure to work to ability (e.g., dropping in test scores), and either a lack of social interaction or experiencing peer problems. Older school age children may manifest similar signs, such as an inability to make or keep friends, poor school performance, or a disinterest in any extracurricular academic activity.

6. b

The purified protein derivative (PPD) test for tuberculosis (TB) is recommended to be administered only once to pediatric patients between 4 and 6 years of age prior to enrolling in school. This minimizes the chance that any children infected with TB will pass it on to their classmates. Although administration of the PPD test was once recommended for all pediatric patients, recent recommendations have suggested applying the PPD test only to populations at a heightened risk for TB, such as children who were born—or have traveled—outside of the United States, or children who have been exposed to individuals with TB. A range of 2–4 years of age is younger than the recommended age at which a child should receive the PPD test. Likewise, children over 6 years of age will not require the PPD test as a matter of course unless certain risk factors are present, such as low socioeconomic status or residence in an area where TB is prevalent.

7. a

A family history of alcoholism is a predisposing psychosocial factor that may lead to attention deficit hyperactivity disorder (ADHD) in children. Perinatal asphyxia is a medical condition that results from an inadequate intake of oxygen that occurs at birth. Although this factor may predispose a child towards ADHD, perinatal asphyxia is a biological, not psychosocial, influence. Depression is a predisposing psychosocial factor for adolescents with eating disorders. Depression may occur simultaneously with ADHD, but it is not a predisposing factor for ADHD. Lastly, a lack of friends is not considered a common psychosocial influence on ADHD, but it may indicate impaired psychosocial development and may occur as a result of ADHD.

8. b

Behavior changes can be identified in children with attention deficit hyperactivity disorder within approximately 30 minutes after ingestion of central nervous system (CNS) stimulants such as methylphenidate. This is important because the goal is for the drug to be in effect by the time the child is interacting with others at school. CNS stimulants commonly do not produce noticeable behavior changes as early as 15 minutes after ingestion, and these drugs typically show effects before 45 or 90 minutes.

9. b

Molars are the last set of permanent teeth to fully erupt; the first molars will come in around 6 years of age, the third molars will typically erupt somewhere between 17 and 21 years of age. Incisors will erupt between 6 and 8 years of age, with the lower central incisors usually developing first. The canines will erupt between 10 and 12 years of age, as will the bicuspids, or premolars.

10. c

Of the choices, it is not necessarily expected that a nurse practitioner (NP) should consider fear of isolation when interviewing a child. Although school age children may have specific fears of the dark or fears of parental separation, there does not tend to be a generalized fear of isolation. The NP should be mindful when interviewing a child that school age children are likely to fear pain, loss of control over personal circumstances or environment, and death.

DISCUSSION

Definition

School age is defined as 6 to 12 years of age.[1]

Focus

Physical

According to Freud's stages of psychosexual development, the latency stage lasts from ages 6 to 12. This stage is marked by repression of sexual urges, as children play mostly with peers of the same sex.[2]

Cognitive

According to Jean Piaget's stages of cognitive development, school age children enter the concrete thinking stage at approximately age 7. During this stage, which lasts until about 11 years of age, children become more organized and rational in their thinking. They become better at conservation tasks and understanding the quantity of something may remain constant even if its appearance changes.[3]

Psychosocial

According to Erik Erikson's stages of psychosocial development, children ages 6 to 12 go through the industry vs. inferiority stage. Children in this stage show a desire to please adults and become capable of performing more complex tasks.[4]

Well Child Checks

Overview

School age children should receive a Well Child Check (WCC) annually.[5] These check-ups measure a child's health by collecting both objective and subjective data. Subjective data in a WCC includes assessing the child for elimination disorders, such as constipation and enuresis, and observing developmental behaviors, such as daily activities and family relationships. Subjective data also includes risk factors and behaviors, such as the use of alcohol, tobacco, and caffeine.[1] Objective data can be gathered from the physical examination.

Immunizations are an important part of a WCC and one of the most successful ways of preventing diseases in children.[5,6] A second dose of the measles, mumps, rubella vaccine is recommended between the ages of 4 and 6 years prior to school entry. Children aged 11 and 12 years should receive a tetanus, diphtheria, pertussis vaccine; human papillomavirus vaccine; and meningococcal conjugate vaccine.[6] A school age child's WCC should also include a discussion of illness management with medications and health promotion strategies. If necessary, the NP should give anticipatory guidance. It is also recommended that pediatric patients receive a dental assessment and cleanings every 6 months.[7]

The Interview

Overview

Measures that can help the nurse practitioner (NP) maximize an interview with a pediatric patient include the use of diagrams, with visual diagrams commonly yielding best results.[1] As previously mentioned, school age children go through the industry vs. inferiority stage; hence, it is important for the NP to remember that children of this age group typically want to be brave. Older school age children should be expected to be more modest than younger children and experience fears related to pain, loss of control, and death.[1]

The Physical Examination: Necessary Elements

Overview

Children should receive a physical examination during each visit. The exam should proceed from head to foot and focus on whether or not the child is reaching normal developmental milestones.[8,9] The child's height and weight should be plotted on standard growth charts.[8] During the school age period, the child's rapid physical growth and development can be expected to level off. The average weight increase of school age children is 5–7 lb per year, and the average height increase is 2–3 inches per year. The average 10-year-old child is 70 lb and 52–56 inches tall; females typically reach peak height velocity at ages 11 and 12 years of age, prior to menarche.[1] It is also important to note the child's body mass index (BMI) in order to diagnose and prevent obesity.[9] Children with a BMI at the 80th percentile are at risk for becoming overweight; obesity is indicated by a BMI over the 95th percentile.[10]

The school age child's vital signs should be measured at each visit; as children get older, pulse and respiration rate decrease and blood pressure increases.[11] Further developments that characterize school age include the eruption of permanent teeth, visual acuity approaching 20/20, and the beginning of breast development in females. Tanner staging can be used to identify precocious puberty, which is puberty in females younger than 8 years of age and boys younger than 9 years of age.[12]

Recommended laboratory screenings in a WCC include a purified protein derivative (PPD) test for tuberculosis; some states require that the test be administered to all children between 4 and 6 years of age prior to school entry. PPD tests should be given annually to children with any of the following risk factors: low socioeconomic status, residence in areas where tuberculosis is prevalent, exposure to tuberculosis, or immigrant status.[1]

According to the American Academy of Pediatrics' (AAP) Bright Futures guidelines, hematocrit assessment is recommended annually during school age because it can be used to detect anemias before the child becomes symptomatic.[13,14]

Lastly, scoliosis is most likely to be identified early by school screening. School screening typically involves use of the Adam's Forward Bend Test or instruments such as a scoliometer. If scoliosis is indicated, radiography may be used in a clinical setting to further assess the degree of curvature.[1,15]

Developmental Monitoring

Motor Skills

School age children's motor skills typically become well developed, with a corresponding increase in muscle strength. Hand dominance can be expected to appear by 5 years of age.[16]

Cognitive Development

According to Erikson's industry vs. inferiority stage, school age children begin to develop a sense of pride in their accomplishments.[17] School age children also go through Piaget's concrete operational thinking stage, during which they develop logical thought and acquire new knowledge.[3]

The language of school age children becomes fluid and descriptive. Also, thought processes expand so that children of this age become capable of reversibility, can grasp the concept of conservation, and can classify objects based upon one characteristic. School age children also begin applying concepts of time and money, develop an understanding of the concept of space, become capable of deductive reasoning, and master the concept of cause and effect.[1]

Psychosocial Development

The psychosocial development of school age children expands markedly to include the outside world. Children during this age often feel competent in abilities such as learning and decision-making. School age children also work to develop self-esteem, which is the belief that they are accepted and valued by those who are important to them.[18]

Typically, school age children socialize through playing with others, such as through organized sports, as they become capable of fully interacting and cooperating in a peer environment and become interested in peer groups and clubs. In late school age, peers usually become extremely important, which can lead children to feel pressure to do what they think their peers are doing.[19]

School age children demonstrate responsibility by being proactive to meet needs and become capable of fulfilling household and school responsibilities (e.g., caring for a pet).[20]

Developmental Discussion/ Guidance

Consistency is critical when disciplining school age children. Adults should act as role models and should emphasize natural and logical consequences. Parents should expect lying and should confront their children in a positive way when disciplining them.[21] Moreover, children should be assigned regular duties and chores.[20] As children develop language skills, their parents should be encouraged to listen and respond. Parents should reinforce honesty and respect their child's need for privacy. Lastly, the AAP recommends that children should be limited to less than 2 hours per day of screen time, which includes television programming, internet activity, video games, and all other digital media.[22]

Nutrition/Feeding

A school age child's diet should conform to the current food recommendations under the MyPlate guidelines. Foods that are high in calories and low in nutrients should be minimized. Also, weight is expected to increase at a steady pace according to height, although height velocity normally decreases prior to prepubertal growth spurts.[23]

Dental Health

School age children should learn to floss and should be encouraged to brush their teeth after meals and before bed. Children should receive a dental cleaning every 6 months, and sealants should be placed on the child's premolars and molars as soon as they come in.[24]

Injury Prevention

To help prevent injuries and other health consequences, communicate with school age children regarding tobacco, drugs, alcohol abuse, and the use of safety devices, such as helmets and seatbelts.[25]

Sexuality

Females should be prepared for menstruation, and males should be prepared for hormonal and bodily changes. Because school age children tend to display an increased curiosity towards sex, communication about sexually transmitted infections should be established, especially regarding HIV and AIDS. Moreover, it is vital for parents to give accurate information about sexual intercourse to ensure the child develops healthy sexuality.[26]

Sleep

According to the National Sleep Foundation, school age children should sleep approximately 10–11 hours per night.[27] The occurrence of nightmares typically peaks during preschool age and decreases during school age.[28]

Developmental Warning Signs

For younger children of school age, developmental warning signs include behaviors that interfere with social interaction and school performance.[29] Frequent illnesses that require a child to stay home from school may indicate a chronic condition.[30] In older school age children, warning signs may include reversion to shy or passive roles.[31] Additional developmental warning signs in older school age children include destructive behavior as a means of self-expression, a lack of interest in any extra academic activity, and poor school performance that leaves the child feeling "left behind."[1]

Obesity

Overview

Obesity is a condition in which a person's body has excess fat because of an imbalance between caloric intake and expenditure.[32] Obesity is determined primarily by a patient's BMI. The BMI does not directly measure body fat, however. It may overestimate adiposity in a child with increased muscle mass, or underestimate adiposity in a child with reduced muscle mass. Pediatric patients are considered overweight when their BMI is at or greater than the 85th percentile.[33] Patients are considered obese when their BMI is at, or greater than, the 95th percentile for their age and gender.[10] Increasing BMI is also a problem. A patient whose BMI is below the 85th percentile but is increasing more than three to four units per year and begins to cross percentile lines is at risk of becoming overweight.[33]

Usually, obesity is caused by a combination of genetic, physiologic, and environmental factors.[1] Environmental factors responsible for almost all cases of obesity include an inactive or sedentary lifestyle combined with a high caloric intake that is greater than the patient's needs.[10] As a result, the patient's body stores unused calories as fat.[34] Certain unhealthy eating habits contribute to weight gain, such as high-fat or high-carbohydrate diets, or the use of food for comfort or control.[1] Obesity can also sometimes be caused by genetic disorders such as Prader-Willi syndrome, or by physical disorders of decreased energy expenditure.[35] Preliminary evidence suggests that viruses and toxins also contribute to childhood obesity. Other environmental factors (e.g., sugar-sweetened beverages, television use, video game use) have been associated with childhood obesity.[36]

Differential Diagnosis

Differential diagnoses of obesity include endocrine diseases and genetic conditions.[1] Certain people with mesomorphic body states may have elevated BMIs as a result of increased muscle mass, rather than fat.[37] Certain types of medications, such as antipsychotics, are also known to produce obesity as a side effect.[1]

Workup

The goal of the evaluation is to identify treatable causes of the patient's obesity and any comorbidities.[33] The NP should begin by taking the patient's history. In order to distinguish between obesity due to overfeeding and obesity due to genetic causes, the age of onset of overweight status should be determined. The patient's eating patterns should also be assessed. The NP should note who feeds the child, what the child eats, and how frequently the child eats.[33] An activity history should also be taken. The NP should note the amount and type of the child's play time, physical exercise, after school activities, and screen time.[36] Medications should also be reviewed, especially weight-promoting medications.[33] A psychosocial history should be taken to assess for depression, school problems, or tobacco use. An overweight parent increases the likelihood of an overweight child becoming an overweight adult. For this reason, a family history is also important.[33]

In addition to taking the patient history, obese patients may undergo other diagnostic studies to rule out physical causes and determine potential complications. The NP should review the patient's body systems to probe for evidence of comorbidities or underlying etiologies, such as type 2 diabetes mellitus, sleep apnea, polycystic ovary syndrome, or vitamin D deficiency.[33]

Management

The safest way for obese patients to lose weight is through a combination of healthy eating and an active lifestyle.[34] The goal for preventative treatment in younger children is to stabilize weight through nutritional planning and increased activity; this will result in compensation through linear growth.[38,39] Patients with a higher degree of obesity may require gradual weight loss. Structured diets are not recommended, but the NP should focus on establishing healthy eating behaviors in the pediatric patient.[33]

Patients should also reduce sedentary activities and minimize screen time. Both the patient and the family should increase levels of physical activity. Young children can increase outdoor play time. Older children may want to participate in structured physical activities.[38,39]

In addition to anticipatory guidance, the NP should treat underlying physical causes and refer the patient for counseling if psychosocial issues are contributing to obesity.[1,40]

Child Abuse and Neglect

Overview

Child abuse is an umbrella term used to describe acts of omission or commission, including emotional, physical, and sexual acts, that pose a clear risk to the development and health of the child.[41] Of these types of acts, the most common type of child abuse is neglect.[42]

Child abuse is believed to occur relatively frequently.[42] A 2011 study estimated that approximately four children die daily in the United States due to child abuse, and the actual number is probably higher due to underreporting.[43] Many abusers are parents. Child abuse amongst Native Americans and African Americans reaches twice the national average of reported incidence.[1] Child abusers may display various personality traits, but these characteristics can generally be traced back to "a breakdown of impulse control."[44] Often, child abusers are former victims themselves and have psychiatric, cognitive, and emotional impairments.[1]

Presentation

When a child presents with injuries, the NP should obtain a detailed history to determine the underlying cause.[45] Obtaining the patient's history is particularly important because adults may bring injured children to the emergency room with explanations that are vague, strange, or incompatible with the injuries.[42] Injuries indicative of child abuse may include soft tissue markings with an outline of an object, weapon, cigarette burn, or hand.[44] Delay in seeking care is suspicious of abuse and may result in bruises and fractures in various stages of healing.[1]

In addition to assessing the child's physical signs and symptoms, the NP should evaluate whether the child's physical and developmental needs are being met. Children with developmental delays have historically had increased rates of abuse and neglect.[1,46] Because unusual parent-child interaction is characteristic of child abuse, the NP should carefully note interactions between the child and members of the child's family.[45]

Differential Diagnosis

Because accidental injuries often occur during childhood, the NP should obtain a history and conduct a physical examination to determine the cause of the child's injuries.[46] Differential diagnoses may include homeopathic or cultural practices. The NP should also consider underlying diseases such as coagulation disorders.[47]

Workup

Diagnostic studies and laboratory tests for an abused child are determined by the child's history and physical examination findings.[48] A coagulation profile is recommended for children who present with bruising and should include a complete blood count, platelet count, prothrombin time, and partial thromboplastin time.[45,49] Serum calcium, alkaline phosphatase, and phosphorus levels may be measured if bone disease is suspected.[45]

During the physical examination, the NP should rule out other conditions that may cause similar symptoms. For example, osteogenesis imperfecta may present with findings similar to those of abused children.[42] A local radiological evaluation is recommended for children who demonstrate bony tenderness or limited range of motion on examination. A skeletal survey is recommended for children with soft tissue findings who are either nonverbal or incapable of giving a clear history.[1] Computed tomography (CT) and magnetic resonance imaging scans are used to detect intracranial injuries; CT scans may also be useful in detecting abdominal trauma.[45,49] Ultrasonography is useful if visceral injuries are suspected.[1] A home assessment may also be requested by the NP, with social services or other local authorities evaluating whether the patient's home is a dangerous environment or not.

Management

In cases of child abuse, care should be aimed at ensuring the child's safety and addressing urgent medical needs. Parents or caregivers may require some type of counseling or intervention as well.[42,44] NPs are required to report suspected child abuse in all 50 states.[50]

Attention Deficit Hyperactivity Disorder (ADHD)

Overview

Attention deficit hyperactivity disorder (ADHD) is a chronic neurodevelopmental disorder that most commonly manifests in school age children.[51] The onset of ADHD is usually no later than 7 years of age, and the peak age of diagnosis is between 8 and 10 years of age.[52,53] Although it is generally acknowledged that ADHD is more common in boys than in girls, the estimated prevalence of ADHD varies depending on the diagnostic criteria and the populations studied.[54] Moreover, ADHD is often overdiagnosed, as some signs and symptoms overlap with other conditions, such as anxiety, depression, and learning disabilities.[53,55]

Patients with ADHD are often overactive and unable to focus or control their behavior.[56] Because of these behavioral inhibitions, the child's developing knowledge of how to self-regulate behaviors is disrupted, and behaviors that are appropriate only for young children continue into school age and adolescence. These behaviors may include inattention, distractibility, impulsivity, and hyperactivity.[55]

The pathology of ADHD is unclear, and there is no single cause responsible for the condition.[52,53] Genetics may play a role in the development of ADHD; there is a noted frequency of the condition among family members.[54] Prenatal exposure to tobacco, alcohol, or cocaine is also a risk factor.[53] Perinatal factors of ADHD include prematurity, prolonged labor, perinatal asphyxia, and signs of fetal distress. Postnatal factors include cerebral palsy, epilepsy, and central nervous system (CNS) trauma or infections.[1]

In addition to these risk factors, environmental influences such as lead are also thought to play a role in the development of the condition.[57] ADHD may also be caused by psychosocial influences, such as disorganized or chaotic environments, child abuse or neglect, a family history of alcoholism, hysterical or sociopathic behaviors, and developmental learning disorders.[1]

Presentation

The fifth edition of the Diagnostic and Statistical Manual of Mental Disorders (DSM-5) classifies the symptoms of ADHD into two categories for diagnosis: (a) inattention, and (b) hyperactivity and impulsivity.[58] To confirm a diagnosis of ADHD in children, at least six symptoms from either category or a combination of both categories must be present.[58] These symptoms must present for at least 6 months to a degree that is inconsistent with

Table 7.1 Clinical Manifestations of Core Signs/Symptoms of ADHD		
Inattention	**Impulsivity**	**Hyperactivity**
Makes careless mistakes	Difficulties awaiting one's turn	Fidgetiness
Fails to pay attention to detail	Frequently blurts out answers	Difficulty remaining seated
Easily distracted	Interrupts or intrudes on others	Difficulty playing quietly
Difficulty concentrating long enough to complete task		Subjective feelings of restless-ness
Difficulty following instructions		Difficulty with social relations
Difficulty organizing tasks and activities		Low frustration tolerance

Used with permission from Barkley TW Jr. Pediatric Primary Care Nurse Practitioner Certification Review/Clinical Update Continuing Education Course. West Hollywood, CA: Barkley and Associates; 2015.

normal development and functioning, and must interfere with the child's functioning in at least two settings, such as home and school.[52] Most children are diagnosed with a combination of both types of ADHD.[57]

Comorbid psychiatric disorders are common in children with ADHD.[54] These disorders include learning disabilities, anxiety, depression, oppositional defiant disorder, and conduct disorder.[59]

Differential Diagnosis

Differential diagnoses of ADHD include sensory impairment, age-appropriate activities, and situational anxiety.[1] Other disorders that should be ruled out include bipolar affective disorders, depression, and sleep disorders, among others.[52] It is important to accurately identify other possible causes of the child's signs and symptoms to avoid overdiagnosis of ADHD and provide accurate treatment.[53]

Workup

Diagnosis is usually made on the basis of the child's pattern of symptoms rather than any one test; the NP should determine whether these symptoms occur in several settings or only in one place.[56,57] Additional factors that should be considered in the child's medical evaluation include family history and the child's prenatal and perinatal history.[60] A variety of standardized tests and questionnaires may be used to assess the child's symptoms, including the Conners' Parent and Teacher Rating Scale, the Achenbach Child Behavior Checklist, and the Vanderbilt Assessment Tool.[61,62,63]

Management

Management of ADHD is multi-modal. The condition is best treated with a combination of medication and behavioral therapy.[64] Treating a child with ADHD likewise requires cooperation between the NP and the child's parents.[56]

Stimulants are the most commonly used medications for ADHD management and are considered to be highly effective.[52,56] CNS stimulants increase the availability of neurotransmitters to strengthen focus and attention.[1] The most widely used stimulant preparations for ADHD management are methylphenidate and amphetamines. Methylphenidate remains relatively consistent across its various brands, which include Ritalin, Concerta, Metadate, and Focalin; amphetamines, on the other hand, come in a variety of formulations, such as lisdexamfetamine (Vyvanse), dextroamphetamine (Dexedrine), and amphetamine/dextroamphetamine (Adderall, Adderall XR).[53,65]

The prescribing principle of ADHD medications is to start low and titrate up slowly.[1] The NP should titrate up at weekly intervals and receive feedback from teachers and parents in order to assess effectiveness. The usual dose of medications is 0.3–0.7 mg/kg, starting with 5–10 mg in the morning. If medications are not effective, the NP should increase dosage in increments of 2.5–5 mg per week until an effective level is reached. Changes in behavior can typically be identified within 30–90 minutes of ingestion.[66]

Short-acting preparations of stimulants are often the initial treatment for children younger than 6 years of age; however, these medications often require re-dosing multiple times per day.[67,68] Long-acting preparations generally last 10–12 hours and are recommended for children who require a duration of action longer than 4 hours.[67]

Because medications can affect children differently, the NP may need to try multiple stimulants, switching between methylphenidate and amphetamines if necessary, before finding the most effective medication with the least side effects.[64] The NP should also avoid evening doses to minimize insomnia.[1]

Pharmacologic treatment of ADHD is contraindicated in children with conditions such as heart disease, hypertension, or glaucoma.[69] Psychiatric contraindications include marked anxiety and increased risk for suicide.[1] Children with comorbid depression should undergo psychiatric evaluation and be assessed by subsequent primary care providers for potential multi-drug interactions. Common side effects of ADHD medications include stomach aches, headaches, anorexia, weight loss, tachycardia, tics, and sleep disturbances. There may also be a temporary decrease in the child's rate of growth and development, although the results of studies on this are not consistent.[53]

Besides medications, children with ADHD benefit from non-pharmacologic measures such as behavior treatment, parent education, and support.[64] In order to assess the patient's symptoms and need for medication, drug holidays may be implemented on occasions such as school breaks or summer vacations.[68]

References

1. Barkley TW Jr. *Pediatric Primary Care Nurse Practitioner Certification Review/Clinical Update Continuing Education Course*. West Hollywood, CA: Barkley and Associates; 2015.

2. Heffner CL. Freud's stages of psychosexual development. AllPsych Web site. http://allpsych.com/psychology101/sexual_development.html. Last updated August 21, 2014. Accessed April 27, 2015.

3. McLeod S. Concrete operational stage. Simply Psychology Web site. http://www.simplypsychology.org/concrete-operational.html. Published 2010. Accessed April 27, 2015.

4. McLeod S. Erik Erikson. Simply Psychology Web site. http://www.simplypsychology.org/Erik-Erikson.html. Published 2008. Updated 2015. Accessed April 27, 2015.

5. American Academy of Pediatrics. Well-child care: A checkup for success. Healthy Children Web site. http://www.healthychildren.org/English/family-life/health-management/pages/Well-Child-Care-A-Check-Up-for-Success.aspx. Last updated August 11, 2014. Accessed April 27, 2015.

6. Drutz JE. Standard immunizations for children and adolescents. In: Basow DS, ed. *UpToDate*. Waltham, MA: UpToDate; 2015. http://www.uptodate.com/contents/standard-immunizations-for-children-and-adolescents. Last updated April 15, 2015. Accessed April 27, 2015.

7. Your child's first dental visit. Cleveland Clinic Children's Web site. https://my.clevelandclinic.org/childrens-hospital/health-info/ages-stages/toddler/hic-your-childs-first-dental-visit. Last reviewed November 23, 2012. Accessed April 27, 2015.

8. Drutz JE. The pediatric physical examination: General principles and standard measurements. In: Basow DS, ed. *UpToDate*. Waltham, MA: UpToDate; 2015. http://www.uptodate.com/contents/the-pediatric-physical-examination-general-principles-and-standard-measurements. Last updated August 13, 2013. Accessed April 27, 2015.

9. Well-child visits. A.D.A.M. Medical Encyclopedia. http://www.nlm.nih.gov/medlineplus/ency/article/001928.htm. Updated January 27, 2013. Accessed April 27, 2015.

10. Klish WJ. Definition; epidemiology; and etiology of obesity in children and adolescents. In: Basow DS, ed. *UpToDate*. Waltham, MA: UpToDate; 2015. http://www.uptodate.com/contents/definition-epidemiology-and-etiology-of-obesity-in-children-and-adolescents. Last updated April 13, 2015. Accessed April 27, 2015.

11. Normal vital signs. School of Health Professions, University of Missouri Health System Web site. https://shp.missouri.edu/pt/pdf/emergency.pdf. Accessed April 27, 2015.

12. Kaplowitz PB. Precocious puberty: Overview. In: Kemp S, ed. Medscape. http://emedicine.medscape.com/article/924002-overview. Updated October 14, 2014. Accessed April 27, 2015.

13. Consolini DM. Health supervision of the well child. In: Porter RS, Kaplan JL, eds. The Merck Manual Online. http://www.merckmanuals.com/professional/pediatrics/health_supervision_of_the_well_child/health_supervision_of_the_well_child.html. Last reviewed April 2014. Accessed April 27, 2015.

14. Minnesota Department of Health, Minnesota Department of Human Services. Child and teen checkups (C&TC) fact sheet. http://www.health.state.mn.us/divs/fh/mch/ctc/factsheets/hgbhct.pdf. Published April 12, 2010. Accessed April 27, 2015.

15. Chowanska J, Kotwicki T, Rosadzinski K, Sliwinski Z. School screening for scoliosis: Can surface topography replace examination with scoliometer? *Scoliosis*. 2012; 7(1): 9. doi: 10.1186/1748-7161-7-9.

16. Brooks A. Physical development in babies and children. Kidspot.com.au Web site. http://www.kidspot.com.au/Development-Development-Physical-development-in-babies-and-children+5367+553+article.htm. Published April 9, 2011. Accessed April 27, 2015.

17. Heffner CL. Erikson's stages of psychosocial development. AllPsych Web site. http://allpsych.com/psychology101/social_development.html. Last updated August 21, 2014. Accessed April 27, 2015.

18. DeBord K. Self-esteem in children. NC State University College of Agriculture and Life Sciences Web site. http://www.ces.ncsu.edu/depts/fcs/pdfs/fcsw_506.pdf. Accessed April 27, 2015.

19. Barker J. Teens and peer pressure. WebMD Web site. http://www.webmd.com/parenting/teenabuse-cough-medicine-9/peer-pressure. Reviewed September 12, 2011. Accessed April 27, 2015.

20. Davis SE, Needlman R. Chores for school aged children. Raising Children Web site. http://raisingchildren.net.au/articles/chores_for_school aged_children.html/context/476. Last updated April 30, 2014. Accessed April 27, 2015.

21. Lehman J. How to deal with lying in children and teens. Empowering Parents Web site. http://www.empoweringparents.com/How-to-Deal-with-Lying-in-Children-and-Teens.php. Accessed April 27, 2015.

22. American Academy of Pediatrics. Managing media: We need a plan. American Academy of Pediatrics Web site. http://www.aap.org/en-us/about-the-aap/aap-press-room/pages/Managing-Media-We-Need-a-Plan.aspx. Published October 28, 2013. Accessed April 27, 2015.

23. Boom JA. Normal growth patterns in infants and prepubertal children. In: Basow DS, ed. *UpToDate*. Waltham, MA: UpToDate; 2015. http://www.uptodate.com/contents/normal-growth-patterns-in-infants-and-prepubertal-children. Last updated April 13, 2015. Accessed April 27, 2015.

24. Drescher S. Dental health: Sealants. WebMD Web site. http://www.webmd.com/oral-health/guide/dental-sealants. Reviewed April 14, 2013. Accessed April 27, 2015.

25. American Academy of Child and Adolescent Psychiatry. Facts for families: Teens: Alcohol and other drugs. American Academy of Child and Adolescent Psychiatry Web site. http://www.aacap.org/App_Themes/AACAP/docs/facts_for_families/03_teens_alcohol_and_other_drugs.pdf. Published July 2013. Accessed April 27, 2015.

26. Mayo Clinic Staff. Sex education: Talking to your teen about sex. Mayo Clinic Web site. http://www.mayoclinic.org/sex-education/art-20044034. Updated July 23, 2014. Accessed April 27, 2015.

27. Children and sleep. National Sleep Foundation Web site. http://www.sleepfoundation.org/article/sleep-topics/children-and-sleep. Accessed April 27, 2015.

28. Lyness D. Nightmares. KidsHealth Web site. http://kidshealth.org/parent/general/sleep/nightmare.html#. Reviewed July 2013. Accessed April 27, 2015.

29. Harris W. Behavioural and developmental paediatrics. In: Harris W. *Examination Paediatrics.* 4th ed. Chatswood, NSW, Australia: Elsevier Churchill Livingstone; 2011: 25–66.

30. Boyse K, Boujaoude L, Laundy J. Children with chronic conditions. University of Michigan Health System Web site. http://www.med.umich.edu/yourchild/topics/chronic.htm. Updated November 2012. Accessed April 27, 2015.

31. Hyson MC, Van Trieste K. Shyness: How to help the shy child and teenager. Child Development Institute Web site. http://childdevelopmentinfo.com/child-psychology/anxiety_disorders_in_children/shy_child. Accessed April 27, 2015.

32. United States Department of Health and Human Services, Centers for Disease Control and Prevention. Childhood obesity facts. http://www.cdc.gov/healthyyouth/obesity/facts.htm. Last updated April 24, 2015. Accessed April 27, 2015.

33. Klish WJ. Clinical evaluation of the obese child and adolescent. In: Basow DS, ed. *UpToDate*. Waltham, MA: UpToDate; 2015. http://www.uptodate.com/contents/clinical-evaluation-of-the-obese-child-and-adolescent?source=search_result&search=clinical+evaluation+of+the+obese+child+and+adolescent&selectedTitle=1~150. Last updated October 9, 2014. Accessed May 11, 2015.

34. Obesity. A.D.A.M. Medical Encyclopedia. http://www.nlm.nih.gov/medlineplus/ency/article/007297.htm. Updated August 17, 2014. Accessed April 27, 2015.

35. Mayo Clinic Staff. Obesity. Mayo Clinic Web site. http://www.mayoclinic.com/health/obesity/DS00314. Updated May 13, 2014. Accessed April 27, 2015.

36. Klish WJ. Definition; epidemiology; and etiology of obesity in children and adolescents. In: Basow DS, ed. *UpToDate*. Waltham, MA: UpToDate; 2015. http://www.uptodate.com/contents/definition-epidemiology-and-etiology-of-obesity-in-children-and-adolescents?source=search_result&search=epidemiology+and+etiology+of+obesity+in+children&selectedTitle=1~150. Last updated April 13, 2015. Accessed May 11, 2015.

37. Hamdy O, Uwaifo GI, Oral EA. Obesity. In: Khardori R, ed. Medscape. http://emedicine.medscape.com/article/123702-overview. Updated February 27, 2015. Accessed April 27, 2015.

38. Skelton JA. Management of childhood obesity in the primary care setting. In: Basow DS, ed. *UpToDate*. Waltham, MA: UpToDate; 2015. http://www.uptodate.com/contents/management-of-childhood-obesity-in-the-primary-care-setting?source=search_result&search=management+of+childhood+obesity+in+primary+care+setting&selectedTitle=1~150. Last updated April 13, 2015. Accessed May 11, 2015.

39. Mayo Clinic Staff. Childhood obesity. Mayo Clinic Web site. http://www.mayoclinic.org/diseases-conditions/childhood-obesity/basics/definition/con-20027428. Accessed May 11, 2015.

40. Schwarz SM. Obesity in children. In: Bhatia J, ed. Medscape. http://emedicine.medscape.com/article/985333-overview. Updated February 27, 2015. Accessed May 11, 2015.

41. Child abuse. A.D.A.M. Medical Encyclopedia. http://www.nlm.nih.gov/medlineplus/childabuse.html. Accessed April 27, 2015.

42. Child abuse – physical. A.D.A.M. Medical Encyclopedia. http://www.nlm.nih.gov/medlineplus/ency/article/001552.htm. Updated November 20, 2014. Accessed April 27, 2015.

43. Mayo Clinic Staff. Child abuse facts and resources. Mayo Clinic Web site. http://www.mayoclinic.org/departments-centers/childrens-center/child-family-advocacy-center/child-abuse-facts-resources. Accessed April 27, 2015.

44. Pekarsky AR. Overview of child maltreatment (child abuse). In: Porter RS, Kaplan JL, eds. The Merck Manual Online. http://www.merckmanuals.com/professional/pediatrics/child_maltreatment/overview_of_child_maltreatment.html?qt=child%20abuse&alt=sh. Last reviewed June 2014. Accessed April 27, 2015.

45. Boos SC, Endom EE. Physical abuse in children: Diagnostic evaluation and management. In: Basow DS, ed. *UpToDate*. Waltham, MA: UpToDate; 2015. http://www.uptodate.com/contents/physical-abuse-in-children-diagnostic-evaluation-and-management. Last updated July 16, 2014. Accessed April 27, 2015.

46. Giardino AP, Giardino ER, Moles RL. Physical child abuse. In: Pataki C, ed. Medscape. http://emedicine.medscape.com/article/915664-overview. Updated June 30, 2014. Accessed April 27, 2015.

47. Segal M. The differential diagnosis of child abuse. SimulConsult Web site. http://www.simulconsult.com/resources/abuse.html. Accessed April 27, 2015.

48. Moles RL, Asnes AG. Has this child been abused?: Exploring uncertainty in the diagnosis of maltreatment. *Pediatr Clin North Am.* 2014; 61(5): 1023–1036. doi: 10.1016/j.pcl.2014.06.009

49. Magana J, Kaufhold M. Child abuse. In: Bechtel KA, ed. Medscape. http://emedicine.medscape.com/article/800657-overview. Updated January 22, 2014. Accessed April 27, 2015.

50. United States Department of Health and Human Services, Administration for Children and Families, Children's Bureau, Child Welfare Information Gateway. Reporting child abuse and neglect. https://www.childwelfare.gov/responding/reporting.cfm. Accessed April 27, 2015.

51. Attention deficit/hyperactivity disorder. American Speech-Language-Hearing Association Web site. http://www.asha.org/public/speech/disorders/adhd. Accessed April 27, 2015.

52. Soreff S. Attention deficit hyperactivity disorder. In: Dunayevich E, ed. Medscape. http://emedicine.medscape.com/article/289350-overview. Updated April 13, 2015. Accessed April 27, 2015.

53. Sulkes SB. Attention-deficit/hyperactivity disorder (ADHD, ADD). In: Porter RS, Kaplan JL, eds. The Merck Manual Online. http://www.merckmanuals.com/professional/pediatrics/learning-and-developmental-disorders/attention-deficit-hyperactivity-disorder-adhd-add. Last reviewed March 2013. Accessed April 27, 2015.

54. Krull KR. Attention deficit hyperactivity disorder in children and adolescents: Epidemiology and pathogenesis. In: Basow DS, ed. *UpToDate*. Waltham, MA: UpToDate; 2015. http://www.uptodate.com/contents/attention-deficit-hyperactivity-disorder-in-children-and-adolescents-epidemiology-and-pathogenesis. Last updated March 27, 2015. Accessed April 27, 2015.

55. United States Department of Health and Human Services, Centers for Disease Control and Prevention. Attention-deficit/hyperactivity disorder (ADHD): Symptoms and diagnosis. http://www.cdc.gov/ncbddd/adhd/diagnosis.html. Last updated September 29, 2014. Last reviewed March 18, 2015. Accessed April 27, 2015.

56. Attention deficit hyperactivity disorder. A.D.A.M. Medical Encyclopedia. http://www.nlm.nih.gov/medlineplus/ency/article/001551.htm. Updated February 24, 2014. Accessed April 27, 2015.

57. United States Department of Health and Human Services, National Institutes of Health, National Institute of Mental Health. Attention deficit hyperactivity disorder (ADHD). http://www.nimh.nih.gov/health/topics/attention-deficit-hyperactivity-disorder-adhd/index.shtml. Accessed April 27, 2015.

58. American Psychiatric Association. DSM-5 Attention deficit/hyperactivity disorder fact sheet. American Psychiatric Association DSM-5 Development Web site. http://www.dsm5.org/documents/adhd%20fact%20sheet.pdf. Published 2013. Accessed April 27, 2015.

59. Wilkes MA, Cobb SM, Spratt EG. Pediatric attention deficit hyperactivity disorder: Differential diagnoses. In: Pataki C, ed. Medscape. http://emedicine.medscape.com/article/912633-differential. Updated December 29, 2014. Accessed April 27, 2015.

60. Krull KR. Attention deficit hyperactivity disorder in children and adolescents: Clinical features and evaluation. In: Basow DS, ed. *UpToDate*. Waltham, MA: UpToDate; 2015. http://www.uptodate.com/contents/attention-deficit-hyperactivity-disorder-in-children-and-adolescents-clinical-features-and-evaluation. Last updated March 12, 2015. Accessed April 27, 2015.

61. Wilkes MA, Cobb SM, Spratt EG. Pediatric attention deficit hyperactivity disorder: Workup. In: Pataki C, ed. Medscape. http://emedicine.medscape.com/article/912633-workup#aw2aab6b5b3. Updated December 29, 2014. Accessed April 27, 2015.

62. Perlstein D. ADHD testing. In: Shiel WC Jr, ed. eMedicineHealth. http://www.emedicinehealth.com/adhd_testing/article_em.htm. Reviewed November 17, 2014. Accessed April 27, 2015.

63. Bhandari S. ADHD tests. WebMD Web site. http://www.webmd.com/add-adhd/guide/adhd-tests-making-assessment?page=2. Reviewed January 20, 2015. Accessed April 27, 2015.

64. United States Department of Health and Human Services, Centers for Disease Control and Prevention. Attention deficit/hyperactivity disorder: Treatment. http://www.cdc.gov/ncbddd/adhd/treatment.html. Last updated April 1, 2015. Accessed April 27, 2015.

65. Wilkes MA, Cobb SM, Spratt EG. Pediatric attention deficit hyperactivity disorder: Medication. In: Pataki C, ed. Medscape. http://emedicine.medscape.com/article/912633-medication#showall. Updated December 29, 2014. Accessed April 27, 2015.

66. Sub-Committee on Attention-Deficit/Hyperactivity Disorder Steering Committee on Quality Improvement Management. ADHD: clinical practice guideline for the diagnosis, evaluation, and treatment of attention-deficit/hyperactivity disorder in children and adolescents: Implementing the key action statements—an algorithm and explanation for process of care for the evaluation, diagnosis, treatment, and monitoring of ADHD in children and adolescents. *Pediatrics.* 2011; 128:1007–1022.

67. Krull KR. Attention deficit hyperactivity disorder in children and adolescents: Treatment with medications. In: Basow DS, ed. *UpToDate*. Waltham, MA: UpToDate; 2015. http://www.uptodate.com/contents/attention-deficit-hyperactivity-disorder-in-children-and-adolescents-treatment-with-medications. Last updated April 15, 2015. Accessed April 27, 2015.

68. O'Brien JM, Christner JG, Biermann B, et al. Guidelines for clinical care: Attention-deficit hyperactivity disorder. University of Michigan Faculty Group Practice Web site. http://www.med.umich.edu/1info/FHP/practiceguides/adhd/adhd.pdf. Published August 2015. Last updated April 2013. Accessed April 27, 2015.

69. Chayer RP. Basic principles in the pharmacologic management of ADHD. Children's Hospital of Wisconsin Web site. http://www.chw.org/~/media/Files/Medical%20Professionals/Medical%20Care%20Guidelines/ADHD.pdf. Approved March 2013. Accessed April 27, 2015.

Chapter 8

Adolescent Health and Issues

QUESTIONS

1. During a physical exam on a 17-year-old female, you note a sore throat, parotid gland enlargement, and dental erosion. You begin to suspect a possible eating disorder. Which of the following findings would most strongly indicate bulimia nervosa in this patient?

   a. Amenorrhea

   b. Russell's sign

   c. Lanugo

   d. Thinning hair

2. Key immunizations to offer during adolescence include all the following <u>except</u>:

   a. Meningococcal

   b. Measles, mumps, and rubella

   c. Tetanus, diphtheria, and attenuated pertussis

   d. Human papillomavirus

3. As a nurse practitioner, you know that the eating disorder mortality rate is about 10% but that a complication from the eating disorder, and not the eating disorder itself, is frequently listed as the cause of death. Which cause of death is most likely to be listed as the cause of an individual who dies from an eating disorder?

   a. Asphyxia

   b. Organ failure

   c. Anemia

   d. Dehydration

4. A Tanner sexual maturity rating of 3 in a male indicates which of the following?

   a. A penis that is adult in shape and appearance with adult pattern pubic hair

   b. A rough, red scrotum with sparse, fine pubic hair

   c. An elongated penis with darker, curlier pubic hair

   d. Development of glans and rugae on the penis and curly, sparse pubic hair

5. Which type of diet practiced by adolescents warrants the closest monitoring by parents?

   a. Vegetarian

   b. High-protein

   c. Lactose-free

   d. Pescetarian

6. When implementing the Guidelines for Adolescent Preventive Services in a Well Child Check with a 16-year-old female, which piece of information would you be most likely to share with her parent?

   a. She mentions that she is depressed and wonders if life is worth living.

   b. She had unprotected sex with her boyfriend last month and is late for her period.

   c. She has three best girlfriends and they have all started experimenting with marijuana.

   d. She thinks her mother's new boyfriend is "creepy."

7. The acronym SAFETEENS provides a checklist of preventive care topics for nurse practitioners. Going by this checklist, which of the following is not a significant concern in preventive care?

   a. Sexual abstinence

   b. Suicide

   c. School performance

   d. Involvement in hobbies

8. After which Tanner stage do males usually begin spermarche or nocturnal emissions?

   a. Stage 1

   b. Stage 2

   c. Stage 3

   d. Stage 4

9. Which of the following are two psychosocial developments that are associated primarily with adolescence?

   a. Sense of identity and narcissism

   b. Narcissism and desire to please adult figures

   c. Sense of identity and development of self-esteem

   d. Development of self-esteem and desire to please adult figures

10. Which test or exam should be performed at every female adolescent Well Child Check regardless of personal or family medical history?

    a. Scoliosis assessment

    b. Blood pressure

    c. Liver function tests

    d. A pelvic exam

RATIONALES

1. b

Russell's sign, characterized by bruises on the knuckles that result from self-induced vomiting, is often an indicator of bulimia. Amenorrhea can indicate either anorexia nervosa or bulimia nervosa. Thinning hair is commonly a sign of anorexia nervosa. Lanugo is more typical of anorexia than bulimia.

2. b

The Centers for Disease Control and Prevention recommend that children 12–15 months old receive the measles, mumps, and rubella vaccination. No booster shot is necessary during adolescence. Children 15–18 months old should receive a diphtheria, tetanus, and pertussis vaccination, and then a booster vaccination should be given to children 11–12 years old. The meningococcal conjugate vaccine and human papillomavirus vaccine should also be administered to children 11–12 years old.

3. b

Organ failure is the most common cause of death in eating disorders, producing as a result of severe malnutrition; cardiac complications, such as arrhythmias and loss of muscle are common, but eating disorders may also result in liver damage and multi-organ failure. Suicide is also a common cause of death in individuals with an eating disorder. Although eating disorders may result in anemia and dehydration, patients are not likely to die from anemia or dehydration. Although asphyxia may result due to improper vomiting, it is rarely the cause of death.

4. c

An elongated penis is a 3 on the Tanner stage of genital development, and darker, curlier pubic hair is also a 3 on the Tanner stage of pubic hair development; the combined average of these scores indicates a sexual maturity rating of 3. A rough, red scrotum and sparse, fine pubic hair are associated with a 2 under each category. Development of glans, rugae, and pubic hair that is adult in character but not volume is associated with a 4 for each category. A penis that is adult in shape and appearance is associated with a 5 in genital development; whereas adult pattern pubic hair is associated with a 5 in pubic hair development.

5. a

Parents should most closely monitor vegetarian diets in adolescents because vegetarian diets may not provide all nutritional requirements. Alternative sources of protein, fatty acids, calcium, zinc, iron, and vitamins B12 and D may need to be incorporated into the diet. Pescetarian diets may not require the level of strict monitoring that is required with vegetarian diets because fish provide a steady source of protein and fatty acids. High-protein diets can be especially helpful in teenage athletes because strength and endurance training requires extra protein. A lactose-free diet may require calcium-intake monitoring, but otherwise the diet would not require extensive parental monitoring.

6. a

Confidentiality should be assured when implementing the Guidelines for Adolescent Preventive Services, but a nurse practitioner is expected to disclose confidentiality when there is concern about a patient hurting herself or someone else. While recreational drug use and a possible pregnancy may require advisement or medical attention, the nurse practitioner does not need to alert the patient's parent. The patient's relationship with her mom's boyfriend should be explored carefully but does not require divulgence at this stage.

7. d

Although SAFETEENS may cover exercise concerns, involvement in hobbies is not a typical concern of preventive care covered under the auspices of SAFETEENS. SAFETEENS is an acronym for Sexuality, Accidents, Firearms/Violence, Emotions, Toxins, Environment, Exercise, Nutrition, and Shots. Sexual abstinence falls under the Sexuality heading. Suicide falls under Emotions, and school performance is included in Environment.

8. c

Spermarche begins shortly after Tanner stage 3 of genital development. Spermarche or nocturnal emissions do not yet begin at Tanner stages 1 and 2, which are distinguished by the initial development and enlargement of the testes, scrotum, and penis. Tanner stage 4 occurs after spermarche or nocturnal emissions begin.

9. a

The two main psychosocial developments during adolescence are sense of identity and narcissism. Unlike pathological narcissism, adolescent narcissism typically focuses on internal reflection and development of a personal identity. Development of self-esteem and the desire to please adult figures usually also occur but are not as strongly definitive. The period of psychosocial development within younger adolescence is characterized by parent and child conflict, which may become resolved during older adolescence.

10. b

The blood pressure of adolescent females should be measured at every Well Child Check. Scoliosis should be assessed at every visit until 2 years after the patient has reached her peak height velocity. Pelvic exams should be performed if clinically warranted, such as if the patient is sexually active or experiences irregular menses. Liver function tests should be performed if the patient has a history of drug use.

DISCUSSION

Definition

Adolescence is considered the bridge from school age to adulthood, ranging from 12 to 20 years of age. The three transitional periods of adolescence are called early adolescence, from 12 to 14 years of age; middle adolescence, from 15 to 17 years of age; and late adolescence, from 18 to 20 years of age.[1]

Focus

Physical

Adolescence is often marked by the onset of difficult changes. Rapid changes in the reproductive, skeletal, muscular, and cardiovascular systems, along with the development of secondary sexual characteristics, occur. Peak height velocity (PHV), or the period where maximum rate of growth occurs, also happens during adolescence.[2]

Cognitive

Adolescents begin to develop logical thinking during this stage of growth. They develop the ability to understand abstract ideas, such as the ability to comprehend higher-level math concepts, and to establish moral philosophies, including rights and privileges.[3]

Psychosocial

Adolescents typically begin to search for a sense of identity and may demonstrate narcissism during this stage.[3]

Well Child Checks

Overview

The framework for Well Child Checks (WCCs) comes from the Guidelines for Adolescent Preventive Services by the American Medical Association. WCCs measure the growth and development of adolescents through stage appropriate screenings. These screenings involve collecting subjective and objective data and creating a management plan for the patient.[4]

Subjective data often include the adolescent's school performance and attendance. Relationships with family and friends are also taken into account, as well as hobbies and work interests. The patient should also be evaluated on how he or she manages or copes with stress and anger. Any history of, or any present inclination, to commit self-inflicted injury or injury to others should be noted.[5] Inquiries should be made into the adolescent's sexual activities, reproductive and gender issues, and any worries or stressors that he or she may have. The nurse practitioner (NP) should also speak to the parents or caregiver and hear their perspectives on the adolescent's communication and relationship with the family. Strengths and weaknesses, as well as any particular attitudes or behaviors, should be discussed. The NP should also inquire about disciplinary practices within the household and how the adolescent responds to those disciplinary measures.

Objective data includes information obtained via a physical examination and laboratory tests. The physical examination may involve observing the interaction between the parent or caregiver and the adolescent.[5] The NP should evaluate whether or not the parent or caregiver is supportive of the adolescent and allows the adolescent to answer questions. The physical examination may include determining blood pressure readings; body mass index (BMI); scoliosis screenings up until 2 years after PHV is attained; Tanner staging; a clinical breast exam and pelvic exam for females; and instructing male and female patients in self-exams of the breasts and testes, respectively. Laboratory tests may include a hematocrit test to assess for risk of anemia. A liver function test may be ordered if the patient has a history of drug use. A cholesterol screening is indicated at least once between 17 and 21 years of age. Cervical cytology (i.e., Pap smear) is routine for female patients after age 21. Testing for sexually transmitted diseases or infections may be required for patients of all genders who are sexually active or who have a history of sexual abuse.[5]

A management plan should be drafted to reflect both existing concerns and findings of the WCC. This often involves immunizations and a completion of vaccine series, such as the meningococcal vaccine; the vaccine for tetanus, diphtheria, and pertussis (Tdap); and the human papillomavirus (HPV) vaccine. If illness is identified, the plan should include a medication regimen aimed at management and treatment. The plan should incorporate health promotion strategies with anticipatory guidance, including recommendations for a dental assessment and cleaning every 6 months.[4]

The Interview

Overview

The interview with the patient and parents or caregivers is an important component of the WCC process to facilitate understanding about their health care. The NP may need to structure part of the interview alone and should be alert for cues that the adolescent does not want to discuss certain issues in front of parents. The NP should encourage expression of feelings and concerns, while being aware that the adolescent is identity-seeking, attempting to establish independence, and may be rebellious. Adolescents are often inflexible and are refining their sex role and sexuality.

Several methods can assist in obtaining the adolescent's history. The HEADSS format, which stands for Home environment, Employment and education, Activities, Drugs, Social, and Sexuality, is a psychosocial interview for adolescents.[6] The PACES format emphasizes the importance of Parents/peers; Accident, alcohol, and/or drugs; Cigarettes; Emotional issues; and School and/or sexuality. SAFETEENS, another commonly used format, typically directs the conversation by the following topics: Sexuality, Accident and/or abuse, Firearms and homicide, Emotions (e.g., suicide/depression), Toxins (e.g., tobacco, alcohol, and others), Environment (e.g., school, home, and friends), Exercise, Nutrition, and Shots (e.g., immunization status and school performance).[7]

The Physical Examination: Necessary Elements

Overview

The adolescent stage is marked by the rapid, dramatic development of secondary sexual characteristics. Vision and hearing screening, along with an assessment of the patient's vitals, should be performed on each visit. The physical examination of adolescents should proceed from head to foot.

Tanner Staging (see figures 8.1–8.3)

Tanner staging is used to rate sexual maturity in adolescents. An adolescent's sexual maturity rating (SMR) is obtained by taking the average of the Tanner stages from the appropriate charts for that adolescent's gender.[8] Precocious puberty is indicated by the onset of puberty before age 8 in girls and before age 9 in boys.

The three charts for the Tanner staging of an adolescent are secondary sexual characteristic development for boys, breast development for girls, and pubic hair development for both genders. Each of these charts has five stages.

The first stage for the secondary sexual characteristic development in boys is marked by the development of preadolescent testes, scrotum, and penis. The second stage is marked by enlargement of the scrotum and testes, with the scrotum roughening and reddening. The third stage is characterized by penis elongation; it is soon after this stage that spermarche typically occurs. Rugae appear and glans develop in the fourth stage while the penis enlarges in breadth. The fifth and final stage is marked by adult shape and appearance.[9]

The first stage for the breast development chart is characterized by preadolescent breasts. Stage 2 is characterized by the breasts budding with areolar enlargement. Stage 3 is marked by breast enlargement but without separate nipple contour. The areola and nipple then project as a secondary mound in the fourth stage, whereas the fifth stage is marked by adult breast appearance with receding areolas and retracting nipples.[9] Menarche typically starts in between stages 3 and 4.

On the Tanner scale regarding pubic hair development, the first stage is characterized by a preadolescent, bare appearance. Sparse, pale, fine hair begins to develop in stage 2, with stage 3 seeing an increased amount of darker, curlier hair. The hair begins to look adult in character in stage

4, but is still not as voluminous. Stage 5 is marked by an adult appearance.

Developmental Monitoring

Physical Development

An adolescent's pubertal growth spurt will account for about 20% of final adult height; it is during this spurt that PHV is typically reached.[10] Musculoskeletal development during this phase commonly results in adolescents progressing from a "long and gangly" frame to adult appearance.

Cognitive Development

Erik Erikson's identity vs. role confusion stage of cognitive development is illustrated during adolescence.[11] During this stage, adolescents assume the roles they are to fill as an adult and attempt to find their sexual and occupational identities.[12] Jean Piaget's

Figure 8.1. Boys: Secondary Sexual Characteristic Development

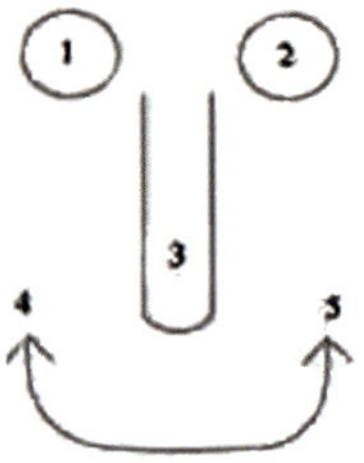

1) Preadolescent testes, scrotum, penis
2) Enlargement of scrotum and testes; scrotum roughens and reddens
3) Penis elongates
4) Penis enlarges in breadth and development of glans; rugae appear
5) Adult shape and appearance

Figure 8.2. Girls: Breast Development

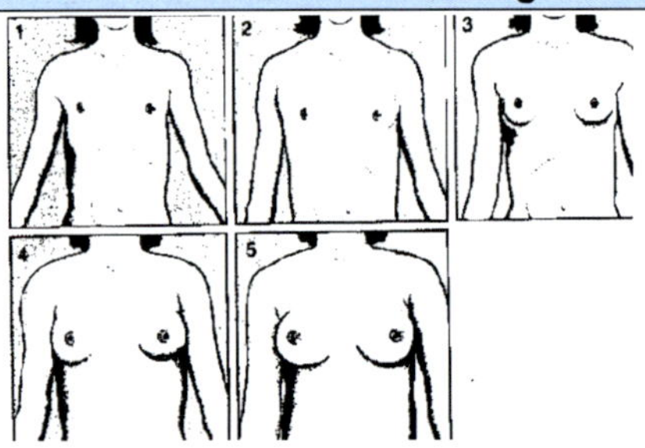

1) Preadolescent breasts
2) Breast buds with areolar enlargement
3) Breast enlargement without separate nipple contour
4) Areola and nipple project as secondary mound
5) Adult breast: areola recedes, nipple retracts

Figure 8.3. Pubic Hair: For Males and Females
1) Preadolescent
2) Sparse, pale, fine
3) Darker, increased amount, curlier
4) Adult in character but not as voluminous
5) Adult pattern

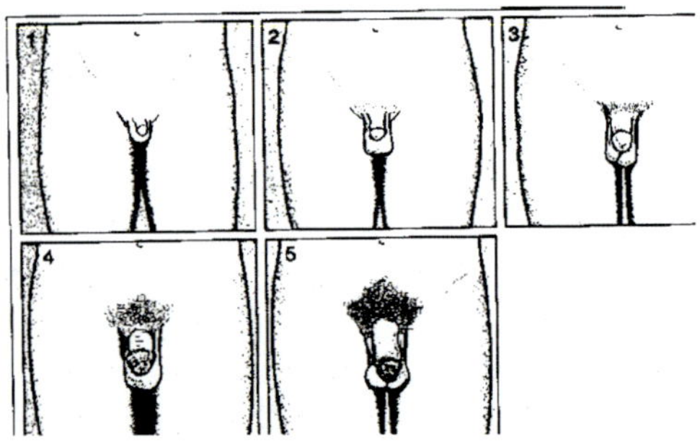

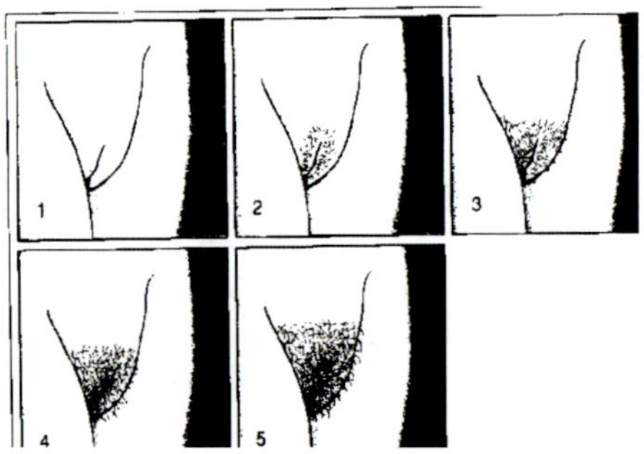

formal operational stage of abstract thinking is also observed during adolescence. During this stage, adolescents demonstrate an expansion in abstract thinking and creativity, begin to enjoy intellectual stimulation and challenge, and start to employ humor and critical thinking on a routine basis.[13]

Psychosocial Development

Different phases of psychosocial development present at different ages in adolescence. Younger adolescence is typically characterized by an increase in parent and child conflict. The child tries to establish a sense of independence and identity and is very influenced by his or her peers. Anger and histrionics are commonly displayed.

Older adolescence is marked by a decrease in emotional lability, usually resulting in a decrease in conflict between parent and child. Although older adolescents are still attempting to develop independence and their own sense of identity, a re-establishment of rapport with parents is often sought. Older adolescents are more likely to have increased self-esteem and confidence than younger adolescents. Furthermore, an increased interest in sex is quite common.

Developmental Discussion/Guidance

Although peer groups become increasingly influential during adolescence, it is the parents who remain the primary influence for guidance. As such, it is of paramount importance that parents and other adults serve as good examples for children. As adolescents grow older and begin to reach young adulthood, it is optimal for parents to begin to treat the children as adults. Honesty in communication should be reinforced, and the adolescent's privacy should be respected. Discipline should begin to incorporate negotiation between parent and child, and should reflect flexibility with trivial matters. The monitoring of television and internet activity should be maintained throughout adolescence.

Nutrition/Feeding

Because adolescents are still physically developing, there are more nutritional requirements for this age group than for adults. High-calorie, low-nutrient food must be minimized, and the regular consumption of balanced meals should be encouraged. Vegetarian or vegan diets, as well as other specific diets that omit certain food groups, should be discussed between parents and adolescents and should be closely monitored to ensure nutritional needs are met.[14]

Eating Disorders

Overview

Eating disorders are chronic disturbances in eating patterns accompanied by a distorted body image. Peak incidence for eating disorders is typically between 14 and 18 years of age. Overall mortality is as high as 10% and is related to both suicide and health consequences, namely organ failure, that arise from the disorders, and may also include severe electrolyte imbalances, such as potassium.

Anorexia nervosa is characterized by eating disturbances such as food restriction and avoidance of eating in public, as well as weight loss and persistent behavior that prevents weight gain.[15] Amenorrhea usually ensues from anorexia. Bulimia nervosa, on the other hand, is characterized by episodic binging and purging.[15] The cause of bulimia is not clearly defined, but it is believed to arise from familial issues, social pressure, low self-esteem, and a desire for control.

Presentation

Presentations of anorexia nervosa may include weight loss, anemia, amenorrhea, constipation, jaundice, cold body temperature, lanugo, and brittle bones, hair, and nails. Presentations of bulimia nervosa may include worn tooth enamel, chronic sore throat, dehydration, swollen salivary glands, and intestinal distress.[16] Bruised and abraded knuckles, known as Russell's sign, may indicate anorexia or bulimia.

Differential Diagnosis

Differential diagnoses for eating disorders include pregnancy, depression, substance abuse, and organic diseases resulting in weight loss, among others.[4]

Workup

Vital signs should be assessed for any patients assumed to be anorexic or bulimic. The level of malnutrition, if any, should also be determined. A patient is considered to be mildly malnourished if he or she weighs less than 20% below their ideal body weight (IDW). A weight 20% to 30% below IDW would indicate moderate malnutrition, whereas a weight that is 30% or more below the IDW would indicate severe malnutrition. Additional diagnostic tests may be necessary to rule out any organic diseases resulting in weight loss, such as cancer or esophageal motility disorders.[17]

Management

An interdisciplinary approach is generally employed in the management of eating disorders in adolescents, aimed at addressing both the psychological underpinnings of the disorder and the physiologic changes resulting from malnutrition. Courses of treatment in adolescents may focus on behavior modification and psychotherapy. In severe cases, adolescents may require hospitalization.[16]

Dental Health

Dental health includes brushing after meals and before bed, having a dental cleaning every 6 months, and flossing.[4]

Sexuality

As adolescents' interest and knowledge in sexuality begins to expand, it is important for them to receive accurate information about sex and sexual maturity. Patients should be prepared for the bodily changes that often come with spermarche and menarche, such as nocturnal emissions and menstruation. Curiosity or conflict with one's gender and sexual identity may present, as adolescents are attempting to develop their sense of identity in various contexts. Adolescents should also receive thorough education in disease and pregnancy prevention measures.[18]

Preventative Health Issues

Preventative health issues for adolescents include mental health care for depression or suicide. Adolescents should be observed for signs indicative of depression, such as behavior changes, self-harm, or sudden weight loss. Treatment for depression centers on psychotherapy, with medications, such as selective serotonin reuptake inhibitors and sometimes tricyclic antidepressants, are prescribed when necessary.[19] Special care must be taken to assess the child for proclivities to violence.

Developmental Warning Signs

Changes in personality, school performance, friendships, or sleeping and eating patterns are often considered to be developmental warning signs.[19] Other signs may include difficulty accepting failure, talk of suicide, and withdrawal from friends or family.

Figures

Figure 8.1. Boys: Secondary sexual characteristic development. Barkley TW Jr. Adolescent health and issues. In: Barkley TW Jr, ed. *Family Nurse Practitioner Certification Review/ Clinical Update Continuing Education Course*. West Hollywood, CA: Barkley and Associates; 2015: 63–71.

Figure 8.2. Girls: Breast development. Barkley TW Jr. Adolescent health and issues. In: Barkley TW Jr, ed. *Family Nurse Practitioner Certification Review/ Clinical Update Continuing Education Course*. West Hollywood, CA: Barkley and Associates; 2015: 63–71.

Figure 8.3. Pubic hair: For males and females. Barkley TW Jr. Adolescent health and issues. In: Barkley TW Jr, ed. *Family Nurse Practitioner Certification Review/Clinical Update Continuing Education Course*. West Hollywood, CA: Barkley and Associates; 2015: 63–71.

References

1. Hagan JF, Shaw JS, Duncan PM, eds. *Bright Futures: Guidelines for Health Supervision of Infants, Children, and Adolescents.* 3rd ed. Elk Grove Village, IL: American Academy of Pediatrics; 2008.

2. The growing child: Adolescent (13 to 18 years). Lucille Packard Children's Hospital Stanford web site. http://www.lpch.org/DiseaseHealthInfo/HealthLibrary/growth/adsct138.html. Accessed April 13, 2015.

3. Adolescent development. A.D.A.M. Medical Encyclopedia. http://www.nlm.nih.gov/medlineplus/ency/article/002003.htm. Updated January 27, 2013. Accessed April 13, 2015.

4. Barkley TW Jr. Adolescent health and issues. In: Barkley TW Jr, ed. *Family Nurse Practitioner Certification Review/Clinical Update Continuing Education Course*. West Hollywood, CA: Barkley and Associates; 2015: 63–71.

5. Sloane PD, Slatt LM, Ebell MH, Jacques LB, Smith MA, eds. *Essentials of Family Medicine.* 6th ed. Philadelphia, PA: Wolters Kluwer Health/Lippincott Williams & Wilkins; 2011.

6. Bradford S, Rickwood D. Psychosocial assessments for young people: A systematic review examining acceptability, disclosure and engagement, and predictive utility. *Adolesc Health Med Ther.* 2012; 3: 111–125. doi: 10.2147/AHMT.S38442

7. Loretz L. *Primary Care Tools for Clinicians: A Compendium of Forms, Questionnaires, and Rating Scales for Everyday Practice.* St. Louis, MO: Elsevier Mosby; 2005.

8. Biro FM, Chan Y-M. Normal puberty. In: Basow DS, ed. *UpToDate*. Waltham, MA: UpToDate; 2015. http://www.uptodate.com/contents/normal-puberty. Last updated March 27, 2015. Accessed April 13, 2015.

9. Ethington MD, Gallagher MR, Wilson D. Health promotion of the adolescent and family. In: Hockenberry MJ, Wilson D, eds. *Wong's Nursing Care of Infants and Children.* 10th ed. St. Louis, MO: Elsevier Mosby; 2015: 651–686.

10. Neinstein LS. Puberty to Normal growth and development (A1). USC web site. https://www.usc.edu/student-affairs/Health_Center/adolhealth/content/a1.html. Accessed April 13, 2015.

11. McLeod SA. Erik Erikson. Simply Psychology web site. http://www.simplypsychology.org/Erik-Erikson.html. Published 2008. Updated 2013. Accessed April 13, 2015.

12. Block M. Identity versus role confusion. In: Goldstein S, Naglieri A, eds. *Encyclopedia of Child Behavior and Development.* New York , NY: Springer; 2011: 785–786.

13. Colyar MR. *Assessment of the School-Age Child and Adolescent.* Philadelphia, PA: F. A. Davis Company; 2011.

14. Demory-Luce D, Motil KJ. Adolescent eating habits. In: Basow DS, ed. *UpToDate*. Waltham, MA: UpToDate; 2015. http://www.uptodate.com/contents/adolescent-eating-habits. Last updated September 25, 2014. Accessed April 14, 2015.

15. Forman SF. Eating disorders: Overview of epidemiology, diagnosis, and course illness. In: Basow DS, ed. *UpToDate*. Waltham, MA: UpToDate; 2015. http://www.uptodate.com/contents/eating-disorders-overview-of-epidemiology-diagnosis-and-course-of-illness. Last updated January 24, 2015. Accessed April 14, 2015.

16. U. S. Department of Health and Human Services, National Institutes of Health, National Institute of Mental Health. Eating disorders: About more than food. http://www.nimh.nih.gov/health/publications/eating-disorders/index.shtml. Revised 2014. Accessed April 14, 2015.

17. Bernstein BE. Anorexia nervosa differential diagnosis. In: Pataki C, ed. Medscape. http://emedicine.medscape.com/article/912187-differential. Updated December 14, 2014. Accessed April 14, 2015.

18. Benson PAS. Patient information: Adolescent sexuality (Beyond the Basics). In: Basow DS, ed. *UpToDate*. Waltham, MA: UpToDate; 2015. http://www.uptodate.com/contents/adolescent-sexuality-beyond-the-basics. Last updated July 7, 2014. Accessed April 14, 2015.

19. Mayo Clinic Staff. Mental illness in children: Know the signs. http://www.mayoclinic.com/health/mental-illness-in-children/MY01915. Updated February 11, 2015. Accessed April 14, 2015.

Chapter 9

Cardiovascular Disorders

QUESTIONS

1. A mother brings her 1-year-old to your practice, claiming that the child has had a fever for 6 days. She thought it was a simple illness at first, but she has noticed recent swelling in the hands and feet. An examination shows that the child has inflammation in the lips and oral cavity, as well as redness in both eyes without exudate. To rule out Kawasaki disease, which test would best help to isolate the child's most likely condition?

   a. Hemoglobin and hematocrit level

   b. Erythrocyte sedimentation rate

   c. White blood cell count

   d. Blood urea nitrogen

2. Which of the following types of congenital heart defects is most likely to present with right-to-left shunting?

   a. Transposition of the great vessels

   b. Coarctation of the aorta

   c. Tetralogy of Fallot

   d. Pulmonary stenosis

3. Which of the following diagnostics is <u>least</u> likely to indicate a diagnosis of rheumatic fever?

   a. Electrocardiogram

   b. Aldosterone level

   c. Echocardiogram

   d. Throat culture

4. How would you best auscultate to confirm a venous hum?

   a. Have the patient lay supine; auscultate the left upper sternal border.

   b. Have the patient stand; auscultate between the left lower sternal border and the apex.

   c. Have the patient sit up; auscultate the right upper sternal border.

   d. Have the patient turn his or her head; auscultate the apex.

5. What feature best distinguishes the characteristic murmur of patent ductus arteriosus?

    a. A holosystolic thrill at the left lower sternal border

    b. A "machinery" noise at the left upper sternal border

    c. An ejection murmur with radiation to the left interscapular area

    d. A click at the left upper sternal border that decreases with inspiration and increases with expiration

6. Which of these heart sounds would most strongly indicate a cardiac disorder in a pediatric patient?

    a. S1

    b. S2

    c. S3

    d. S4

7. Which of the following types of heart murmurs is <u>not</u> typically considered an innocent heart murmur?

    a. Continuous humming murmur

    b. Radiating murmur

    c. Murmur that may vary with position changes

    d. Musical systolic murmur

8. During auscultation of a newborn, a grade IV murmur is heard with a holosystolic thrill at the left lower sternal border. You suspect a congenital heart defect and order an x-ray. What findings would be most consistent with a suspected diagnosis of ventricular septal defect?

    a. A normal chest x-ray

    b. Cardiomegaly with rib notching

    c. Boot-shaped heart

    d. Cardiomegaly with increased pulmonary vascular markings

9. What finding is <u>not</u> a classic characteristic of a 3-month-old with congenital heart disease and signs of heart failure?

    a. Failure to thrive

    b. Irritability

    c. Rales upon lung auscultation

    d. Frequent vomiting with feeding

10. Which of the following patients, all of whom have a known history of congenital heart disease, is <u>least</u> likely to require prophylactic antibiotics prior to a dental procedure?

    a. A patient with a heart transplant

    b. A patient with a ventricular septal defect with a patch repair

    c. A patient with a previous history of endocarditis

    d. A patient with a partially repaired cyanotic heart defect

RATIONALES

1. b

An erythrocyte sedimentation rate test can help to rule out a diagnosis of Kawasaki disease, which, although rare, most commonly manifests in children younger than 2 years of age and typically produces a fever that lasts at least 5 or more days. Kawasaki disease also often causes changes in the extremities, such as erythema, edema, and desquamation. Other common presentations include inflammatory changes in the lips and oral cavity, bilateral conjunctivitis without exudate, and cervical lymphadenopathy. Patients with the cardinal signs should have a pediatric cardiac referral to evaluate for latent adverse outcomes associated with Kawasaki disease. Hemoglobin and hematocrit levels are more confirmatory for anemia, whereas a blood urea nitrogen test may help to identify abnormalities in the kidneys. White blood cell count may be elevated in patients with Kawasaki disease, but this finding is not confirmatory.

2. c

Cyanotic cardiac defects, such as tetralogy of Fallot, are congenital heart defects that typically present with right-to-left shunting. Both pulmonary stenosis and a large ventricular septal defect are commonly seen with tetralogy of Fallot; however, pulmonary stenosis on its own is considered an obstructive lesion, whereas ventricular septal defect is typically considered an acyanotic cardiac defect (i.e., left-to-right shunting). Coarctation of the aorta is commonly considered an obstructive lesion.

3. b

Plasma aldosterone levels are least likely to provide an indication of rheumatic fever, as the condition does not typically produce altered plasma aldosterone levels. Plasma aldosterone levels may be ordered when hypertension is present in order to rule out aldosteronism. Throat culture is a key diagnostic for rheumatic fever when used to confirm prior streptococcal infection; other common diagnostics include a rapid strep assay and a strep antibody titer. An echocardiogram may reveal cardiomegaly in patients with rheumatic fever, whereas an electrocardiogram may show a prolonged PR interval.

4. c

A venous hum is typically considered benign and is best auscultated at the right upper sternal border just below the clavicle while the patient is sitting upright during diastole. Asking the patient to either lay supine or turn his or her head may eliminate the venous hum. Still's murmur, rather than a venous hum, is best auscultated between the left lower sternal border and the apex.

5. b

Patent ductus arteriosus is commonly characterized by a grade II to IV/VI holosystolic murmur at the left upper sternal border (LUSB) with a distinguishing "machinery" noise. Pulmonic stenosis is also typically auscultated at the LUSB, but is more often characterized by an ejection click that increases in intensity with expiration and decreases with inspiration. A holosystolic thrill at the lower left sternal border would commonly indicate ventricular septal defect. Coarctation of the aorta is commonly characterized by an ejection murmur that radiates to the left interscapular area.

6. d

The S4 heart sound is best heard at the apex and is almost always considered to be pathological. S4, characterized by a cadence similar to "Ten-ne-ssee," is produced by stiff ventricular walls, which cause increased resistance to inflow within the ventricle. The S1 and S2 heart sounds are normal and associated with the opening and closing of the atrioventricular and semilunar valves, respectively. The S3 heart sound may be considered an indicator of heart failure in older patients but is usually considered normal in children.

7. b

A radiating murmur is not typically associated with an innocent heart murmur, as this type of murmur may be indicative of an obstructive defect. Congenital innocent heart murmurs may be indicated by a continuous humming murmur (i.e., venous hum), a murmur that may vary with position changes, or a musical systolic murmur (commonly called a Still's murmur).

8. d

Ventricular septal defect commonly presents with a grade II to V/VI systolic ejection murmur with holosystolic thrill in the left lower sternal border, as well as a chest x-ray that shows cardiomegaly with increased pulmonary vascular markings. Rib notching due to collateral circulation is a distinguishing feature of coarctation of the aorta, which also commonly presents with cardiomegaly. A heart that appears normal on x-rays may appear with aortic and pulmonic stenosis, though congestive heart failure may be visible if the aortic stenosis is severe. A boot-shaped heart is a characteristic x-ray finding of tetralogy of Fallot.

9. d

While infants with congestive heart failure (CHF) may have some feeding intolerance, vomiting is not commonly considered a cardinal sign of CHF. Irritability and restlessness are common in infants with CHF. Rales typically derive from pulmonary congestion; as the congestion progresses, there is often leaking into the alveoli and interstitium of the lung from increased intracardiac pressure. Failure to thrive is one of the common hallmarks for CHF; feeding becomes exhaustive as coordination of sucking, swallowing, and breathing taxes the ill infant.

10. a

A heart transplant patient does not typically require prophylactic antibiotics prior to dental work unless they have developed valvular disease post-transplant. Any patch repair for a cardiac defect, a partially repaired cyanotic congenital heart defect, or a previous incidence of endocarditis would indicate a need for antibiotics prior to dental procedures to prevent infective endocarditis. Premedication with a penicillin, such as amoxicillin, is recommended 30–60 minutes prior to the procedure.

DISCUSSION

Cardiovascular

Overview

The cardiovascular system consists of the heart, vessels, and blood. The purpose of the system is to transport blood throughout the body. Components of the cardiovascular system, in the order of blood flow, include the following: the superior and inferior vena cava; right atrium; tricuspid valve; right ventricle; pulmonic valve; pulmonary artery; lungs; pulmonary veins; left atrium; mitral valve; left ventricle; aortic valve; and the aorta. From the aorta, blood is pumped to the rest of the body.[1,2]

Nurse practitioners (NPs) commonly use four different heart sounds to determine the anatomic and physiologic state of the heart. One heart sound is the S1, which is produced by mitral and/or tricuspid atrioventricular valve closure. The S2 heart sound is produced by aortic and pulmonic, or semilunar, valve closure. Systole occurs in the period between the S1 and S2 sounds, whereas diastole occurs in the period between the S2 and S1 sounds. The S3 heart sound is known as the "Ken-tuck-y" gallop. It is heard during the rapid entry of blood from the atrium to the ventricle; on the left side, it is best heard at the apex, whereas a right ventricular S3 sound is best audible at the left lower sternal border (LLSB). Lastly, the S4 heart sound is the "Ten-ne-ssee" sound. The S4 sound occurs when active atrial contraction leads to late ventricular filling; like the S3, the S4 sound is best heard at the apex in the left ventricle and at the LLSB in the right ventricle.[1,3]

There are five main auscultatory areas of the cardiovascular system. The aortic area is the right upper sternal border (RUSB). The pulmonic area is the left upper sternal border (LUSB). The mitral area is located in the fifth intercostal space at the apex. Erb's point is located in the third intercostal space at the left sternal border. The ventricular septal defect (VSD) or tricuspid area is the fourth intercostal space at the LLSB.[1]

Congenital Heart Diseases/Defects

Overview

Congenital heart diseases and defects are cardiovascular malformations resulting from abnormal structural development in the first trimester. The etiology of these conditions is multifactorial and often includes chromosomal abnormalities and adverse environmental conditions.[1] Congenital heart disease occurs in 6–13 per 1,000 births.[4] VSDs comprise up to 30% of all congenital heart defects.[5] Congenital heart defects include acyanotic lesions (left to right shunting), cyanotic lesions (right to left shunting), and obstructive lesions.[4]

Presentation

Infants with cardiovascular defects may present with feeding intolerance, sweating during feeding, or poor growth.[4] Older children may also present with poor growth, as well as repeated infections or activity intolerance.[6]

Acyanotic Defects (left to right shunting)

Overview

Acyanotic defects occur when a shunt causes blood to flow from the left side to the right side of the heart. This condition is due to a structural defect of the heart, such as a hole in the interventricular septum. There are three types of acyanotic defects: atrial septal defect (ASD), VSD, and patent ductus arteriosus (PDA).[7]

Presentation

ASD typically presents with a murmur. The murmur is characterized as a grade II/VI to III/VI systolic ejection, which is heard best at the LUSB. VSD usually presents with a grade II/VI to V/VI regurgitant systolic murmur, and a systolic thrill may be palpated at the LLSB. PDA often presents with a grade II to IV/VI continuous murmur at the LUSB that produces a characteristic machinery sound.[8]

Workup

Electrocardiograms (ECGs), x-rays, and echocardiograms are often used to diagnose acyanotic defects. X-rays commonly show the same results—cardiomegaly and increased pulmonary vascular markings—for all three acyanotic defects. With ASD, an ECG typically shows right ventricular hypertrophy (RVH), whereas left ventricular hypertrophy (LVH) would indicate a VSD. An ECG would typically show an LVH progressing to biventricular hypertrophy in cases of PDA, as well as in cases of large VSD.[8] Final diagnosis of these types of lesions is best done through consultation and evaluation with a pediatric cardiologist.

Cyanotic Defects (right to left shunting)

Overview

Cyanotic heart defects, characterized by right to left shunting, are structural defects of the heart that cause deoxygenated blood to bypass the lungs and enter the systemic circulation. Cyanotic defects can also cause a mixing of oxygenated and unoxygenated blood, which then enters the systemic circulation.[9]

Two major cyanotic defects are transposition of the great arteries and tetralogy of Fallot. Transposition of the great arteries can be either dextrotransposition of the great arteries or levotransposition of the great arteries. Tetralogy of Fallot consists of the following defects: large VSD, pulmonary stenosis, an overriding aorta, and RVH.[8]

Presentation

Transposition of the great arteries and tetralogy of Fallot both commonly present with a murmur. VSD usually occurs alongside transposition of the great arteries. Therefore, a loud, harsh systolic murmur characteristic of VSD is often present.[10,11] In tetralogy of Fallot, the murmur is characterized by a loud systolic ejection click at the middle and upper left sternal border.[12]

Workup

Both transposition of the great arteries and tetralogy of Fallot can be diagnosed with an ECG and x-rays. However, an echocardiogram will likely also be done to more definitively visualize all structures within the heart. Radiographs of transposition of the great arteries show an "egg on a string" heart with cardiomegaly and increased pulmonary vascular markings.[13] An ECG shows a right axis deviation and RVH.[13] Abnormal origins of great arteries from the ventricles can be identified on an echocardiogram.[8] Radiographs of tetralogy of Fallot will show decreased or increased heart size, decreased pulmonary vascularity, and a boot-shaped heart.[8] Large VSD and an overriding aorta can usually be seen in an ECG of patients with tetralogy of Fallot.[12] Echocardiograms typically show right atrial enlargement and RVH.[12]

Obstructive Lesions

Overview

Obstructive cardiac lesions involve the narrowing of the pathways or major vessels where blood flows in the heart, which increases blood pressure (BP). Aortic stenosis, pulmonic stenosis, and coarctation of the aorta are three types of obstructive cardiac lesions.[6]

Presentation

Aortic stenosis, pulmonic stenosis, and coarctation of the aorta all commonly present with a murmur. Aortic stenosis is characterized by a grade II/VI to IV/VI systolic ejection murmur at the second right or left intercostal space.[8] A thrill at the RUSB is also commonly present.[14] Pulmonic stenosis is characterized by a grade II/VI to V/VI systolic murmur with ejection click that is loudest at the LUSB.[8] The intensity of the click commonly decreases with inspiration and increases with expiration. A left parasternal systolic thrill can be felt at the 2nd intercostal space.[15] Coarctation of the aorta is characterized by a systolic thrill that can be felt in the suprasternal notch.[8] A grade II/VI to III/VI systolic ejection murmur may be heard in the left interscapular area.[8,16] Additionally, with coarctation of the aorta, the provider may note diminished pulses in the lower extremities.[8] Diminished growth may be noted if the coarctation is not critical.

Workup

Aortic stenosis is primarily diagnosed through an echocardiogram, although x-rays and an ECG can also be beneficial.[14] An echocardiogram shows prominent thickening of the septum and abnormal mitral valve motions.[8] Radiographs are typically normal but may show a dilated ascending aorta or cardiomegaly.[8,14] An ECG is also likely to be normal, but mild LVH may be detected.[8]

Pulmonic stenosis is diagnosed through an ECG and x-rays, but an echocardiogram is typically used to confirm the diagnosis.[17] In mild cases, an ECG will be normal. In moderate cases, the ECG will show right axis deviation or RVH.[8] Radiographs typically show a normal heart size but occasionally may show dilated pulmonary arteries.[8,17] An echocardiogram can confirm the diagnosis by showing decreased motion of the pulmonary valve leaflets and poststenotic dilation of the main pulmonary artery segment.[8]

Coarctation of the aorta may show cardiomegaly on x-rays, but some patients may have normal x-rays.[8] X-rays may also show increased pulmonary venous congestion.[18] An ECG may also be normal, but some patients may show LVH.[18] An echocardiogram will show the localized area of coarctation by demonstrating increased velocities and turbulence.[18] With coarctation of the aorta, BP in lower extremities will usually be lower than in upper extremities.[1]

Common Genetic Syndromes and Associated Cardiac Defects

Overview

Numerous genetic syndromes, such as DiGeorge syndrome, trisomies, Marfan syndrome, and Turner syndrome, typically present with cardiac defects.[19] For instance, DiGeorge syndrome is associated with conotruncal defects, such as interrupted aortic arch, truncus arteriosus, and tetralogy of Fallot. These defects often cause cyanotic heart disease in newborns.[20] Marfan syndrome is associated with aortic root disease, which can lead to aneurysmal dilation, aortic regurgitation, and dissection. Mitral valve prolapse is also common.[21] Turner syndrome is associated with coarctation of the aorta and aortic valve abnormalities, primarily bicuspid aortic valve.[22] Trisomy 18 (i.e., Edward's syndrome) is characterized by acyanotic heart defects (e.g., VSD, ASD, PDA).[23] Approximately half of all patients with Trisomy 21 (i.e., Down syndrome) have congenital heart disease. Complete atrioventricular septal defects and VSD are the two most common primary lesions.[24]

Presentation

Assessment for cardiovascular disorders should begin with a careful history and physical examination. A family history of hereditary diseases or congenital heart defects is significant and suggests further evaluation. The neonatal history should include a history of frequent respiratory infections, color changes, cyanosis, tachypnea during sleep, feeding problems, diaphoresis, abnormal heart sounds, edema, clubbing, and congestive heart failure. The physical examination should include inspection, palpation, and auscultation.[8]

Workup

Referral to a pediatric cardiologist is the standard of care for patients with significant cardiac defects. Additionally, the NP should ensure optimal primary care and provide anticipatory guidance.[1]

Innocent Murmurs (Functional, Benign, or Physiologic)

Overview

Innocent murmurs, which occur in more than 50% of all children, are heart murmurs mostly due to physiological conditions (e.g., extra blood flow), not structural defects of the heart.[25,26] Innocent murmurs are most common in children 3 to 7 years old. The murmur can be easily heard because of the child's thin chest and may become louder when the child is scared or febrile.

The murmur may vary with position, often presenting with greater intensity in the sitting position compared to the standing position. Typically, innocent murmurs do not radiate to the neck or back.[27] Most innocent murmurs are grade I/VI or grade II/VI.[28]

Presentation

The most common innocent murmur is the Still's murmur.[28] This type of murmur is musical, systolic, and heard best between LLSB and the apex due to vibrations of the left outflow tract.[28,29] The murmur is often more difficult to hear when patients are sitting or lying on their stomach.[27]

A venous hum is a continuous murmur at the RUSB that can be heard as blood flows into the jugular veins.[27] This presentation is heard best in the sitting position and commonly disappears in the supine position or when the child's head is turned.[28]

Hypertension

Overview

Hypertension is a persistent elevation of BP that is greater than or equal to the 95th percentile for age and sex. In children, secondary hypertension, frequently from renal parenchymal disease or renovascular disease, is more common than primary hypertension.[30]

Presentation

Patients with hypertension are typically asymptomatic.[31] Signs and symptoms of hypertensive emergencies may include headaches, visual problems, dizziness, respiratory distress, irritability, and nosebleeds. Cardiovascular complaints of heart failure, such as chest pain, palpitations, cough, and shortness of breath, are also consistent with a hypertensive emergency.[32]

Workup

Hypertension is diagnosed after the child has three elevated BP readings over the course of at least three doctor's visits.[31] Once hypertension is confirmed, several laboratory tests are used in conjunction with other diagnostic criteria to determine the cause of hypertension. X-rays are used to check the posteroanterior and lateral chest for an enlarged heart or other significant markings.[33] A plasma aldosterone level is often used to rule out aldosteronism.[32] Urinalysis, basic metabolic panel, and complete blood count (CBC) are also helpful in determining the etiology.[31,32] An echocardiogram can be used to detect LVH.[32]

Treatment

Management of patients with primary hypertension can be conducted by the primary care providers. Patients with secondary hypertension typically require a referral to a cardiologist or nephrologist. BP goals for these patients should be based on etiology. Most children with primary and secondary hypertension will require antihypertensive medications and lifestyle modifications.[30]

Rheumatic Fever/Heart Disease

Overview

Rheumatic fever is a post-infectious inflammatory disease that can negatively impact the heart, joints, and central nervous system. Rheumatic fever follows an upper respiratory tract infection that derives from a group "A" streptococcal infection and is most common in ages 6 to 15 years.[1,34] Rheumatic heart disease may develop years after one or more episodes of rheumatic fever.[35]

Presentation

Common signs and symptoms of rheumatic fever include abdominal pain, fever, and joint pain and swelling. Patients may experience arthritis in the knees, elbows, ankles, and wrists. A ring-shaped rash may also appear on the trunk and upper part of the arms or legs. Sydenham chorea, which is a neurologic disorder characterized by muscle weakness, may also present.[36] Children with rheumatic heart disease may experience the same symptoms of rheumatic fever, but do not typically experience symptoms from heart damage.[37]

Workup

Rheumatic fever is diagnosed by using the Jones criteria. A diagnosis necessitates one required criteria and either two major criteria or one major criteria and two minor criteria.[38] The required criteria is evidence of an antecedent Strep infection.[38] Major criteria include carditis, polyarthritis, chorea, erythema marginatum, and subcutaneous nodules. Minor criteria include arthralgia without objective inflammation, fever higher than 102.2 °F (39 °C), elevated levels of acute phase reactants (e.g., erythrocyte sedimentation rate [ESR] and C-reactive protein), and a prolonged PR interval.[1,38]

In diagnosing rheumatic heart disease, the NP should check for signs of a recent Strep infection. Indications of rheumatic fever, such as joint pain and inflammation, should also be noted. A chest x-ray and echocardiogram are beneficial in assessing the size of the heart and the presence of any excess fluid.[37]

Treatment

Rheumatic fever is primarily treated by antibiotics and antiinflammatory agents. Antibiotics, primarily penicillin, are used to eradicate the group A beta-hemolytic streptococcus carriage.[36,39] Antiinflammatory agents are used in treating arthritis.[39] Bed rest is recommended if acute carditis is present.[1]

Patients with rheumatic heart disease are typically prescribed penicillin for many years to prevent the recurrence of rheumatic fever. If the patient has a severe valve leak, surgery is required to either repair or replace the valve.[37]

Kawasaki Disease

Overview

Kawasaki disease is an acute febrile vasculitic syndrome that involves inflammation of the blood vessels.[40] This condition often causes cardiac complications in children by damaging the coronary arteries that supply oxygen to the heart.[41] Kawasaki disease is most prevalent in children of Asian ethnicities.[42]

Presentation

Kawasaki disease has three stages: the acute, subacute, and convalescent phases. Prior to the onset of fever, patients may be irritable or vomit. The acute phase is characterized by fever lasting 7 to 14 days. Other findings include nonexudative bilateral conjunctivitis, anterior uveitis, perianal erythema, and lymphadenopathy.[40]

The subacute phase begins once fever abates and lasts until about week four. Findings include desquamation of the digits, thrombocytosis, and development of coronary aneurysms. Risk of sudden death is highest during the subacute phase.[40] The convalescent phase is characterized by the resolution of clinical signs of illness. Patients typically enter this phase within 3 months of presentation.[40]

Workup

Diagnosis of Kawasaki disease requires presentation of fever and four of the following criteria: bilateral bulbar conjunctival injection, oral mucous membrane changes, peripheral extremity changes, polymorphous rash, and cervical lymphadenopathy.[43]

Acute-phase reactants (i.e., erythrocyte sedimentation rate, C-reactive protein levels, alpha1-antitrypsin levels) are typically elevated at the start of the illness.[36,44] A CBC will often show mild anemia.[44] ECG changes indicative of Kawasaki disease include prolonged PR or QT intervals.[44] An echocardiogram should be conducted periodically throughout the phases of the illness to evaluate for coronary artery aneurysms.[40]

Treatment

Immediate referral to a pediatric cardiologist is recommended. Inpatient therapy should be initiated with a high dose of aspirin and a single infusion of intravenous immune globulin. Once fever has been absent for 48 hours, a low dose of aspirin should be administered daily for its antiplatelet effect. Aspirin therapy should be continued until laboratory markers indicate an absence of acute inflammation. The NP should discontinue aspirin therapy in collaboration with a cardiologist.[42,45]

References

1. Barkley TW Jr. Cardiovascular issues and disorders. In: Barkley TW Jr, ed. *Pediatric Primary Care Nurse Practitioner*. West Hollywood, CA: Barkley & Associates, Inc.; 2015: 72–81.

2. Cardiovascular. A.D.A.M. Medical Encyclopedia. http://www.nlm.nih.gov/medlineplus/ency/article/002310.htm. Updated January 21, 2013. Accessed April 14, 2015.

3. Mangla A. Heart sounds. In: Lang RA, ed. Medscape. http://emedicine.medscape.com/article/1894036-overview#showall. Updated April 24, 2014. Accessed June 2, 2015.

4. Altman CA. Congenital heart disease (CHD) in the newborn: Presentation and screening for critical CHD. In: Basow DS, ed. *UpToDate*. Waltham, MA: UpToDate; 2015. http://www.uptodate.com/contents/congenital-heart-disease-chd-in-the-newborn-presentation-and-screening-for-critical-chd. Last updated February 4, 2015. Accessed April 14, 2015.

5. Ashraf A. Ventricular septal defects. University of Texas Medical Branch Web site. http://www.utmb.edu/pedi_ed/core/cardiology/page_06.htm. Accessed June 2, 2008.

6. Singh RK, Singh TP. Etiology and diagnosis of heart failure in infants and children. In: Basow DS, ed. *UpToDate*. Waltham, MA: UpToDate; 2015. http://www.uptodate.com/contents/etiology-and-diagnosis-of-heart-failure-in-infants-and-children. Last updated May 28, 2014. Accessed April 14, 2015.

7. Webb GD, Smallhorn JF, Therrien J, Redington AN. Congenital heart disease. In: Zipes DP, Libby P, Bonow RO, eds. *Braunwald's Heart Disease: A Textbook of Cardiovascular Medicine*. 9th ed. Philadelphia, PA: Elsevier Saunders; 2011: 1411–1467.

8. Lott JW. Cardiovascular system. In: Kenner C, Lott JW, eds. *Comprehensive Neonatal Nursing Care*. 5th ed. New York, NY: Springer Publishing Company; 2014: 152–188.

9. Cyanotic heart disease. A.D.A.M. Medical Encyclopedia. http://www.nlm.nih.gov/medlineplus/ency/article/001104.htm. Updated November 5, 2013. Accessed April 14, 2015.

10. Bernstein D. Cyanotic congenital heart disease: Evaluation of the critically ill neonate with cyanosis and respiratory distress. In: Kliegman RM, Behrman RE, Jenson HB, Stanton BF, eds. *Nelson Textbook of Pediatrics*. 19th ed. Philadelphia, PA: Elsevier Saunders; 2011: 1572.

11. Fulton DR, Kane DA. L-transposition of the great arteries. In: Basow DS, ed. *UpToDate*. Waltham, MA: UpToDate; 2015. http://www.uptodate.com/contents/l-transposition-of-the-great-arteries?source=search_result&search=L-transposition+of+the+great+arteries&selectedTitle=1~6. Last updated September 26, 2014. Accessed June 2, 2015.

12. Doyle T, Kavanaugh-McHugh A. Pathophysiology, clinical features, and diagnosis of tetralogy of Fallot. In: Basow DS, ed. *UpToDate*. Waltham, MA: UpToDate; 2015. http://www.uptodate.com/contents/pathophysiology-clinical-features-and-diagnosis-of-tetralogy-of-fallot?source=search_result&search=pathophysiology%2C+clinical+features%2C+and+diagnosis+of+tetralogy+of+fallot&selectedTitle=1~115. Last updated May 6, 2015. Accessed June 2, 2015.

13. Geggel RL. Diagnosis and initial management of cyanotic heart disease in the newborn. In: Basow DS, ed. *UpToDate*. Waltham, MA: UpToDate; 2015. http://www.uptodate.com/contents/diagnosis-and-initial-management-of-cyanotic-heart-disease-in-the-newborn. Last updated June 17, 2014. Accessed April 14, 2015.

14. Brown DW. Valvar aortic stenosis in children. In: Basow DS, ed. *UpToDate*. Waltham, MA: UpToDate; 2015. http://www.uptodate.com/contents/valvar-aortic-stenosis-in-children. Last updated March 31, 2015. Accessed April 14, 2015.

15. Armstrong GP. Pulmonic stenosis. In: Porter RS, Kaplan JL, eds. Merck Manual Professional Version. http://www.merckmanuals.com/professional/cardiovascular-disorders/valvular-disorders/pulmonic-stenosis. Last reviewed July 2014. Accessed April 14, 2015.

16. Frank JE, Jacobe KM. Evaluation and management of heart murmurs in children. *Am Fam Physician.* 2011; 84(7): 793–800. http://www.aafp.org/afp/2011/1001/p793.html

17. Peng LF, Perry S. Pulmonic stenosis (PS) in neonates, infants, and children. In: Basow DS, ed. *UpToDate*. Waltham, MA: UpToDate; 2015. http://www.uptodate.com/contents/pulmonic-stenosis-ps-in-neonates-infants-and-children?source=search_result&search=pulmonic+stenosis+in+neonates&selectedTitle=1~52. Last updated July 22, 2014. Accessed June 2, 2015.

18. Agarwala BN, Bacha E, Cao QL, Hijazi ZM. Clinical manifestations and diagnosis of coarctation of the aorta. In: Basow DS, ed. *UpToDate*. Waltham, MA: UpToDate; 2015. http://www.uptodate.com/contents/clinical-manifestations-and-diagnosis-of-coarctation-of-the-aorta?source=search_result&search=clinical+manifestations+and+diagnosis+of+coarctation+of+the+aorta&selectedTitle=1~124. Last accessed February 9, 2015. Accessed June 2, 2015.

19. Wiesmann-Günzler S. Congenital syndromes with malformations of the heart. Corience Web site. http://www.corience.org/about-heart-defects/syndromes. Last updated March 13, 2014. Accessed April 14, 2015.

20. Seroogy CM. DiGeorge (22q11.2 deletion) syndrome: Clinical features and diagnosis. In: Basow DS, ed. *UpToDate*. Waltham, MA: UpToDate; 2015. http://www.uptodate.com/contents/digeorge-22q11-2-deletion-syndrome-clinical-features-and-diagnosis?source=search_result&search=digeorge+syndrome+clinical+features&selectedTitle=1~66. Last updated April 29, 2015. Accessed June 2, 2015.

21. Wright MJ, Connolly HM. Genetics, clinical features, and diagnosis of Marfan syndrome and related disorders. In: Basow DS, ed. *UpToDate*. Waltham, MA: UpToDate; 2015. http://www.uptodate.com/contents/genetics-clinical-features-and-diagnosis-of-marfan-syndrome-and-related-disorders?source=search_result&search=genetics%2C+clinical+features%2C+and+diagnosis+of+marfan+syndrome&selectedTitle=1~150. Last updated March 18, 2015. Accessed June 2, 2015.

22. Saenger P. Clinical manifestations and diagnosis of Turner syndrome (gonadal dysgenesis). In: Basow DS, ed. *UpToDate*. Waltham, MA: UpToDate; 2015. http://www.uptodate.com/contents/clinical-manifestations-and-diagnosis-of-turner-syndrome-gonadal-dysgenesis?source=search_result&search=clinical+manifestations+and+diagnosis+of+turner+syndrome&selectedTitle=1~144. Last updated September 17, 2014. Accessed June 2, 2015.

23. Chan H. Trisomy 18 clinical presentation. In: Rohena LO, ed. Medscape. http://emedicine.medscape.com/article/943463-clinical. Updated August 27, 2014. Accessed June 2, 2015.

24. Ostermaier KK. Down syndrome: Clinical features and diagnosis. In: Basow DS, ed. *UpToDate*. Waltham, MA: UpToDate; 2015. http://www.uptodate.com/contents/down-syndrome-clinical-features-and-diagnosis?source=search_result&search=down+syndrome%3A+clinical+features+and+diagnosis&selectedTitle=1~150. Last updated April 28, 2015. Accessed June 2, 2015.

25. Innocent heart murmur. Congenital & Children's Heart Centre Web site. http://www.childrensheartcentre.com/selectedheart-conditions/innocentmurmur.html. Accessed June 2, 2015.

26. U.S. Department of Health and Human Services, National Institute of Health (NIH), National Heart, Lung, and Blood Institute. What causes heart murmurs? National Heart, Lung, and Blood Institute Web site. http://www.nhlbi.nih.gov/health/health-topics/topics/heartmurmur/causes. Updated September 20, 2012. Accessed June 2, 2015.

27. Punnoose AR, Burke AE, Golub RM. Innocent (harmless) heart murmurs in children. *JAMA*. 2012; 308(3): 305. doi: 10.1001/jama.2012.6223

28. McConnell ME, Adkins SB III, Hannon DW. Heart murmurs in pediatric patients: When do you refer? *Am Fam Physician*. 1999; 60(2): 558–564. http://www.aafp.org/afp/1999/0801/p558.html

29. Gersh BJ. Auscultation of cardiac murmurs. In: Basow DS, ed. *UpToDate*. Waltham, MA: UpToDate; 2015. http://www.uptodate.com/contents/auscultation-of-cardiac-murmurs. Last updated April 23, 2014. Accessed April 14, 2015.

30. Riley M, Bluhm B. High blood pressure in children and adolescents. *Am Fam Physician*. 2012; 85(7): 693–700. http://www.aafp.org/afp/2012/0401/p693.html

31. Mayo Clinic Staff. High blood pressure. Mayo Clinic Web site. http://www.mayoclinic.org/diseases-conditions/high-blood-pressure-in-children/basics/symptoms/con-20033799. Updated December 18, 2012. Accessed June 2, 2015.

32. Mattoo TK. Evaluation of hypertension in children and adolescents. In: Basow DS, ed. *UpToDate*. Waltham, MA: UpToDate; 2015. http://www.uptodate.com/contents/evaluation-of-hypertension-in-children-and-adolescents?source=search_result&search=evaluation+of+hypertension+in+children+and+adolescents&selectedTitle=1~150. Last updated January 21, 2014. Accessed June 2, 2015.

33. Berger S. Pediatric primary pulmonary hypertension. In: Bye MR, ed. Medscape. http://emedicine.medscape.com/article/1004828-overview. Updated December 31, 2013. Accessed June 2, 2015.

34. Gibofsky A, Zabriskie JB. Clinical manifestations and diagnosis of acute rheumatic fever. In: Basow DS, ed. *UpToDate*. Waltham, MA: UpToDate; 2015. http://www.uptodate.com/contents/clinical-manifestations-and-diagnosis-of-acute-rheumatic-fever?source=search_result&search=clinical+manifestations+and+diagnosis+of+acute+rheumatic+fever&selectedTitle=1~110. Last updated October 4, 2013. Accessed June 2, 2015.

35. Mayosi B. Natural history, screening, and management of rheumatic heart disease. In: Basow DS, ed. *UpToDate*. Waltham, MA: UpToDate; 2015. http://www.uptodate.com/contents/natural-history-screening-and-management-of-rheumatic-heart-disease?source=search_result&search=natural+history%2C+screening%2C+and+management+of+rheumatic+heart+disease&selectedTitle=1~85. Last updated January 8, 2014. Accessed June 2, 2015.

36. Rheumatic fever. A.D.A.M. Medical Encyclopedia. http://www.nlm.nih.gov/medlineplus/ency/article/003940.htm. Updated May 11, 2014. Accessed April 14, 2015.

37. Rheumatic heart disease diagnosis. UCSF Benioff Children's Hospital San Francisco Web site. http://www.ucsfbenioffchildrens.org/conditions/rheumatic_heart_disease/diagnosis.html. Accessed June 2, 2015.

38. Jones criteria for diagnosis of rheumatic fever. Medscape. http://reference.medscape.com/calculator/jones-criteria-diagnosis-rheumatic. Accessed June 2, 2015.

39. Gibofsky A, Zabriskie JB. Treatment and prevention of acute rheumatic fever. In: Basow DS, ed. *UpToDate*. Waltham, MA: UpToDate; 2015. http://www.uptodate.com/contents/treatment-and-prevention-of-acute-rheumatic-fever?source=-search_result&search=treatment+and+prevention+of+acute+rheumatic+fever&selectedTitle=1~110. Last updated October 7, 2013. Accessed June 2, 2015.

40. Scheinfeld NS. Kawasaki disease. In: Steele RW, ed. Medscape. http://emedicine.medscape.com/article/965367-overview. Updated January 12, 2015. Accessed April 14, 2015.

41. Kawasaki disease. American Heart Association Web site. http://www.heart.org/HEARTORG/Conditions/More/CardiovascularConditionsofChildhood/Kawasaki-Disease_UCM_308777_Article.jsp. Last reviewed March 22, 2013. Accessed April 14, 2015.

42. Porth CM. Disorders of cardiac function. In: Porth CM, ed. *Essentials of Pathophysiology: Concepts of Altered Health States.* 3rd ed. Philadelphia, PA: Wolters Kluwer Health/Lippincott Williams & Wilkins; 2011: 447–485.

43. Sundel R. Kawasaki disease: Clinical features and diagnosis. In: Basow DS, ed. *UpToDate*. Waltham, MA: UpToDate; 2015. http://www.uptodate.com/contents/kawasaki-disease-clinical-features-and-diagnosis?source=search_result&search=kawasaki+disease+clinical+features+and+diagnosis&selectedTitle=1~150. Last updated May 5, 2015. Accessed June 2, 3015.

44. Horeczko T, Inaba AS. Cardiac disorders. In: Marx JA, Hockberger RS, Walls RM, eds. *Rosen's Emergency Medicine: Concepts and Clinical Practice.* 8th ed. Philadelphia, PA: Elsevier Saunders; 2014: 2139–2167.

45. Sundel R. Kawasaki disease: Initial treatment and prognosis. In: Basow DS, ed. *UpToDate*. Waltham, MA: UpToDate; 2015. http://www.uptodate.com/contents/kawasaki-disease-initial-treatment-and-prognosis?source=search_result&search=kawasaki+disease+in+pediatrics&selectedTitle=2~150. Last updated November 18, 2014. Accessed June 2, 2015.

Chapter 10

Gastrointestinal Disorders

QUESTIONS

1. You are evaluating a 4-month-old, whose mother says, "She's been vomiting and doesn't seem to be taking any milk or fluids. She's also been sleeping a lot more than usual." You note that the patient's fontanel is slightly sunken, and that her skin is cool to the touch and has poor turgor. These findings are <u>least</u> likely to be an initial indication of which condition?

   a. Intussusception

   b. Gastroenteritis

   c. Pyloric stenosis

   d. Hirschsprung's disease

2. Which test would provide the most definitive diagnosis of neuroblastoma?

   a. Physical exam

   b. Low levels of urine catecholamines

   c. Abdominal computed tomography scan

   d. Surgical biopsy

3. A mother brings her 18-month-old daughter to your practice with complaints of watery diarrhea. The mother says that she has noticed her child "has not looked too well." She also says that her daughter has been refusing to eat and has been unable to keep her food down. The mother also reports hearing loud rumbling noises coming from the child's stomach. Based on these findings, which finding would you most expect to see in this patient during your exam?

   a. Enlarged abdominal mass

   b. Visible peristaltic waves

   c. Abdominal distention

   d. Positive psoas sign

4. Vitamin deficiency resulting from malabsorption is most likely to present with:

   a. Vomiting

   b. Chronic diarrhea

   c. Fatigue

   d. Thin stools

5. A 6-month-old male is brought to your clinic with complaints of vomiting. His mother says that her son was fine, but then "he just got really irritable and started crying, and then just started throwing up green barf." The mother says that she noticed her son has not been as energetic as usual, and that there was "jelly-like poop" when changing his diaper. Based on these findings, which gastrointestinal disorder would you most likely suspect?

   a. Gastroenteritis

   b. Hirschsprung's disease

   c. Pyloric stenosis

   d. Intussusception

6. How and where does the obturator sign present in pediatric patients with appendicitis?

   a. Sharp pain in the right lower quadrant of the abdomen

   b. Pain with internal rotation of the right hip

   c. Pain with extension of the right hip

   d. Tenderness one-third the distance from the anterior superior iliac spine to the umbilicus

7. You are teaching the parents of an 8-month-old infant with gastroesophageal reflux disease. Which of the following actions should you advise the parents to perform immediately after meals specifically to decrease reflux activity?

   a. Position the infant in a semi-supine position

   b. Assist the newborn to burp after meals

   c. Elevate the newborn's head

   d. Administer a histamine 2-receptor antagonist

8. Incidence of viral gastroenteritis in pediatric patients usually peaks during which season?

   a. Spring

   b. Summer

   c. Autumn

   d. Winter

9. Management of symptoms in infants with gastroesophageal reflux disease is more likely to include which of these in non-severe cases?

   a. Thickening of feedings

   b. Histamine 2-receptor antagonist

   c. A diet that either reduces or eliminates protein

   d. Switching to hydrolyzed or amino acid-based formula

10. Which test can be used to diagnose either Hirschsprung's disease or intussusception?

   a. Barium enema

   b. Rectal biopsy

   c. Ultrasound

   d. Colon biopsy

RATIONALES

1. c

Decreased skin turgor and a slightly sunken fontanel are signs of dehydration; however, pyloric stenosis is least likely to result in an infant who remains hungry after vomiting. Dehydration and poor feeding may accompany Hirschsprung's disease, intussusception, pyloric stenosis, and gastroenteritis.

2. d

A surgical biopsy is the most definitive diagnosis for neuroblastoma. Elevated urinary catecholamine levels, rather than low urinary catecholamine levels, may be used to diagnose neuroblastoma. Imaging studies, such as a computerized tomography scan and physical exams, may strongly suggest the presence of this condition, but are unable to confirm a diagnosis.

3. c

Abdominal distention is an expected finding of gastroenteritis, which often produces watery diarrhea, hyperactive bowel sounds, non-bilious vomiting, and anorexia in infants. An enlarged abdominal mass, on the other hand, may be a sign of neuroblastoma, but this condition is accompanied by profuse sweating and tachycardia. Although gastroenteritis may present with peristaltic rushes, peristaltic waves are more likely a sign of pyloric stenosis. A positive psoas sign indicates appendicitis, not gastroenteritis.

4. c

Fatigue is most likely to be associated with vitamin deficiency due to malabsorption because it may be a sign of anemia resulting from malabsorption of vitamin B12, folate, and iron. Vomiting and chronic diarrhea are also symptoms of malabsorption, but are not directly caused by vitamin deficiency. Thin stools usually are not indications of an abnormal condition, but may result from irritable bowel syndrome.

5. d

Intussusception is a medical emergency that presents with sudden onset of bilious vomiting, progressive lethargy, and acute colicky pain, which may be indicated in infants by crying. A “currant-jelly” stool is a hallmark symptom of the latter stages of the condition as the intestine sheds its mucosa. Hirschsprung’s disease also presents in infancy with pain and bilious vomiting, but may produce bloody diarrhea. Pyloric stenosis is associated with non-bilious, projectile vomiting, as opposed to bilious vomiting. Gastroenteritis, which also may present with vomiting, would produce watery diarrhea rather than a “currant-jelly” stool.

6. b

The obturator sign presents as pain with internal rotation of the right hip, as the inflamed appendix comes into contact with the obturator internus muscle. Although psoas sign also produces through action on the right thigh, it produces through extension of the thigh rather than rotation. Appendicitis presents with tenderness at McBurney’s point, which is found one-third of the distance from the anterior superior iliac spine to the umbilicus. Sharp stomach pain that originates around the navel and shifts to the right lower quadrant after several hours may indicate a perforation, which is much more common in pediatrics due to age-related communication barriers.

7. c

Parents of infants with gastroesophageal reflux disease (GERD) should be advised to elevate the infant's head after feeding to decrease reflux activity. Parents should also be told that burping should be performed frequently during the infant's feeding session, not after. Positioning the infant in a semi-supine position is not advised because it would increase reflux, rather than decrease it. Histamine 2-receptor antagonists should be reserved only for severe or complicated cases, because symptoms of GERD typically resolve in infants without medical intervention.

8. d

Incidence of viral gastroenteritis in pediatric patients usually peaks during the winter. Viral causes of gastroenteritis include the norovirus and the rotavirus, which is particularly more active during the winter, from November to February.

9. a

Management of symptoms in infants with non-severe gastroesophageal reflux disease (GERD) is more likely to include small, frequent feeds that are thickened with cereal. Conservative management with optimization of positioning, feeding, and nutrition is often sufficient to manage healthy and thriving infants with symptoms due to physiological GERD. Severe cases of GERD, rather than non-severe cases, may require pharmacologic intervention with histamine 2-receptor antagonists, with proton pump inhibitors (PPIs) co-administered to block gastric acid secretion caused by histamine or other PPIs, but the administration of these drugs may lead to malabsorption of B12. Because an allergy to cow's milk protein may mimic symptoms of GERD, formula-fed infants with persistent vomiting may benefit from a 2–4 week trial of a hydrolyzed or amino acid-based formula. Although some breast-fed infants with symptoms may benefit from a maternal diet excluding all dairy and egg, a diet that either reduces or eliminates protein is more often used to manage symptoms associated with pediatric viral hepatitis than GERD.

10. a

A barium enema is a diagnostic for both Hirschsprung's disease and intussusception. Rectal and colon biopsies are only useful for diagnosis of Hirschsprung's disease. Ultrasounds, on the other hand, are useful in the diagnosis of intussusception but not for Hirschsprung's disease.

DISCUSSION

Gastroenteritis

Overview

Gastroenteritis is a broad term applied to a syndrome of acute vomiting, nausea, and diarrhea that stems from acute irritation and inflammation of the gastric mucosa. Although gastroenteritis has many causes, the condition is most commonly caused by viruses, which are particularly active in the months of winter.[1] Gastroenteritis may also be caused by bacterial or parasitic infections which can be transmitted by food, water, dirty surfaces, or contact with infected persons.[2] Moreover, inorganic food content and emotional stress may lead to gastroenteritis.[3]

The majority of viral gastroenteritis cases are due to rotavirus and norovirus. Astrovirus and adenoviruses are also common viral causes of the condition.[4] The three leading causes of bacterial diarrhea are bacteria in the *Salmonella*, *Campylobacter*, and *Shigella* genera.[5] Although *Salmonella* bacteria do not tend to produce distinctive symptoms, *Campylobacter* bacteria often cause malodorous stool, whereas *Shigella* bacteria can be distinguished by fever spikes, bloody stools, and febrile seizures. *Escherichia coli* bacteria, another common cause of bacterial gastroenteritis, may produce loose stools.[3]

Presentation

Characteristic findings include abdominal distention, nausea and vomiting, cramping abdominal pain, and diarrhea.[6] Patients may also present with a fever, hyperactive bowel sounds, and anorexia.

Diarrhea and vomiting may lead to dehydration.[2] Dehydration can appear in mild, moderate, or severe forms. These forms can be classified by assessing the patient's signs and symptoms according to table 10.1.[3]

Workup

In most cases, gastroenteritis is diagnosed clinically. No diagnostic tests are indicated for gastroenteritis unless the patient's symptoms persist for more than 72 hours, bloody stool is present, or the patient has a fever.[3] A complete blood count (CBC) can be performed to help determine a possible bacterial etiology, whereas a blood urea nitrogen test can be performed to note dehydration.[7] A stool culture can be used to determine the specific bacterial etiology after 72 hours.[4]

Treatment

The mainstay of supportive care focuses on drinking fluids to maintain hydration.[2,8] Infants should continue to be breastfed or formula fed. Older children can gradually resume a regular diet once rehydrated. The BRAT diet, which consists of bananas, rice, applesauce, and toast, is often recommended because these foods are well

Table 10.1 Signs and Symptoms of Dehydration

Variable	Mild (3%–5%)	Moderate (6%–9%)	Severe (≥ 10%)
Blood Pressure	Normal	Normal	Normal, decreased
Pulse/Heart Rate	Normal	Increased	Severe, decreased
CAP Refill	WNL	WNL	Prolonged (> 3 seconds)
Skin Turgor	Normal	Decreased	Decreased
Fontanel	Normal	Sunken (slightly)	Sunken
Urine	Slightly decreased	< 1 ml/kg/hour	< 1 ml/kg/hour

Used with permission from Barkley TW Jr. *Pediatric Primary Care Nurse Practitioner Certification Review/Clinical Update Continuing Education Course.* West Hollywood, CA: Barkley and Associates; 2015.

tolerated by most people and are easy to digest.[9] However, virtually any food or drink that a child would normally partake in is acceptable to maintain hydration and avoid electrolyte imbalance.

Children with gastroenteritis should be excluded from daycare, particularly if their condition is caused by rotavirus, *E. coli*, or *Shigella spp.* In bacterial cases caused by *E. coli* and *Shigella spp.*, two negative stool cultures collected consecutively at least 24 hours apart are required prior to the child's return to daycare.[3,10]

In-patient pediatric patients should be treated by oral rehydration therapy at 50–100 ml/hr to remedy their fluid deficit.[11] Antidiarrheal medications are not recommended because it may prolong symptoms.[2,3]

Gastroesophageal Reflux Disease (GERD)

Overview

Gastroesophageal reflux disease (GERD) is a condition where gastric contents pass from the stomach into the esophagus due to incompetence of the lower esophageal sphincter.[12] GERD frequently presents in premature infants and infants with low birth weight but typically resolves by 18 months of age.[13]

The three classes of GERD are physiological, functional, and pathological.[3] Physiological GERD is characterized by infrequent, episodic vomiting. Functional GERD, on the other hand, presents with painless, effortless vomiting with no physical sequelae. Pathological GERD presents with frequent vomiting with alteration in physical functioning, which may include failure to thrive (FTT) or aspiration pneumonia.

Presentation

The most common and prominent symptom of GERD is heartburn, which may be accompanied by other findings such as acid regurgitation and dysphagia.[14] Heartburn usually occurs after eating, or when the patient is bending over or lying supine. Conditions that cause issues with the ear or teeth, such as otitis media and dental erosion, may result from abnormal reflux.[15] Vomiting and irritability are common symptoms of GERD in infants, whereas coughing and wheezing may appear in infants and adults alike.[12] Patients may also experience additional signs and symptoms affecting the throat such as pharyngitis, choking, and painful belching. Weight loss, abdominal pain, and stool pattern changes may also present.[3]

Workup

Most cases of GERD are made clinically.[16] However, when a patient's signs and symptoms are longstanding or do not improve with conservative management, an endoscopy may be helpful.[12] Additional studies that may be considered include ambulatory 24-hour pH monitoring,[15] a CBC, and urinalysis. When the diagnosis is not clear, an abdominal ultrasonography can help to rule out pyloric stenosis.[3]

Treatment

Infant cases of GERD can usually be treated with dietary and behavioral modifications, but more severe cases may require a referral to a gastrointestinal specialist.[17] Infant GERD patients should receive small, frequent feedings and should be burped frequently during feedings. The pediatric patient's head should be elevated for 60 minutes after feeding.[18] Breastfeeding should continue, and formula changes should be avoided. For pediatric patients who require thickened formula in GERD management, one tablespoon of rice cereal may be added per ounce of formula.[3,17]

When dietary and behavioral modifications do not provide relief, pharmacological measures may be instituted. Treatment should begin with over-the-counter antacids to control heartburn.[19] Other medications that may be ordered to treat GERD include histamine H2-receptor antagonists, such as ranitidine (Zantac) and famotidine (Pepcid AC). If histamine H2-receptor antagonists prove ineffective, proton pump inhibitors such as omeprazole (Prilosec) may be ordered to inhibit gastric acid secretion produced by acetylcholine, histamine, or gastrin.[19]

Pyloric Stenosis

Overview

Pyloric stenosis is a rare obstruction disorder in which the stomach is unable to empty into the small intestine because of the thickening of the circular muscles of the pylorus.[20] The cause of pyloric stenosis is unclear, although the condition may involve genetic or familial predisposition as well as environmental factors.[21] Males are more often affected than females, and the condition is more common in Caucasians. Pyloric stenosis most often affects children younger than 6 months of age.[20]

Presentation

Pyloric stenosis typically presents in children between 3 weeks and 4 months of age.[3] Projectile non-bilious vomiting occurs after eating. Afterward, the patient remains apparently hungry.[22] A palpable olive-shaped mass may be observed in the right side of the patient's abdomen. As the condition progresses, the patient may become dehydrated and either loses weight or fails to gain weight.[23] The appearance of peristaltic waves in the patient's abdomen is also a sign of pyloric stenosis.[24]

Workup

Pyloric stenosis is diagnosed by an abdominal ultrasound that shows increased thickness and elongation of the pylorus.[23] An upper gastrointestinal imaging (GI) test can be useful when an ultrasound or other imaging tests are not conclusive.[22] An upper GI study commonly shows delayed gastric emptying and a "string sign," a thin strip of contrast material in the lumen which indicates the narrowing of the pyloric channel.[23]

Treatment

Patients usually need a surgical procedure known as a pyloromyotomy, which opens the thickened area of the pylorus and allows food to pass through.[24] Surgery typically relieves all of the patient's symptoms. Within a few hours post-surgery, the patient can often tolerate small, frequent feedings.[20]

Intussusception

Overview

Intussusception is a disorder in which one part of the intestine experiences an acute inversion into an adjacent segment of the intestine. This process, known as telescoping, often blocks food or fluids.[14] Most cases of intussusception occur prior to 2 years of age, and the condition is more common in males.[3] Intussusception commonly occurs in children who are otherwise healthy. Although the cause of intussusception is unknown, the condition is associated with viral triggers such as adenovirus.[25] Patients with celiac disease and cystic fibrosis also have an increased incidence of intussusception.[3]

Presentation

Acute colicky pain, usually accompanied by vomiting, is often the first sign of intussusception.[26] This vomiting is initially non-bilious but becomes bilious when the patient's intestine becomes obstructed.[27] Progressive lethargy is also a common symptom and in some cases may be the patient's sole presenting symptom.[27] As intussusception progresses, a palpable, sausage-shaped mass may develop in the right side of the patient's abdomen.[25] The patient's stool may be mixed with blood and mucus, which gives the appearance of currant jelly.[25] Patients may present with progressive abdominal distention and tenderness, which may indicate intestinal perforation.[3]

Workup

An ultrasonography is the preferred diagnostic test to detect intussusception.[25] If the ultrasonography is not clear, a radiograph of the patient's abdomen should be considered to exclude intussusception, but should not be relied upon to confirm a diagnosis.[25,27] A barium enema is both diagnostic and therapeutic because it can reduce the telescoped segments of the patient's intestine. However, barium enemas have fallen out of favor as a diagnostic, as the barium may enter a clinically unsuspected perforation and produce peritonitis.[26]

Treatment

When a diagnosis of intussusception is confirmed, the patient should be treated with a non-operative reduction, if possible.[25] Enemas are the primary non-operative treatments.[25] If these treatments are not successful, the patient will require emergent surgery because intussusception is fatal if not treated urgently.[3,28]

Hirschsprung's Disease (Aganglionic Megacolon)

Overview

Hirschsprung's disease, or aganglionic megacolon, is a developmental disorder in which functional bowel obstruction is caused by improper muscle movement in the bowel and the absence of ganglion cells in the distal colon.[29] Although the cause of Hirschsprung's disease is unknown, the disease sometimes occurs in families or develops spontaneously from genetic mutations.[3,30] If untreated, enterocolitis, an inflammation of the colon with potentially fatal results, may develop in patients. Hirschsprung's disease is rare, more common in boys than girls, and may present both in infancy and in older children.[29]

Presentation

Infants with Hirschsprung's disease frequently fail to pass meconium shortly after birth.[31] Newborns and infants may also present with abdominal distention, bilious vomiting, FTT, jaundice, and infrequent and explosive bowel movements.[32] Older children often present with abdominal distention, constipation, and malnutrition.[32]

Workup

A rectal biopsy, which confirms an absence of ganglion cells, is the standard for diagnosing Hirschsprung's disease.[29,33] A barium enema and abdominal x-ray may also be helpful, but an abdominal x-ray is only suggestive of the disease and a barium enema is less sensitive.[29]

Treatment

Patients should be referred to a gastroenterologist for management and surgery.[29] Surgical treatment of Hirschsprung's disease typically involves a one-stage procedure focused on resecting the aganglionic portion of the colon.[31,33]

Appendicitis

Overview

Appendicitis is an acute inflammation of the vermiform appendix.[34] Typically, appendicitis is precipitated by obstruction of the appendix by fecalith, foreign bodies, or neoplasms.[35] If the condition remains untreated, perforation and gangrene may develop within 36 hours. Appendicitis affects approximately 10% of the general population and most commonly occurs in males 10–30 years of age.[3]

Presentation

Appendicitis typically begins with vague, colicky umbilical pain, which shifts to the right lower quadrant of the abdomen within several hours. The pain often worsens, localizes with coughing, and is followed by nausea, vomiting, fever, and anorexia.[36]

Nausea accompanied by one to two episodes of vomiting is characteristic of appendicitis, but more vomiting may suggest another diagnosis.[3] Diarrhea is a less common finding.[34]

Although more difficult to elicit in children than adults, the psoas sign, the obturator sign, McBurney's point tenderness, and Rovsing's sign each have a high specificity for appendicitis.[37] Psoas sign is pain with right thigh extension. Obturator sign occurs when the right thigh is rotated internally. McBurney's point can be found by tracing a line from the anterior superior iliac spine to the umbilicus, then finding a point at one-third of the line starting from the iliac spine; tenderness at this point commonly indicates appendicitis. Lastly, Rovsing's sign, also known as indirect tenderness, is pain in the right lower quadrant upon palpation of the left lower quadrant.[37]

Workup

A diagnosis of appendicitis can be made clinically in patients who present with the classic signs and symptoms of anorexia, periumbilical pain, migration of pain to the right lower quadrant, fever, and vomiting.[36] Along with a history and physical exam, a possible elevated erythrocyte sedimentation rate and an elevated white blood cell count between 10,000 and 20,000 cells/μL will further support a diagnosis of appendicitis.[3] An ultrasound or computed tomography (CT) are diagnostic.[37]

Treatment

An appendectomy is the only curative treatment for appendicitis.[34] The prognosis is very good in patients experiencing the early stages of the condition.[38] The prognosis for advanced appendicitis is also good, but special attention must be given to postoperative care to reduce wound infection and other possible complications.[38]

Malabsorption

Overview

Malabsorption is a state where the intestine is unable to fully absorb essential nutrients and electrolytes.[39] Celiac disease and cystic fibrosis can cause malabsorption, as can infection, inflammation, and other conditions that may result in damage to the intestine.[40]

Presentation

Severe, chronic diarrhea is the most common finding of malabsorption.[41] Bulky, foul stool (i.e., steatorrhea) occurs in patients who excrete more than 7 grams of fat per day.[42] Other common signs and symptoms may include FTT, vomiting, abdominal pain, and a protuberant abdomen. Patients with vitamin deficiencies may also present with pallor, fatigue, hair and dermatological abnormalities, cheilosis, and peripheral neuropathy.[3]

Workup

Although a diagnosis of malabsorption is often apparent based on the patient's clinical presentation, this diagnosis may be further established by iron and folate tests.[39,41] Other diagnostic tests for malabsorption include a stool assessment for ova and parasites, liver function tests, and tests to assess serum calcium, phosphorus, alkaline phosphatase, and total protein levels.[3]

Further diagnostic tests can be done to determine the etiology. Differential diagnoses of malabsorption include conditions such as FTT, cystic fibrosis, immune deficiency, hepatic disease, inflammatory bowel disease, chronic diarrhea, and celiac disease.[3]

Treatment

Patients should be referred to a gastroenterologist for treatment. Treatment should be aimed at correcting nutritional deficiencies and managing causative diseases.[41] Dietary modifications are useful, particularly in treating diarrhea due to malabsorption.[43] The appropriate dietary treatment depends on the patient's underlying condition. For example, patients with celiac disease should avoid wheat, oat, rye, and barley. Cystic fibrosis patients should be treated with pancreatic enzyme replacement and fat soluble vitamins.[3]

Neuroblastoma

Overview

Neuroblastoma is a malignant tumor that arises from the neural tissue. Most cases of neuroblastoma are in the adrenal gland or abdomen and can expand to the bone marrow, lymph nodes, skin, liver, and orbits of the eyes.[44] Neuroblastoma is the most common cancer in infants and most always occurs in children younger than 5 years of age.[45]

Presentation

Signs and symptoms vary depending on the location of the tumor and the extent of metastasis.[46] Children with localized disease are typically asymptomatic, but systemic manifestations appear in children with disseminated neuroblastoma.[47] The most common findings are an abdominal mass, abdominal pain, and discomfort.[41] Other common findings include FTT, general malaise, and bone pain.[47]

Workup

After referring to a pediatric oncologist, neuroblastoma may be diagnosed by a surgical biopsy and elevated urinary catecholamine levels. An abdominal CT scan may also be used as a diagnostic study.[3] Once neuroblastoma is diagnosed, staging of the disease is determined by the patient's age, the location of the tumor, and the extent of tumor spread.[44]

Treatment

The NP should refer the patient to a pediatric oncologist for treatment. Surgery is used to treat low-stage neuroblastoma. More advanced stages are treated with multiple-agent chemotherapy and surgery.[47]

Hepatitis

Overview

Hepatitis is an inflammation of the liver that results in liver dysfunction.[48] Manifestation of symptoms can range anywhere from mild and self-limiting to profound and life-threatening. Hepatitis may be caused by a variety of viral subtypes; in pediatric patients, the most common subtypes are A, B, and C.[49]

The hepatitis A virus is an enteral virus transmitted via the oral-fecal route. The mortality rate of this condition is very low, and almost all patients recover completely.[50] Common sources of the hepatitis A virus are contaminated water and food, particularly shellfish.[51] Symptoms of hepatitis A typically manifest 2–6 weeks after infection, but patients' blood and stool are infectious 2 weeks before symptoms appear and 1 week after the onset of clinical illness.[52] Because many patients are asymptomatic, infections frequently go unnoticed or unreported.[52]

The hepatitis B virus is found in blood and all body fluids. The virus has an incubation period of 30–180 days.[54] Hepatitis B may be transmitted perinatally or via blood or sexual activity.[55] Hepatitis A and B share similar clinical features, but onset tends to be more insidious in cases of hepatitis B. Although the risk of fulminant hepatitis B is less than 1%, the mortality rate is high when it does occur.[56,57]

Hepatitis C is traditionally associated with blood transfusions; however, in the United States, donated blood is now screened for the disease.[58] The virus is most commonly transmitted through intravenous drug use.[59] Hepatitis C may also be transmitted through sexual intercourse with an infected person, but the risk of sexual transmission is lower than that of intravenous drug use transmission.[60] The incubation period of hepatitis C is variable and ranges from 4 to 12 weeks.[59]

Presentation

Hepatitis presents with different signs and symptoms in its pre-icteric and icteric states. Signs and symptoms of the pre-icteric phase include malaise, anorexia, fever, nausea, and vomiting.[59] The icteric phase, characterized by jaundice, also features weight loss, itching, right upper quadrant abdominal pain, mild splenomegaly, clay-colored stool, and dark urine.[61]

Workup

Depending on the type of hepatitis, diagnostics may include a CBC, urinalysis, and serology tests. Both alanine aminotransferase (ALT) and aspartate aminotransferase (AST) levels increase prior to the onset of jaundice and decrease after jaundice presents. If ALT and AST levels indicate acute viral hepatitis, a prothrombin time test may be used, with slightly elevated results further indicating the disease. Urinalysis may reveal bilirubinuria and proteinuria, with urinary bilirubin typically preceding jaundice.[62]

Once the likelihood of hepatitis has been established, serology is the primary means of isolating the particular strain. Patients with acute hepatitis A will present with immunoglobulin M (IgM) hepatitis A antibodies (anti-HAV), whereas the presence of immunoglobulin G (IgG) anti-HAV will indicate a patient who has recovered from hepatitis A. Acute hepatitis B is indicated by hepatitis B virus surface antigen (HBsAg), hepatitis B e antigen (HBeAg), antibodies to the hepatitis B c antigen (anti-HBc), and IgM. If IgG and antibodies to HBeAg present alongside HBsAg, the patient has chronic hepatitis B; if anti-HBc and antibodies to HBsAg are present, the patient has likely recovered from hepatitis B. Both acute and chronic cases of hepatitis C will show hepatitis C antibodies (anti-HCV) and hepatitis C virus RNA. A patient who has recovered from hepatitis C will typically show anti-HCV but no hepatitis C virus RNA.[62]

Table 10.2	Hepatitis Serology
Virus	**Serology**
Active hepatitis A	Anti-HAV, IgM
Recovered hepatitis A	Anti-HAV, IgG
Active hepatitis B	HBsAg, HBeAg, Anti-HBc, IgM
Chronic hepatitis B	HBsAg, Anti-HBc, Anti-Hbe, IgM, IgG
Recovered hepatitis B	Anti-HBc, Anti-HBsAg
Acute hepatitis C	Anti-HCV, HCV RNA
Chronic hepatitis C	Anti-HCV, HCV RNA

Barkley TW Jr. *Pediatric Primary Care Nurse Practitioner Certification Review/Clinical Update Continuing Education Course.* West Hollywood, CA: Barkley and Associates; 2015.

Treatment

As there is no established antiviral therapy for hepatitis, management is generally supportive. Patients should be encouraged to rest during the active phase of the condition.[59] The NP should encourage fluid intake to prevent electrolyte or fluid imbalances, with the goal of increasing the patient's fluids to 3,000–4,000 ml per day. Vitamin K is recommended for patients with a prolonged prothrombin time longer than 15 seconds.[3] Patients with hepatitis should avoid excessive protein, alcohol, and medications detoxified by the liver.[61]

Vaccines exist for hepatitis A and hepatitis B. The hepatitis A vaccine should be administered at 1 year of age, and hepatitis A immune globulin is recommended as a short-term protection for those exposed to the virus. Once a pediatric patient recovers from hepatitis A, the vaccine is typically not necessary, as anti-HAV remains in the patient's system for life.[52] Hepatitis B vaccine should be administered within 12 hours of birth, with follow-up doses at 1 and 6 months of age. Patients who have not received the hepatitis B vaccine may receive it as prophylaxis within 24 hours of exposure to the virus; however, there is little benefit to administering the vaccine to someone who has already developed hepatitis B.[63]

References

1. Mayo Clinic Staff. Viral gastroenteritis (stomach flu). Mayo Clinic web site. http://www.mayoclinic.org/diseases-conditions/viral-gastroenteritis/basics/risk-factors/con-20019350. Updated December 2, 2014. Accessed April 15, 2015.

2. Cleveland Clinic Foundation. Diseases and conditions: Gastroenteritis. Cleveland Clinic web site. http://my.clevelandclinic.org/disorders/gastroenteritis/hic_gastroenteritis.aspx. Last reviewed April 4, 2012. Accessed April 15, 2015.

3. Barkley TW Jr. *Pediatric Primary Care Nurse Practitioner Certification Review/Clinical Update Continuing Education Course*. West Hollywood, CA: Barkley and Associates; 2015.

4. Boyce TG. Overview of gastroenteritis. In: Porter RS, Kaplan JL, eds. The Merck Manual Online. http://www.merckmanuals.com/professional/gastrointestinal_disorders/gastroenteritis/overview_of_gastroenteritis.html?qt=gastroenteritis&alt=sh. Last reviewed July 2014. Accessed April 15, 2015.

5. Bonheur JL, Arya M, Tarner MA. Bacterial gastroenteritis. In: Anand BS, ed. Medscape. http://emedicine.medscape.com/article/176400-overview#showall. Updated October 2, 2014. Accessed April 15, 2015.

6. Mayo Clinic Staff. Gastroenteritis: First aid. Mayo Clinic web site. http://www.mayoclinic.com/health/first-aid-gastroenteritis/FA00030. Updated February 7, 2015. Accessed April 15, 2015.

7. Patient information: Viral gastroenteritis (the basics). In: Basow DS, ed. *UpToDate*. Waltham, MA: UpToDate; 2015. http://www.uptodate.com/contents/viral-gastroenteritis-the-basics. Accessed April 15, 2015.

8. Gastroenteritis. WedMD web site. http://www.webmd.com/digestive-disorders/gastroenteritis. Reviewed April 25, 2014. Accessed April 15, 2015.

9. Stöppler MC. The BRAT diet. In: Doerr S, ed. MedicineNet. http://www.medicinenet.com/the_brat_diet/article.htm. Reviewed February 18, 2015. Accessed April 15, 2015.

10. Minnesota Department of Health. Specific disease exclusion guidelines for childcare and preschool. http://www.health.state.mn.us/divs/idepc/dtopics/foodborne/exclusions.html. Accessed April 15, 2015.

11. Prescilla RP. Pediatric gastroenteritis. In: Steele RW, ed. Medscape. http://emedicine.medscape.com/article/964131-overview#showall. Updated September 29, 2014. Accessed April 15, 2015.

12. DiMarino MC. Gastroesophageal reflux disease (GERD). In: Porter RS, Kaplan JL, eds. The Merck Manual Online. http://www.merckmanuals.com/professional/gastrointestinal_disorders/esophageal_and_swallowing_disorders/gastroesophageal_reflux_disease_gerd.html?qt=gastroesophageal%20reflux%20disease&alt=sh. Last reviewed May 2014. Accessed April 15, 2015.

13. Schwarz SM. Pediatric gastroesophageal reflux. In: Cuffari C, ed. Medscape. http://emedicine.medscape.com/article/930029-overview#aw2aab6b2b5. Updated April 26, 2014. Accessed April 23, 2015.

14. Mayo Clinic Staff. Intussusception. Mayo Clinic web site. http://www.mayoclinic.com/health/intussusception/DS00798. Updated December 14, 2012. Accessed April 15, 2015.

15. Patti MG. Gastroesophageal reflux disease. In: Katz J, ed. Medscape. http://emedicine.medscape.com/article/176595-overview. Updated April 16, 2014. Accessed April 15, 2015.

16. Kahrilas PJ. Clinical manifestations and diagnosis of gastroesophageal reflux in adults. In: Basow DS, ed. *UpToDate*. Waltham, MA: UpToDate; 2015. http://www.uptodate.com/contents/clinical-manifestations-and-diagnosis-of-gastroesophageal-reflux-in-adults. Last updated March 11, 2015. Accessed April 15, 2015.

17. Lightdale JR. Gastroesophageal reflux: Management guidance for the pediatrician. *Pediatrics*. 2013; 131(5): e1684–e1695. doi: 10.1542/peds.2013-0421

18. Schwarz SM. Pediatric gastroesophageal reflux treatment & management. In: Cuffari C, ed. Medscape. http://emedicine.medscape.com/article/930029-treatment#aw2aab6b6b2. Updated April 26, 2014. Accessed April 23, 2015.

19. Mayo Clinic Staff. GERD. Mayo Clinic web site. http://www.mayoclinic.org/diseases-conditions/gerd/basics/treatment/con-20025201. Updated July 31, 2014. Accessed April 16, 2015.

20. Pyloric stenosis. A.D.A.M. Medical Encyclopedia. http://www.nlm.nih.gov/medlineplus/ency/article/000970.htm. Updated August 22, 2013. Accessed April 16, 2015.

21. Olivé AP, Endom EE. Infantile hypertrophic pyloric stenosis. In: Basow DS, ed. *UpToDate*. Waltham, MA: UpToDate; 2015. http://www.uptodate.com/contents/infantile-hypertrophic-pyloric-stenosis. Last updated April 10, 2015. Accessed April 16, 2015.

22. Singh J. Pediatric pyloric stenosis. In: Bechtel KA, ed. Medscape. http://emedicine.medscape.com/article/803489-overview. Updated October 9, 2014. Accessed April 16, 2015.

23. Cochran WJ. Hypertrophic pyloric stenosis. In: Porter RS, Kaplan JL, eds. The Merck Manual Online. http://www.merckmanuals.com/professional/pediatrics/gastrointestinal_disorders_in_infants/hypertrophic_pyloric_stenosis.html?qt=pyloric%20stenosis&alt=sh. Last reviewed October 2014. Accessed April 16, 2015.

24. Mayo Clinic Staff. Pyloric stenosis. Mayo Clinic web site. http://www.mayoclinic.com/health/pyloric-stenosis/DS00815/DSECTION=tests-and-diagnosis. Updated November 16, 2012. Accessed April 16, 2015.

25. Kitagawa S, Miqdady M. Intussusception in children. In: Basow DS, ed. *UpToDate*. Waltham, MA: UpToDate; 2015. http://www.uptodate.com/contents/intussusception-in-children. Last reviewed April 6, 2015. Accessed April 16, 2015.

26. Cochran WJ. Intussusception. In: Porter RS, Kaplan JL, eds. The Merck Manual Online. http://www.merckmanuals.com/professional/pediatrics/gastrointestinal_disorders_in_infants/intussusception.html?qt=intussusception&alt=sh. Last reviewed October 2014. Accessed April 16, 2015.

27. Blanco F. Intussusception. In: Cuffari C, ed. Medscape. http://emedicine.medscape.com/article/930708-overview. Updated April 22, 2014. Accessed April 16, 2015.

28. Intussusception – children. A.D.A.M. Medical Encyclopedia. http://www.nlm.nih.gov/medlineplus/ency/article/000958.htm. Updated May 14, 2014. Accessed April 16, 2015.

29. Wesson DE. Congenital aganglionic megacolon (Hirschsprung disease). In: Basow DS, ed. *UpToDate*. Waltham, MA: UpToDate; 2015. http://www.uptodate.com/contents/congenital-aganglionic-megacolon-hirschsprung-disease. Last updated January 29, 2015. Accessed April 16, 2015.

30. Mayo Clinic Staff. Hirschsprung's disease. Mayo Clinic web site. http://www.mayoclinic.com/health/hirschsprungs-disease/DS00825/DSECTION=causes. Updated March 28, 2013. Accessed April 16, 2015.

31. Cochran WJ. Hirschsprung disease. In: Porter RS, Kaplan JL, eds. The Merck Manual Online. http://www.merckmanuals.com/professional/pediatrics/congenital_gastrointestinal_anomalies/hirschsprung_disease.html?qt=megacolon&alt=sh. Last reviewed March 2013. Accessed April 16, 2015.

32. Hirschsprung's disease. A.D.A.M. Medical Encyclopedia. http://www.nlm.nih.gov/medlineplus/ency/article/001140.htm. Updated December 4, 2013. Accessed April 16, 2015.

33. Wagner JP. Hirschsprung disease. In: Katz J, ed. Medscape. http://emedicine.medscape.com/article/178493-overview. Updated May 30, 2014. Accessed April 16, 2015.

34. Craig S. Appendicitis. In: Brenner BE, ed. Medscape. http://emedicine.medscape.com/article/773895-overview#showall. Updated July 21, 2014. Accessed April 16, 2015.

35. Appendicitis. A.D.A.M. Medical Encyclopedia. http://www.ncbi.nlm.nih.gov/pubmedhealth/PMH0001302. Accessed April 16, 2015.

36. Ansari P. Appendicitis. In: Porter RS, Kaplan JL, eds. The Merck Manual Online. http://www.merckmanuals.com/professional/gastrointestinal_disorders/acute_abdomen_and_surgical_gastroenterology/appendicitis.html. Last reviewed June 2014. Accessed April 16, 2015.

37. Wesson DE. Acute appendicitis in children: Clinical manifestations and diagnosis. In: Basow DS, ed. *UpToDate*. Waltham, MA: UpToDate; 2015. http://www.uptodate.com/contents/acute-appendicitis-in-children-clinical-manifestations-and-diagnosis. Last updated December 4, 2014. Accessed April 16, 2015.

38. Wesson DE. Acute appendicitis in children: Management. In: Basow DS, ed. *UpToDate*. Waltham, MA: UpToDate; 2015. http://www.uptodate.com/contents/acute-appendicitis-in-children-management?source=-search_result&search=appendicitis+in+children&selectedTitle=2~150. Last updated February 6, 2015. Accessed April 24, 2015.

39. Ruiz AR Jr. Malabsorption syndromes. In: Porter RS, Kaplan JL, eds. The Merck Manual Online. http://www.merckmanuals.com/professional/gastrointestinal_disorders/malabsorption_syndromes/overview_of_malabsorption.html?qt=malabsorption&alt=sh. Last reviewed May 2014. Accessed April 16, 2015.

40. Kerr M. Malabsorption syndrome. Healthline web site. http://www.healthline.com/health/malabsorption. Published June 14, 2012. Accessed April 16, 2015.

41. Goebel SU. Malabsorption. In: Katz J, ed. Medscape. http://emedicine.medscape.com/article/180785-clinical#showall. Updated December 16, 2014. Accessed April 16, 2015.

42. Malabsorption. A.D.A.M. Medical Encyclopedia. http://www.nlm.nih.gov/medlineplus/ency/article/000299.htm. Updated August 10, 2012. Accessed April 16, 2015.

43. Mason JB, Milovic V. Overview of the treatment of malabsorption. In: Basow DS, ed. *UpToDate*. Waltham, MA: UpToDate; 2015. http://www.uptodate.com/contents/overview-of-the-treatment-of-malabsorption. Last updated April 14, 2014. Accessed April 16, 2015.

44. Neuroblastoma. A.D.A.M. Medical Encyclopedia. http://www.nlm.nih.gov/medlineplus/ency/article/001408.htm. Updated October 30, 2013. Accessed April 16, 2015.

45. United States Department of Health and Human Services, National Institutes of Health, National Cancer Institute. Neuroblastoma treatment. http://www.cancer.gov/cancertopics/pdq/treatment/neuroblastoma/HealthProfessional/page1. Updated December 15, 2014. Accessed April 16, 2015.

46. Shohet JM, Nuchtern JG. Clinical presentation, diagnosis, and staging evaluation of neuroblastoma. In: Basow DS, ed. *UpToDate*. Waltham, MA: UpToDate; 2015. http://www.uptodate.com/contents/clinical-presentation-diagnosis-and-staging-evaluation-of-neuroblastoma. Last updated December 30, 2013. Accessed April 17, 2015.

47. Joyner BD. Neuroblastoma. In: Kopell BH, ed. Medscape. http://emedicine.medscape.com/article/439263-overview#showall. Updated March 27, 2015. Accessed April 17, 2015.

48. Rutherford AE. Overview of hepatitis. In: Porter RS, Kaplan JL, eds. The Merck Manual Online. http://www.merckmanuals.com/professional/hepatic_and_biliary_disorders/hepatitis/overview_of_hepatitis.html?qt=hepatitis&alt=sh. Last reviewed February 2014. Accessed April 17, 2015.

49. Ben Joseph EP. Hepatitis. KidsHealth web site. http://kidshealth.org/teen/sexual_health/stds/hepatitis.html#. Reviewed February 2014. Accessed April 17, 2015.

50. United States Department of Health and Human Services, Centers for Disease Control and Prevention. Hepatitis A FAQs for the public. http://www.cdc.gov/hepatitis/A/aFAQ.htm#overview. Last updated March 6, 2015. Accessed April 17, 2015.

51. Bennett NJ, Domachowske J. Pediatric hepatitis A. In: Steele RW, ed. Medscape. http://emedicine.medscape.com/article/964575-overview#showall. Updated March 3, 2014. Accessed April 17, 2015.

52. United States Department of Health and Human Services, Centers for Disease Control and Prevention. Hepatitis A information for health professionals. http://www.cdc.gov/hepatitis/HAV/. Updated April 14, 2014. Accessed April 24, 2015.

53. Hepatitis A. A.D.A.M. Medical Encyclopedia. http://www.nlm.nih.gov/medlineplus/ency/article/000278.htm. Updated October 13, 2013. Accessed April 17, 2015.

54. World Health Organization. Hepatitis B. World Health Organization web site. http://www.who.int/mediacentre/factsheets/fs204/en. Updated March 2015. Accessed April 17, 2015.

55. United States Department of Health and Human Services, Centers for Disease Control and Prevention. Hepatitis B FAQs for the public. http://www.cdc.gov/hepatitis/b/bFAQ.htm#overview. Last updated March 6, 2015. Accessed April 17, 2015.

56. Rapti IN, Hadziyannis SJ. Chronic hepatitis B infection: Treatment of special populations: HBV prophylaxis following liver transplantation. http://www.medscape.org/viewarticle/743845_6. Updated June 8, 2011. Accessed April 17, 2015.

57. Government of Canada, Canadian Centre for Occupational Health and Safety. Hepatitis B. http://www.ccohs.ca/oshanswers/diseases/hepatitis_b.html. Last updated August 28 ,2013. Accessed April 17, 2015.

58. United States Department of Health and Human Services, Centers for Disease Control and Prevention. Hepatitis C information for the public. http://www.cdc.gov/hepatitis/C/index.htm. Updated May 6, 2013. Accessed April 24, 2015.

59. United States Department of Health and Human Services, Centers for Disease Control and Prevention. The ABCs of hepatitis. http://www.cdc.gov/hepatitis/resources/professionals/pdfs/abctable.pdf. Updated 2014. Accessed April 17, 2015.

60. World Health Organization. Hepatitis C. World Health Organization web site. http://www.who.int/mediacentre/factsheets/fs164/en. Updated April 2014. Accessed April 17, 2015.

61. Hepatitis C. A.D.A.M. Medical Encyclopedia. http://www.nlm.nih.gov/medlineplus/ency/article/000284.htm. Updated October 13, 2013. Accessed April 18, 2015.

62. Rutherford AE. Acute viral hepatitis. In: Porter RS, Kaplan JL, eds. The Merck Manual Online Web site. http://www.merckmanuals.com/professional/hepatic-and-biliary-disorders/hepatitis/acute-viral-hepatitis. Last reviewed February 2014. Accessed April 24, 2015.

63. United States Department of Health and Human Services, Centers for Disease Control and Prevention. Hepatitis B FAQs for health professionals. http://www.cdc.gov/hepatitis/HBV/HBVfaq.htm. Last updated March 6, 2015. Accessed April 18, 2015.

Chapter 11

Dermatological Disorders

QUESTIONS

1. You are examining Ryan, a 17-year-old male, and note inflamed papules on his face and upper trunk. He admits to using steroids in order to keep up with his teammates in baseball; these steroids appear to have exacerbated the symptoms. Of the following, which dermatological disorder is the most likely diagnosis?

   a. Acne

   b. Psoriasis

   c. Atopic dermatitis

   d. Pityriasis rosea

2. Which of these dermatological disorders is most commonly associated with elevated serum immunoglobulin E (IgE) levels?

   a. Atopic dermatitis

   b. Acne

   c. Pityriasis rosea

   d. Varicella zoster virus

3. Which of these treatments is primarily recommended for management of tinea capitis?

   a. Oral acyclovir

   b. Aluminum subacetate solution

   c. Neem shampoo

   d. Griseofulvin

4. The most common findings of impetigo include all of the following choices <u>except</u>:

   a. Pain

   b. Pruritic rash

   c. Honey-crusting lesions

   d. Regional lymphadenopathy

5. A 5-month-old infant's parent describes him as being recently irritable and constantly rubbing at his skin. Your examination reveals red-brown vesiculopapular lesions on his soles. Which drug would be the best choice to manage the most likely condition?

   a. Lindane lotion (Kwell)

   b. Calamine with topical diphenhydramine (Ivarest)

   c. Permethrin (Nix) 5% rinse

   d. Griseofulvin (Grifulvin V)

6. An infant presents to the clinic with an angry red diaper rash with satellite lesions. A potassium hydroxide preparation used to examine the lesion is negative. Your treatment would consist of which of these methods?

   a. Hydrocortisone 1% cream

   b. Zinc oxide ointment

   c. Acyclovir 5% cream

   d. Nystatin 100,000 units/gram

7. A 14-year-old patient presents to your clinic with complaints of stiff joints and pain that starts in her shoulders before traveling down her arms. She reports that, following a recent nature hike, she found a tick on her leg. Within a few days, a lesion that "looks like a bull's eye" had developed at the tick site. She also tells you that she has been experiencing severe headaches, and that her heart occasionally "races like a drum." Which stage of the most likely diagnosis is the patient experiencing?

   a. Stage 1

   b. Stage 2

   c. Stage 3

   d. Stage 4

8. Of the following, which viral infection most commonly presents with Koplik spots?

   a. Rubeola

   b. Roseola infantum

   c. Rubella

   d. Lyme disease

9. A 5-year-old patient is brought to your clinic with extensive second-degree burns. The burns cover the entirety of the back of his head but do not extend any further than that. Approximately how much of his body has been burned?

   a. Approximately 6%

   b. Approximately 7%

   c. Approximately 9%

   d. Approximately 10%

10. While assessing a patient during a physical, you find a small elevated area on her lower back. The area is a firm lesion of approximately 1.5 cm; it feels smooth to the touch, is not filled with fluid, and does not appear to extend below the epidermis. This morphology best describes which type of lesion?

    a. Wheal

    b. Tumor

    c. Cyst

    d. Nodule

RATIONALES

1. a

Because the patient presents with papules and cysts on his face and upper trunk and has a history of steroid use, he is most likely experiencing acne. Psoriasis typically presents as lesions with red, sharply defined plaques with silvery scales, not comedones or pustules, and commonly occurs due to genetic predisposition, not steroid use. Atopic dermatitis often involves dry scaly skin rather than comedones or papules, and commonly presents with intense pruritus along the face, neck, trunk, wrists, hands, and antecubital and popliteal folds. Lastly, although pityriasis rosea also typically manifests on the upper trunk, it usually manifests as a pruritic rash, not comedones and cysts, and is often treated with, not exacerbated by, steroids.

2. a

Atopic dermatitis commonly presents with elevated serum immunoglobulin E (IgE) and eosinophilia. Allergic rhinitis, asthma, and parasitic diseases are also typically associated with elevated IgE, but pityriasis rosea, acne, or varicella zoster virus are not.

3. d

Primary treatment for tinea capitis often utilizes griseofulvin, given in doses of 20 mg/kg/day for 6 weeks. Oral acyclovir is a common primary treatment for the varicella zoster virus, not tinea capitis. Aluminum subacetate solution often treats both tinea manuum and pedis. Neem shampoo is a common treatment for scabies.

4. b

Pruritic rash is not a standard sign or symptom of impetigo, and is more commonly associated with pityriasis rosea. Honey-crusting lesions are a classic symptom of impetigo, and the bacterial infection of the skin often produces pain and regional lymphadenopathy.

5. c

Permethrin (Nix) 5% rinse is a common primary treatment for scabies, which is indicated by the infant's irritability, itching, and red-brown vesiculopapular lesions on his soles. Lindane lotion is also a common treatment of choice for scabies; however, as the patient in the scenario is younger than 6 months old, it should be avoided, as lindane is often neurotoxic to this population and can cause seizures or death. As scabies is easily spread among family members, it is important to treat the household in order to reduce the incidence of reacquisition and retreatment. Calamine with a topical antihistamine, such as diphenhydramine, may relieve the patient's pruritus, but it will not typically affect the mites that cause scabies. Griseofulvin is meant to remedy fungal, not parasitic, skin infections.

6. a

Irritant diaper dermatitis presenting with satellite lesions is typically treated with 1% hydrocortisone cream in order to reduce inflammation. Nystatin may be called for if secondary *Candida albicans* infection is suspected; however, as the patient's potassium hydroxide preparation turned up negative for the fungus, this medication is not necessarily indicated. Zinc oxide ointment functions as a barrier emollient and is typically recommended for more mild cases of irritant diaper dermatitis. Acyclovir cream is commonly reserved for viral lesions stemming from the herpes simplex virus or other viral skin infections.

7. b

Headache, stiff joints, migratory pains, and cardiac irregularities all typically characterize Stage 2 of Lyme disease, as would aseptic meningitis, Bell's palsy, and peripheral neuropathy. Although muscle and joint pain may present in Stage 1, this stage is more commonly characterized by flu-like symptoms, fatigue, and erythema migrans. Stage 3 is also often characterized by pain, stiffness, and swelling in the joints, but these symptoms would typically evolve into clear manifestations of arthritis, usually presenting in the knees. Furthermore, other symptoms such as acrodermatitis chronicum atrophicans, characterized by bluish-red discoloring of the distal extremity with edema, or subacute encephalopathy may produce in Stage 3. There is no Stage 4 for Lyme disease.

8. a

Rubeola (measles) commonly presents with Koplik spots, which are small, white, granular spots surrounded by red rings found inside the oro-pharynx. Small, pink, and flat to raised bumps often appear in roseola infantum (Sixth disease), rather than white spots. Rubella typically presents with a fine, erythematous maculopapular rash that first manifests on the face before spreading to the trunk and extremities. Lyme disease is characterized by erythema migrans in a distinctive "bulls-eye" pattern, not Koplik spots.

9. b

For a 5-year-old child, the back of the head is commonly considered 7% of the surface area of the skin. The surface area of a child's head, thighs, and legs changes during early development, and thus has varying values based on age. The back of the head would typically be considered 10% of total skin surface area in a newborn, 9% in a 1-year-old, and 6% in a 10-year-old.

10. d

Nodules are classified as elevated, firm lesions that extend beyond 1 cm. Although tumors are also firm and elevated, they commonly take on the appearance of lumps, which are masses of indefinite size, rather than lesions, which are more circumscribed. A wheal typically appears both above the surface of the skin and extends below the epidermis; many times, it is a sign of an allergic reaction. A cyst is often filled with either air, fluid, or semi-solid material, such as in the case of a pilonidal cyst.

DISCUSSION

Burns

Overview

Burns are traumatic injuries to the skin and underlying tissues caused by exposure to or contact with thermal or non-thermal sources.

Burn injuries can be thermal, chemical, electrical, or radiological.[1,2]

Burn injuries are categorized as first-degree, second-degree, third-degree, and fourth-degree burns. Healing time depends on the depth and size of the burn area, care given, and a timely treatment.

Presentation

Superficial or first-degree burns are burns that affect only the epidermis. Typically, the site of injury is dry and red, with later development of moisture. These injuries are painful and include severe sunburns and burns caused by scalding hot water.[3]

Partial-thickness or second-degree burns extend beyond the epidermis. These burns may be described as superficial or deep, and may present with a variety of findings, such as moist wounds, blisters, and pain, among others.[3,4]

Full-thickness or third-degree burns extend beyond the dermis to the underlying subcutaneous tissues. Third-degree burns result in eschar, leaving a dry, hard, leathery surface. The site may be black, pearly, or red and waxy. As with partial-thickness burns, the skin appears flat and dehydrated, and may be peeled with ease. The patient feels no pain due to destruction of pain sensors.[3,4]

Fourth-degree burns are full-thickness burns affecting the deeper tissues. These types of burns involve total destruction of the skin, subcutaneous tissue, tendons, muscle, and/or bone, and the damaged areas are typically black and charred in appearance.[2,3,4]

Workup (see figures 11.1–11.2 and table 11.1)

Burns to certain parts of the body warrant special consideration.[5] Burns to the eyes should be immediately assessed by an ophthalmologist. Burns to the face may be accompanied by inhalation injury and facial edema, which may affect the airway. Burns to the genitalia and surrounding region (i.e., the perineum) require immediate hospitalization.

Assessing the extent of a burn injury, which is expressed as a percentage of the total body surface area (TBSA), is necessary to determine severity, estimate fluid resuscitation requirements, and assess whether or not the patient should be transported to emergency care. The TBSA is calculated by using either the "Rule of Nines" or the Lund and Browder Chart. Inhalation injuries can increase the TBSA estimate.

The "Rule of Nines" is an estimation of TBSA measured in multiples of 9, but is calculated differently for pediatric patients than in adult patients.[6] In pediatrics, a larger

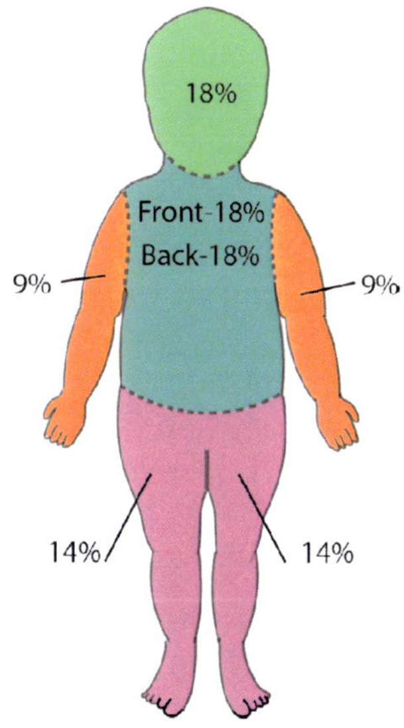

Figure 11.1. Rule of Nines diagram for a pediatric patient

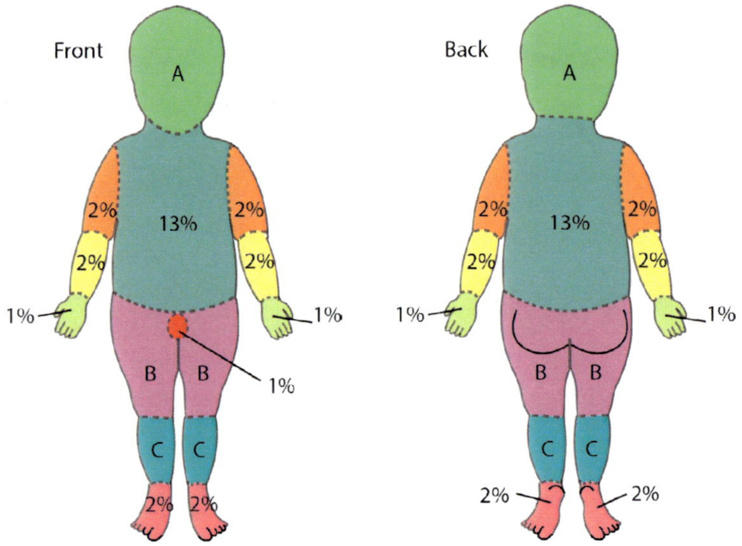

Figure 11.2. Lund and Browder diagram for pediatric patients

Table 11.1	Relative Percentage of Body Surface Area for Lund and Browder Chart			
Area	**Age 0**	**1 year**	**5 years**	**10 years**
A=1/2 of head	10%	9%	7%	6%
B=1/2 of one thigh	3%	3%	4%	5%
C=1/2 of one leg	2%	3%	3%	3%

Used with permission from Barkley TW Jr. *Adult-Gerontology Primary Care Nurse Practitioner Certification Review/Clinical Update Continuing Education Course.* West Hollywood, CA: Barkley and Associates; 2015.

percentage is assigned to the surface area of the head, whereas the legs are assigned a smaller percentage. For example, the TBSA of an infant's head ranges from 18% to 20% and the legs range from 13% to 14% for each leg—half the percentage is attributed to the anterior and posterior surface areas. For adults, the head and neck are 9%, and each leg equals 18% of TBSA.[7]

The Lund and Browder chart is the preferred method in most burn units, as it correlates TBSA with age-related proportions, while also further subdividing the areas of the body and taking the patient's age and TBSA into account.[8]

Treatment

As the first 6 hours following a burn injury are critical, children with severe burns should be transported to the emergency department as soon as possible. For all burns, patients should be assessed for the ABCs—airway, breathing, and circulation—and for signs that warrant prophylactic intubation (e.g., singed nares or eyebrows, soot and/or black mucous in nares or mouth).[5] In minor burns, all burnt clothing should be removed, and the burn should be immersed in cool, not iced, water for 30 minutes to prevent further damage and reduce pain. Once this is done, a clean wrap should be applied to the wound. The burn should not be covered with lotion, butter, or other products.

According to guidelines established by the American College of Surgeons, pediatric patients with severe and major burns should be referred to a burn center for treatment and recovery.[11] This includes patients with partial-thickness burns covering more than 10% of the TBSA, burns that involve areas especially prone to damage (e.g., face, hands, feet, genitalia, perineum, major joints), full-thickness burns, electrical or chemical burns, inhalation injury, burn injuries in patients with preexisting conditions that may complicate management, and burns with concomitant trauma where the burn poses the highest risk of mortality. Pediatric patients should also be referred to a burn center if the hospital lacks qualified personnel or equipment for the care of children, or if the patient requires special social, emotional, or rehabilitative intervention.[11]

Evaluation of Skin Disorders

Overview

The systematic approach to evaluating skin disorders consists of identifying the morphology, configuration, and distribution of lesions. A macule is a flat discoloration on the surface of the skin.[12] A patch is a flat discoloration that appears as a collection of multiple, tiny pigment changes. Papules are elevated, firm skin lesions smaller than 1 cm in diameter. A nodule is an elevated, firm lesion greater than 1 cm in diameter.[13] A tumor is a firm, elevated mass of tissue. Wheals, which are caused by either a contact or systemic allergic reaction, are raised above the skin surface and extend slightly below the epidermis.[14] Plaques are scaly, elevated lesions, which are classically associated with psoriasis. Vesicles are lesions smaller than 1 cm that are filled with serous fluid; bullae are serous fluid-filled vesicles greater than 1 cm in diameter.[15] A pustule is a small pus-filled lesion smaller than 1 cm in diameter, whereas an abscess is a pus-filled lesion greater than 1 cm in diameter.[16] Lastly, cysts are large, raised lesions filled with serous fluid, blood, and/or pus.[17]

Presentation

Skin lesions are grouped into two categories: primary and secondary. Primary lesions are lesions that develop on previously unaltered skin as a result of disease, trauma, or insult. Secondary lesions result from changes over time to primary lesions or may develop as a consequence of insult to the lesion (e.g., infection, scratching, etc.).[18] Furthermore, solitary or discrete lesions present as individual or distinct lesions that remain separate. Grouped lesions form a linear cluster, whereas confluent lesions run together.[18] Linear lesions may resemble scratches, streaks, lines, or stripes. Annular lesions present in a circular pattern, beginning in the center and spreading to the periphery. In some patients, annular lesions may merge to form polycyclic lesions.[19] Usually, lesions develop on the face, trunk, upper extremities, groin, feet, axilla, and dermatomal regions.

Acne

Overview

Acne vulgaris is a common skin disorder characterized by the formation of comedones, papules, pustules, and cysts. The onset is both more common and more severe in males.[20] Although exact causes of acne are unknown, androgens play a role in genetically predisposed individuals.[21] Acne is also exacerbated by the use of steroids and anticonvulsants.[22]

Presentation (see figure 11.3)

Patients with acne present with comedones on the face and upper trunk. Comedones can be either open or closed.[23] Open comedones, also known as blackheads, are openings in the skin capped with blackened skin debris. Closed comedones, also known as whiteheads, are obstructed openings capped with white skin debris. Depending on the severity of acne, papules, pustules, nodules, cysts, or a combination of the four may also present. More severe acne lesions may result in atrophic (i.e., depressed) or hypertrophic scars.[24] In adolescents, acne may be exacerbated by hormonal fluctuations related to menses.[25]

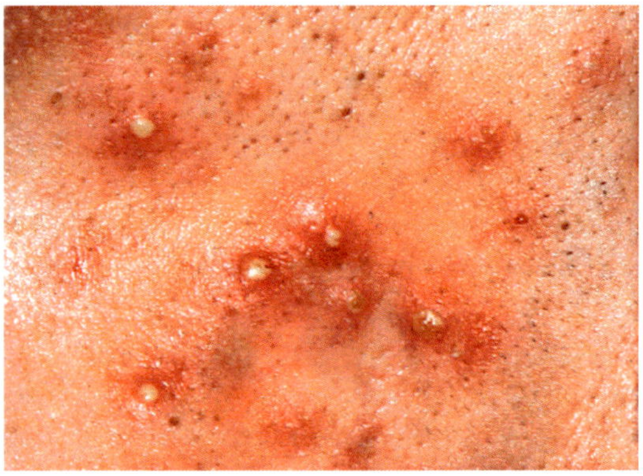

Figure 11.3. Acne

Workup

The diagnosis of acne is based on clinical appearance.[26]

Treatment

Patients with acne should first be encouraged to wash their face several times per day. Non-pharmacologic management of acne focuses on avoidance of topical, oil-based products and use of oil-free mild soaps, cleansers, and moisturizers. Pharmacologic management options include salicylic acid preparations and topical antibiotics such as erythromycin and clindamycin.[27] For patients with mild acne, topical treatment with benzoyl peroxide (2.5%–10%) is first recommended. If not effective, others agents may be considered, such as retinoic acid (0.025%–0.1%) cream or gel. Retinoic acid should be prescribed with caution in females, as it is classified as a Pregnancy Category C drug.[28] Topical tretinoin is also highly effective in the treatment of acne.[29]

Moderate and severe pustular acne often requires topical treatments with systemic antibiotics, such as doxycycline (Vibramycin), erythromycin (Erythrocin), or minocycline (Minocin).[30] Patients with severe acne that does not respond to antibiotics should be referred to a dermatologist.

Fungal Infections

Overview

The various types of fungal infections are distinguished by the causal species of fungi and the location of affected areas of the body. Fungal infections are classified based on location on the body.[31]

Many fungal infections in pediatric patients are caused by dermatophytes, including tinea capitis, located on the scalp; tinea corporis, or ringworm (usually the legs, arms, and trunk), tinea cruris (groin), tinea pedis (feet), and tinea versicolor (trunk and legs).[32,33] Tinea pedis may be accompanied by tinea manuum (surfaces of the palms).[34]

Presentation

Some fungal infections, such as tinea capitis, may be asymptomatic at first; eventually, however, tinea capitis presents with papules, pruritus, and detachment of hair from the scalp. Pruritus is common, but may be more severe in tinea cruris and tinea pedis.[35] Tinea corporis is characterized by erythematous rings.[36] Tinea versicolor is distinguished by the appearance of solitary areas of hypopigmented or hyperpigmented macules.[34,37]

Workup

The diagnosis of fungal infections is determined via a clinical examination.[38] A potassium hydroxide (KOH) microscopy may also be necessary; on a KOH preparation, fungal infections are distinguished by a "spaghetti and meatballs" pattern.[39,40]

Treatment

Tinea capitis is treated with antifungal shampoo, but may require systemic management. The traditional choice for systemic treatment is griseofulvin (Gris-PEG), 20–25 mg/kg/day for approximately six weeks. Newer therapeutic options with shorter courses of treatment include oral terbinafine, itraconazole, and fluconazole.[41]

Like most other fungal infections, tinea corporis responds well to topical antifungals, including miconazole 2% and ketoconazole 2%.[42] Griseofulvin may be ordered for severe cases. Terbinafine cream is effective in more than 80% of all cases when prescribed twice a day for 7 days.[43]

The treatment regimen for tinea manuum and tinea pedis depends on the stage of infection. In the macerated stage of infection, aluminum subacetate solution is used for 20 minutes twice a day.[44] The dry, scaly stage is treated with topical antifungals.

The standard treatment for tinea versicolor is selenium sulfide for 5–15 minutes daily over 7 days. Itraconazole, given at 200 mg every day by mouth, may serve as an alternative treatment in patients 3 years of age or older.[40]

Varicella Zoster Virus (Chickenpox)

Overview

Varicella zoster is an acute, contagious disease caused by primary infection of the varicella zoster virus, transmitted through direct contact with lesions.[45] Patients are contagious 48 hours before the outbreak of the disease, with contagion persisting until lesions have crusted over.[46] Varicella zoster is most common in children between 5 and 10 years of age.[47]

Presentation (see figure 11.4)

Varicella zoster is characterized by the outbreak of erythematous macules and subsequent development of papules.[48] In most cases, vesicles initially appear on the trunk before developing on the scalp and face, accompanied by intense pruritus, low-grade fever, and generalized lymphadenopathy.[48]

Workup

Typically, a clinical examination is sufficient to diagnose varicella zoster.[49] Lab tests may be required in cases with immunocompromised patients or atypical lesions.[49]

Treatment

Varicella zoster may be prevented with varicella vaccine; the initial dose is administered to infants at 12–15 months of age, followed by a second dose at 4–6 years of age.[50] The standard treatment for varicella zoster is oral acyclovir, 20 mg/kg every 6 hours for 5 days, not to exceed 800 mg; this dosage may need to be adjusted based on age, weight, and immunocompetence.[51] Supportive treatment may include antihistamine and calamine (Caladryl) for pruritus, as well as acetaminophen for fever.[52,53] Aspirin should be avoided, however, as children given acetylsalicylic acid during cases of varicella zoster may develop Reye's syndrome.

Molluscum Contagiosum

Overview

Molluscum contagiosum is a benign viral skin infection, causing small pearly or flesh-colored papules that may disappear within 6–12 months without treatment.[54]

Presentation (see figure 11.5)

Patients with molluscum contagiosum present with pruritus and very small, firm, pink or flesh-colored discrete papules.[55] Lesions develop on the face, axillae, antecubital fossa, trunk, and extremities. Although not easily treated, these lesions frequently disappear over the course of a few months.[56,57,58]

Workup

The diagnosis of molluscum contagiosum can be determined based on clinical presentation.[59]

Treatment

Because molluscum contagiosum is self-limiting, treatment may not be necessary. Curettage is a useful treatment but should

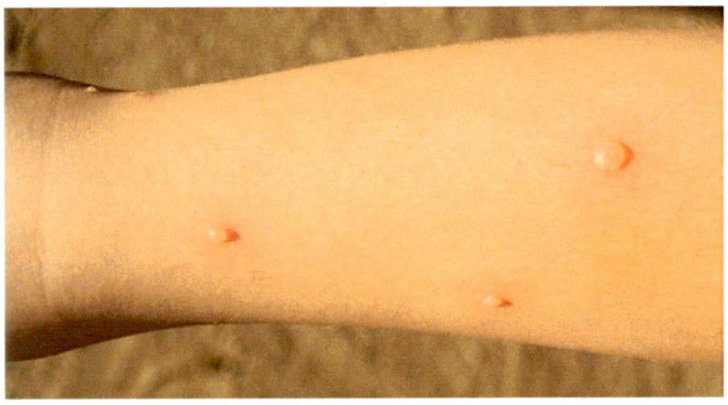

Figure 11.4. Chickenpox

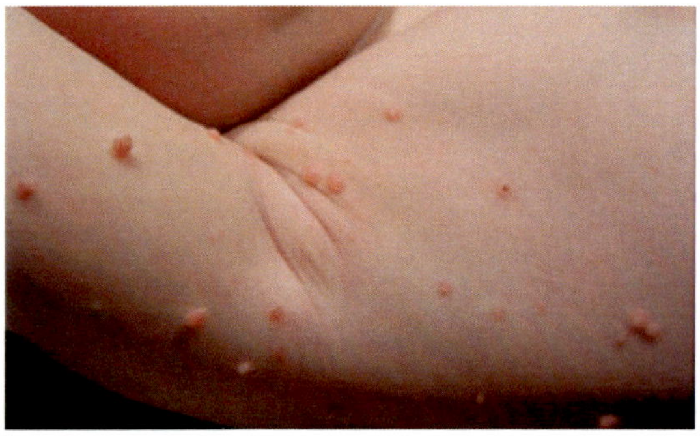

Figure 11.5. Molluscum contagiosum

not be used on sensitive areas due to risk of scarring.[12]

Molluscum contagiosum is treated with agents such as tretinoin, salicylic acid, liquid nitrogen, trichloroacetic acid, podofilox, silver nitrate, or electrocautery.[60,61] Cantharidin 0.7% may be applied to individual lesions and covered with clear tape.[62] Cantharidin should, however, be avoided on facial lesions since it may cause blistering within 24 hours.

Scratching and touching lesions should be avoided to prevent further spread.[63]

Atopic Dermatitis (Eczema)

Overview

Atopic dermatitis, also known as eczema, is a chronic skin condition characterized by intense pruritus, as well as plaques with a typical pattern of distribution and periods of remission and exacerbation. In infants and young children, plaques commonly appear on facial and extensor surfaces. This condition is particularly sensitive to low humidity and often worsens in the winter.[64]

Presentation (see figure 11.6)

Patients with atopic dermatitis have plaques that may appear along the face, neck, trunk, wrists, and/or antecubital and popliteal folds.[65] These patches are often inflamed or scabbed and exhibit diffuse erythema and scaling, followed by dry, leathery lichenification. Acute flare-ups show red, shiny, or thickened patches.[66]

Workup

The patient's personal or family history of asthma, allergic rhinitis, atopic dermatitis, and predisposition to skin infections should be considered during the diagnostic evaluation. Laboratory tests may reveal eosinophilia and elevated serum immunoglobulin E levels.[67] A radioallergosorbent (RAST) test or allergy tests may be used to determine the causative allergen.[44]

Treatment

Treatment of eczema focuses on managing dry skin. Patients should blot themselves dry after every bath or shower prior to applying medication or moisturizing cream to the area.[68]

Topical steroids, such as hydrocortisone cream, fluocinonide cream 0.05%, desonide, and triamcinolone 0.1%, among others, may be thinly applied 2–4 times daily and should only be used for exacerbations.[69,70] Systemic steroids such as prednisone should only be used in extremely severe cases. For acute weeping lesions that are moist, either saline, aluminum subacetate solution, or colloidal oatmeal baths (e.g., Aveeno) are beneficial. Ultraviolet therapy may also see use, and immune modulators may be used in immunocompetent patients over the age of 2 years with severe atopic dermatitis.[71]

Allergic Contact Dermatitis

Overview

Allergic contact dermatitis is a condition characterized by inflammation that results from direct skin contact with chemicals or allergens.[72]

Presentation

A variety of findings, including redness, pruritus, and scabbing, among others, are seen in patients with allergic contact dermatitis. The acute phase is characterized by small vesicles and oozing, encrusted lesions. The chronic phase involves scaling, erythema, and thickened, lichenified skin.[71] Affected areas may appear inflamed and swollen.

Workup

Diagnosis of allergic contact dermatitis is made by clinical evaluation and, sometimes, by patch testing.[73]

Treatment

Management depends on the severity of findings and the offending agent. Supportive treatment consists of compresses applied locally. Patients should avoid scrubbing the affected area with soap and water. High potency topical steroids applied locally are considered first-line treatment for localized allergic contact dermatitis.[74] If severe, management may incorporate prednisone, 60 mg daily on a 14-day tapered course for older children and adolescents. Younger children should be dosed based on weight.[75] Antihistamines may also be used.

Irritant (Diaper) Dermatitis

Overview

Diaper dermatitis is a common skin irritation of the genital-perianal region in infants, caused by exposure to chemical irritants or prolonged contact with urine or feces. This exposure can lead to infection by bacteria or *Candida albicans*.[76] Irritant dermatitis occurs at some time in 95% of all infants, with the incidence peaking at 9–12 months.[77]

Presentation (see figure 11.7)

A fiery red rash with papules, vesicles, crusts, and ulcerations is common in cases of irritant diaper dermatitis.[78]

Workup

The diagnosis for irritant diaper dermatitis is made clinically, with a focus on ruling out other conditions. A KOH test may be used to confirm the presence of a *Candida* infection.[78]

Treatment

In mild cases, barrier emollients improve skin condition.[79] When erythema and papules are present, 1% hydrocortisone is recommended to reduce skin inflammation.[80]

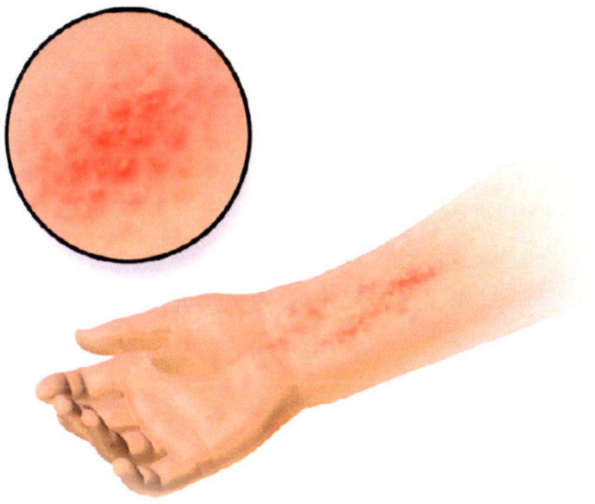

Figure 11.6. Allergic contact dermatitis

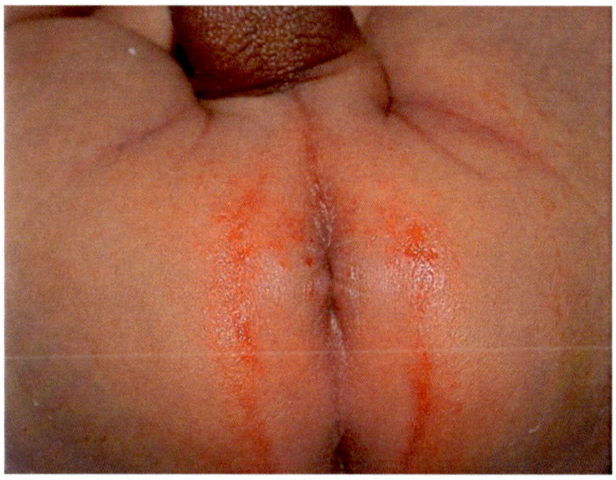

Figure 11.7. Irritant diaper dermatitis

Burow's (Domeboro) compresses may be used to relieve severe erythema and vesicles.[77]

Cases with secondary bacterial or fungal infection require topical antibiotics or antifungal cream, respectively.[42] The NP should also educate parents about preventive measures, such as allowing the diaper area to be open to air several times daily.[77]

Psoriasis

Overview

Psoriasis is a benign hyperproliferative inflammatory skin disease that affects the protective function of the epidermis. The disorder may be either acute or chronic, and may be associated with more serious diseases. The development of psoriasis is dependent upon a genetic predisposition affecting approximately 2%–3% percent of the population, although environmental and immunologic factors may play a role.[81,82]

In most cases of psoriasis, normal maturation of the skin cells cannot take place, keratinization is faulty, the epidermis is thickened, and immature nucleated cells are seen on the stratum corneum (i.e., the horny layer).[83]

Presentation

Some patients may present with no more than pruritus, whereas others experience red, sharply defined plaques with silvery scales.[84] Lesions commonly develop on the scalp, elbows, knees, palms, soles, and nails.[85] Fine pitting of the nails and separation of the nail plate from the bed are additional findings commonly noted in psoriasis.[86] Pink or red lines may be seen in the intergluteal fold. Auspitz sign is another common finding, consisting of pinpoint bleeding spots that appear when scales are removed.[87]

Workup

Psoriasis can be clinically diagnosed through a physical exam and medical history. In rare cases, skin biopsy may be used to determine the exact type of psoriasis.[88]

Treatment

Common management options for psoriasis include topicals for the scalp, such as coal tar or salicylic acid shampoo and medium potency topical steroid oil.[89] Coal tar shampoo is not approved for use in patients under 2 years of age. Topical steroids may be applied to affected regions twice a day for 2 weeks.[90] Following treatment with steroids, management of psoriasis is usually resumed with calcipotriene (Dovonex).[91] Alternatively, the treatment may be continued with either betamethasone dipropionate 0.05% (Diprolene AF) or triamcinolone acetonide 0.5% (Aristocort). Moisturizers may be used for supportive treatment. Ultraviolet B phototherapy may be combined with topical or systemic agents to increase efficacy of treatment, especially if more than 30% of the body surface is involved.[92]

Pityriasis Rosea

Overview

Pityriasis rosea is a mild, acute self-limiting inflammatory disorder, lasting 3–8 weeks. According to current theories, this disorder is viral in origin, although the causes remain unknown.[93] Pityriasis rosea is more common in the spring and fall seasons, presents more often in females than in males, and has an age-related onset. Patients with pityriasis rosea often have a history of recent upper respiratory infections.[94]

Presentation

A "herald patch" is commonly seen as the initial finding of pityriasis rosea.[95] This patch is usually 2–10 cm in diameter and is macular, oval, and fawn-colored with a crinkled appearance and collarette scale. A mild pruritic rash follows within 1–2 weeks of onset, often developing in a "Christmas tree pattern" that runs along the trunk and proximal extremities.[96]

Workup

A diagnosis of pityriasis rosea is made by considering the clinical distribution and appearance of the patient's lesions. A serologic test for syphilis should also be performed if the patient's lesions are small in number, perfectly-shaped, not pruritic, or located on the palmar or plantar surfaces.[52]

Treatment

Cases of pityriasis rosea with pruritus may require hydroxyzine hydrochloride (Atarax), topical antipruritic lotions, or oral antihistamines.[97] Medium-strength topical steroids (e.g., triamcinolone 0.1%), cool compresses, and baths—either with or without colloidal oatmeal—may also be used for pruritus.[98]

Daily sunlight exposure is also known to hasten the healing process. Another option is ultraviolet B treatment, which is most effective when administered daily over the course of 1 week.[99]

Impetigo

Overview

Impetigo is a bacterial infection of the skin caused by gram-positive streptococcal or staphylococcal (e.g., *Staphylococcus aureus*) organisms. This disorder predominantly affects the face but can occur anywhere on the body.[52,100] Impetigo occurs most often in the summer and is highly contagious and autoinoculable.

Presentation

Impetigo is characterized by thin-walled vesicles that can easily rupture and honey-crusting lesions.[101] Satellite lesions commonly spread to remote areas of the skin. Other findings include inflammation, pain, swelling, warmth, systemic infection, fever, chills, malaise, and anorexia, among others.[52]

Workup

Impetigo is diagnosed through a clinical exam. In some cases, a culture test may be called for to confirm the causative organism.[102]

Treatment

Systemic treatment of impetigo should be directed at the offending organism. Minor infections may be treated with topical antimicrobials (e.g., bacitracin, mupirocin, etc.).[103] Depending on the offending organism, the NP should consider prescribing oral beta-lactamase resistant antibiotics (e.g., dicloxacillin, cephalexin, erythromycin, clindamycin).[104] In cases of severe cellulitis, intravenous agents (e.g., nafcillin, vancomycin, and doxycycline) may be ordered in an acute care facility.[105] Burow's (Domeboro) solution should be applied to clean lesions.[106] Lastly, a patient with impetigo should abstain from school and other community events until the completion of 48 hours of treatment.

Scabies

Overview

Scabies is a highly contagious skin infestation caused by a parasitic mite that burrows into the stratum corneum. The outbreak of the infestation is usually preceded by an incubation period of 4–6 weeks. Scabies spreads through direct skin-to-skin contact, but can also be transmitted indirectly through contact with an infected patient's personal items.[96]

Presentation

Clinical findings of scabies in infants include linear or curved burrows, intense itching, and irritability. Infants with scabies may present with red-brown vesiculopapular lesions on the head, neck, palms, or soles.[107] Red papules on the umbilicus, abdomen, or skin folds frequently present in older children. Regional adenopathy may be observed in some cases.

Workup

To confirm a diagnosis, skin scrapings are examined for mites, ova, or feces.[34]

Treatment

For patients older than 2 months of age, permethrin (Nix) 5% rinse is the standard management option for scabies. Permethrin should be left on overnight for 8–12 hours upon the first treatment, and then repeated in 1 week.[108] Ivermectin may also be used to treat scabies, but is contraindicated in certain patients (e.g., pregnant/lactating mothers, children under 15 kg). Lindane lotion (Kwell) may be used with caution in children over 6 months of age.[109]

Antihistamines may be used for pruritus. Because a scabies rash may persist, it is recommended that washable items be washed in hot water and dried.[110]

Lyme Disease

Overview

Lyme disease, the most common vector-borne disease in the United States, is caused by the spirochete bacterium *Borrelia burgdorferi*. The majority of cases are concentrated in the Northeast and Upper Midwest regions, and less commonly on the Pacific West Coast; incidence peaks during the summer months.[111]

Deer ticks (*Ixodes scapularis*) are the source of transmission for Lyme disease. After latching onto a host, ticks carrying the pathogen typically take 36–48 hours to transmit the bacteria via feeding.[112,113]

Presentation (see figure 11.8)

Clinical manifestation of Lyme disease occurs in three stages. The first stage is characterized by erythema migrans, a rash that is the hallmark sign of Lyme disease.[114] The rash begins as a flat or slightly raised annular, erythematous lesion that gradually grows to assume a characteristic "bulls eye" shape. An erythema migrans lesion usually appears 1 week after the host has been infected. Although most tick bites occur in areas of tight clothing, they can present anywhere on the body.

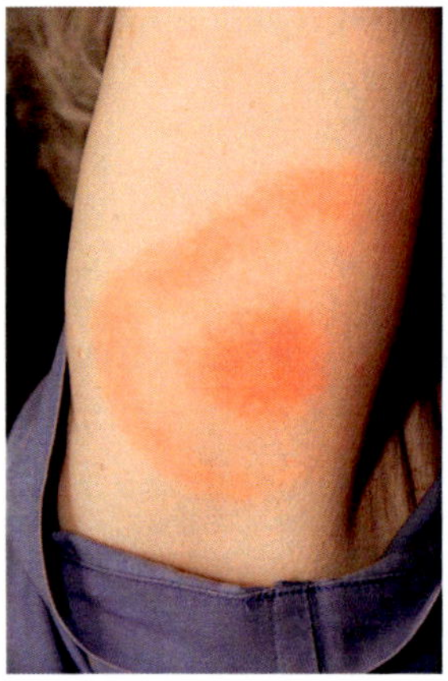

Figure 11.8. Lyme disease

About 50% of all patients present with non-specific, virus-like findings during the first stage, including fever, fatigue, headache, neck pain, arthralgia, and myalgia.[115] Asymptomatic cases during the first stage are rare. Erythema migrans and associated symptoms generally resolve within 3–4 weeks.

Findings and complications associated with the second and third stages include headache, stiff and painful joints, migratory and periarticular pain, Bell's palsy, peripheral neuropathy, acrodermatitis chronicum atrophicans (bluish-red discoloration of the distal extremity with edema), aseptic meningitis, and subacute encephalopathy.[116]

Workup

A clinical diagnosis of Lyme disease should take into account whether the patient was exposed to a tick habitat within the last 30 days.

Initial diagnosis of Lyme disease involves ELISA screening for *B. burgdorferi* antibodies. A Western blot assay is then used to confirm the diagnosis.[117] A complete blood count may also be ordered to check for elevated erythrocyte sedimentation rate.

Treatment

In cases of infection confined to the skin, patients younger than 7 years of age should be given either amoxicillin or cefuroxime axetil. Patients older than age 7 should be prescribed doxycycline.[68] Patients with second or third stage Lyme disease may need to be referred to an infectious disease specialist.

Rubeola

Overview

Rubeola, commonly known as ordinary measles, is an acute viral disease that is transmitted through inhalation of infective droplets and person-to-person contact. Although rubeola usually causes a mild illness, it may produce serious complications. Rubeola is a leading cause of death in young pediatric patients globally, and is more prevalent in non-vaccinated populations.[118]

Because of strict vaccination and prevention measures, rubeola was previously declared to be eliminated in the United States. However, the disease is highly contagious, can be imported, and may spread in unvaccinated communities.[49] In most cases, infected individuals are contagious about four days prior to and four days following the onset of rash.[119]

Complications can be life-threatening, including pneumonia, encephalitis, and pericarditis, among others.[120]

Presentation

Characteristic findings of rubeola include high-grade fever, maculopapular rash, and/or signs and symptoms similar to a respiratory illness.

Rubeola infections generally occur in four stages, beginning with an incubation period that lasts from 7 to 21 days. The incubation stage is followed by a prodromal stage, exanthema, and recovery.[119,121]

Initial findings during the prodromal stage, which can last from 2 to 10 days, commonly include a high fever, malaise, and anorexia. Within 2 days, additional findings may include coryza (i.e., rhinitis and sore throat); a productive, persistent cough; and conjunctivitis, which may be accompanied by photophobia, discharge or lacrimation, and swelling. In severe cases, patients may develop generalized lymphadenopathy and splenomegaly.[120,121,122]

A characteristic finding is Koplik's spots, 1–3 mm elevations that manifest as granular spots surrounded by red rings with an erythematous base. These spots may be white, gray, or blue in color, and are found on the buccal mucosa, opposite the first and second upper molars, but may spread to the hard and soft palate.[121]

The exanthema stage typically manifests a few days after the appearance of fever, and begins with a deep red, irregular maculopapular rash on the face, consisting of small papules the size of a pinhead. After originating around the hairline, the rash typically spreads to the face and neck, the trunk, and then to the extremities. This stage may be accompanied by additional findings, such as respiratory complications and hyperpigmentation in fair-skinned patients. The rash begins to fade after a couple days and resolves within a week.[118,120]

During the recovery period, a cough may persist for up to 2 weeks. Patients diagnosed with rubeola develop an immunity to the virus after recovery.

Workup

A clinical diagnosis of rubeola is determined from the presence of a rash lasting 3 or more days, high fever, and either cough or coryza.[119]

If required, diagnostic labs may be useful. Thrombocytopenia is a common finding, and a white blood cell count may show leukopenia. Other diagnostic findings include serologic assays showing rubeola antibodies, or a polymerase chain reaction that shows measles virus RNA.[120,121]

Treatment

Rubeola resolves within 2–3 weeks, and mainly requires supportive treatment. However, the patient may need to be hospitalized if complications manifest.

Vaccination is indicated in young pediatric patients, as severe complications are more commonly seen in children younger than age 5.[118] In the United States, the two combination vaccines approved for use are the measles-mumps-rubella (MMR) and measles-mumps-rubella-varicella (MMRV) vaccines. The MMR vaccine is administered to infants younger than age 1, and the MMRV vaccine is administered to children between 12 months and 12 years of age. Although the MMR and MMRV vaccines rarely cause fever and febrile seizures, neither vaccine has been linked to cases of hearing deficits or autism.[119]

Rubella

Overview

Rubella, also known as German measles or 3-day measles, is a contagious disease that causes a mild illness and characteristic rash. Transmission of the rubella virus occurs through contact with an infected patient's fluids (e.g., coughing, sneezing).

Although rubella manifests as an acute illness in pediatric patients and adults, the disease can cause birth defects or fetal death in pregnant women if the virus is transmitted through the placenta. The effects of infection on the fetus are most severe in the early weeks of gestation, particularly within the first 12 weeks. Additionally, infants infected in utero may be born with congenital rubella syndrome (CRS), which can lead to congenital heart disease, developmental delays, and hearing impairment.[123]

The incidence of rubella is virtually non-existent in the Unites States due to strict prevention measures, which include early vaccination programs and surveillance; however, there is a chance for cases to be imported from international travel or other countries that do not implement strict measures to control the disease.[124]

Presentation

Patients who are pregnant and have a history of inadequate immunization or show signs of infection are referred for further management.

The incubation period for rubella lasts 14–21 days after transmission.[125]

Characteristic findings of rubella include low-grade fever and a fine, erythematous, non-pruritic maculopapular rash that is red to light pink in color. The rash begins on the face, then rapidly spreads to the extremities and trunk. The rash fades rapidly and is gone within 3 days.[120,123]

About one to five days prior to onset of rash, patients may develop signs and symptoms that include malaise, joint pain or general body aches, and lymphadenopathy. A reddish maculopapular eruption on the soft palate (i.e., the Forchheimer sign) may also develop. Signs and symptoms generally last no more than 3 days and are seen in only about half of all rubella cases.[123,125] Less common complications of rubella include postinfectious encephalopathy, thrombocytopenia, vascular damage, duodenal stenosis, and mild hepatitis.[120]

Workup

An enzyme immunoassay (EIA) is the most common method used to detect rubella-specific immunoglobulin M (IgM) antibodies. Adolescents who may be pregnant or are considering pregnancy should be tested for antibodies following exposure.[120]

Diagnostic testing also includes an analysis of the patients' nasal, throat, urine, and blood specimens.[124]

Treatment

Vaccination against rubella requires 2 doses: The first dose is administered to infants between 12 and 15 months of age, and the second dose is administered to children between the ages of 4 and 6 years.[123]

Infants born with CRS are considered to be infectious until 1 year of age. To prevent spreading the virus, it is important to restrict contact with others. Surveillance of CRS should be implemented in cases involving suspected or confirmed rubella infection in the fetus.[124]

Erythema Infectiosum (Fifth Disease)

Overview

Erythema infectiosum, also known as fifth disease, is a mild contagious disease caused by human parvovirus B19, which is usually benign and peaks in incidence in the spring. The virus is mainly seen in children between 5 and 14 years of age, but can affect adults as well.[68,126] Erythema infectiosum can be transmitted through respiratory secretions, blood transfusions, and blood-derived products, and has an incubation period that typically lasts for 4–14 days. Adolescents who are pregnant and infected with erythema infectiosum may also transmit the virus to the fetus.[127]

Presentation (see figure 11.9)

Initial findings during the prodromal stage are usually non-specific and vary according to each patient. Headache, fever, and sore throat may manifest, as well as malaise, pruritus on the palms and soles, coryza, and arthralgias.[127,128] After the initial findings subside, a characteristic facial exanthema manifests with a sudden onset, producing the appearance of fiery red, flushed cheeks (i.e., "slapped cheek" appearance).[120] The facial exanthema fades within 2–4 days and is followed by onset of a lacy, erythematous maculopapular rash that spreads to the upper arms, legs, trunk, and dorsum of the hands and feet. On average, the rash lasts one-and-a-half weeks, but may persist up to 40 days.[67]

Workup

Diagnosis of erythema infectiosum in pediatrics can be determined through clinical observation. If further confirmation is necessary, a diagnostic analysis of the patient's blood may be performed to detect parvovirus B19 antibodies.[129] Diagnostic testing is commonly required if infection is suspected in pregnant adolescents.[128]

Treatment

Erythema infectiosum is a self-limiting disease that usually does not require treatment in children.[128]

Roseola Infantum (Sixth Disease)

Overview

Roseola infantum, often referred to as sixth disease, is a mild contagious disease caused by human herpesvirus type 6 (HHV-6) that occurs in infants between 6 months and 2 years of age. Roseola infantum is a major cause of febrile seizures in infants, and the incidence is rare in children older than 4 years of age.[68]

Presentation (see figure 11.10)

Roseola infantum is characterized by a high fever that is followed by a distinctive maculopapular rash. The initial high fever onsets abruptly and can last from 3 to 8 days. During this time, infants are susceptible to febrile seizures. Additional findings may include inflammation of the tympanic membrane and cold-like signs and symptoms. After the fever resolves, a rash initially manifests on the trunk and then spreads to the extremities, characterized by papules that are small, pink, flat, or slightly raised.[68,130]

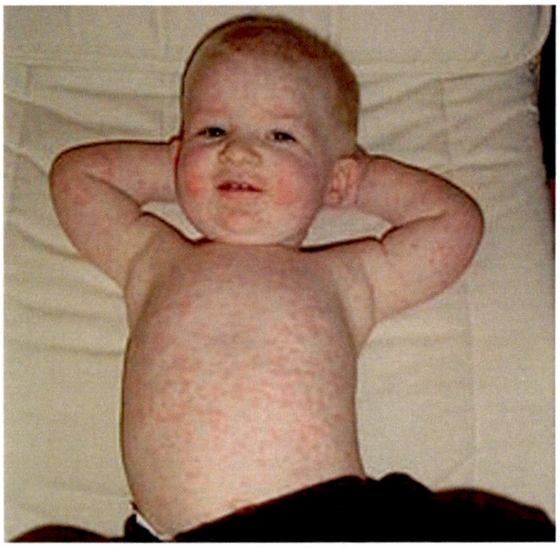

Figure 11.9. Fifth disease

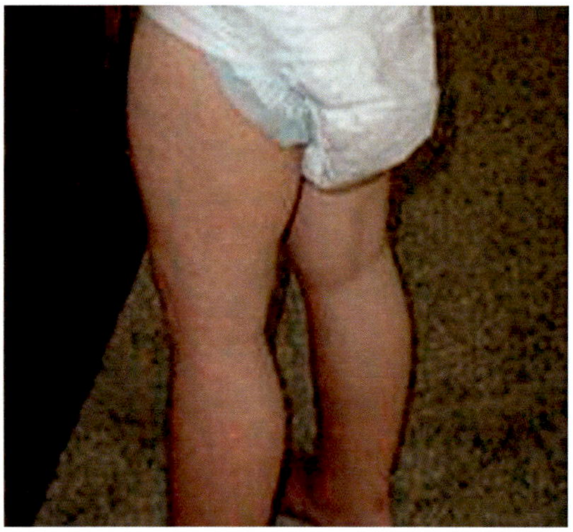

Figure 11.10. Sixth disease

Workup

Diagnosis is determined through clinical observation, with a particular focus on the presentation of the rash.[131] A lab diagnostic is rarely required, but blood antibody titers and viral cultures may be performed to confirm a diagnosis, if necessary.[130]

Treatment

Roseola infantum resolves on its own. Management is mainly supportive, as there is no cure. Antipyretics may be used for fever reduction.[131,132]

Coxsackie Virus (Hand, Foot, and Mouth Disease)

Overview

The coxsackie virus is an RNA enterovirus that resides in the digestive tract. There are several strains of the coxsackie virus, but the one most commonly seen in pediatric patients younger than age 10 is hand, foot, and mouth disease (HFMD).[133,134]

Pediatric patients with HFMD are most contagious within the first week of infection, and transmission occurs through contact with the infected patient's fluids (e.g., oral and respiratory secretions, vesicle fluid) or the fecal-oral route.[135] Viral coxsackie infections are rare in adults, but women are more susceptible to infection during pregnancy.[136] Transmission of infection from the pregnant mother to the fetus is extremely rare, but neonates are highly susceptible to infection.[137] In rare cases, referral is necessary for complications.[133,135]

Presentation

Findings of HFMD include soreness in the mouth or throat, loss of appetite or refusal to eat, and malaise. A low-grade fever is also present, lasting 24–48 hours.[138]

The most characteristic features of HFMD are oral enanthema or exanthema. Oral sores initially appear as erythematous macules that progress to vesicles surrounded by an erythematous halo, which characteristically appear on the tongue and buccal mucosa but may manifest anywhere in the mouth or throat.[138] Skin rashes manifest on the palms of the hands, soles of the feet, buttocks, legs, and arms, and present with similar appearance to oral sores.[135,139]

Workup

Diagnosis of HFMD is determined through clinical observation of the patient's findings, with special focus on the characteristic oral sores and exanthema. Labs and diagnostics are usually unnecessary.[136]

Treatment

Treatment of HFMD is supportive, as HFMD typically resolves within a week. Management consists of antipyretics (e.g., acetaminophen) for fever reduction and mouthwash for mouth sores and pain.[135]

Figures

Figure 11.1. Rule of Nines diagram for a pediatric patient. Barkley & Associates, Inc. Published 2015.

Figure 11.2. Lund and Browder diagram for pediatric patients. Barkley & Associates, Inc. Published 2015.

Figure 11.3. Acne vulgaris. In: Cavallini J. Phototake. Reproduced with permission.

Figure 11.4. Chickenpox. In: Ager-Wick R. http://commons.wikimedia.org/wiki/File:Bem_chickenpox_vannkopper_20140318.jpg. Reproduced with permission.

Figure 11.5. Molluscum contagiosum. In Herk E. http://commons.wikimedia.org/wiki/File:Mollusca1klein.jpg. Reproduced with permission.

Figure 11.6. Allergic contact dermatitis. In: Blausen.com staff. *Blausen gallery 2014*. Wikiversity Journal of Medicine. DOI:10.15347/wjm/2014.010. ISSN 20018762. Reproduced with permission.

Figure 11.7. Diaper dermatitis. http://commons.wikimedia.org/wiki/File:Irritant_diaper_dermatitis.jpg. Reproduced with permission.

Figure 11.8. Lyme disease. In: J. Gathany. http://upload.wikimedia.org/wikipedia/commons/0/01/Erythema_migrans_-_erythematous_rash_in_Lyme_disease_-_PHIL_9875.jpg. Copyright by CDC. Reproduced with permission.

Figure 11.9. Fifth disease. In: Kerr A. http://commons.wikimedia.org/wiki/File:Fifth_disease.jpg. Reproduced with permission.

Figure 11.10. Sixth disease. In: Davis A. http://commons.wikimedia.org/wiki/File:Roseola_on_a_21-month-old_girl.jpg. Reproduced with permission.

References

1. Burn Classification. The University of New Mexico Hospitals Web site. http://hospitals.unm.edu/burn/classification.shtml. Accessed April 23, 2015.

2. Huether SE, McCance KL, eds. *Understanding Pathophysiology*. 5th ed. St. Louis, MO: Elsevier Mosby; 2012.

3. Deshaies L. Burns. In: Cooper C, ed. *Fundamentals of Hand Therapy: Clinical Reasoning and Treatment Guidelines for Common Diagnoses of the Upper Extremity*. 2nd ed. Philadelphia: Elsevier; 2014: 479–490.4.

4. Rice PL Jr, Orgill DP. Classification of burns. In: Basow DS, ed. *UpToDate*. Waltham, MA: UpToDate; 2015. http://www.uptodate.com/contents/classification-of-burns?detectedLanguage=en&source=search_result&search=burns&selectedTitle=2~150&provider=noProvider. Updated January 16, 2014. Accessed April 23, 2015.

5. County of Los Angeles Department of Health Services, Emergency Medical Services Agency, Disaster Services. Burn resource manual. http://file.lacounty.gov/dhs/cms1_206654.pdf. Published June 2010. Accessed April 24, 2015.

6. Sharma RK, Parashar A. Special considerations in paediatric burn patients. *Indian J Plast Surg*. 2010; 43(Suppl): S43–S50.

7. United States Department of Health and Human Services, Office of the Assistant Secretary for Preparedness and Response, National Library of Medicine. Burn triage and treatment – thermal injuries. Chemical Hazards Emergency Medical Management Web site. http://chemm.nlm.nih.gov/burns.htm. Updated June 25, 2011. Accessed April 24, 2015.

8. Hinkle JL, Cheever KH. *Brunner & Suddarth's Textbook of Medical-Surgical Nursing*. 13th ed. Philadelphia, PA: Wolters Kluwer Health/Lippincott Williams & Wilkins; 2014.

9. LeMone P, Burke K, Levett-Jones T, et al. *Medical-Surgical Nursing: Critical Thinking for Person-Centered Care.* 2nd ed. Frenchs Forest, NSW, Australia: Pearson Australia; 2014.

10. Trauma/burn clinical guidelines: A quick guide for the management of trauma/burn disasters for emergency department personnel. Yale New Haven Health Web site. http://yalenewhavenhealth.org/emergency/PDFs/TraumaBurn_ClinicalGuidelines_Final.pdf. Updated August 2013. Accessed April 27, 2015.

11. Burn center referral criteria. American Burn Association Web site. http://www.ameriburn.org/BurnCenterReferralCriteria.pdf. Accessed April 27, 2015.

12. Usatine, RP. Anesthesia. In: Usatine RP, Pfenninger JL, Stulberg DL, Small R, eds. *Dermatologic and Cosmetic Procedures in Office Practice.* Philadelphia, PA: Elsevier Saunders; 2012: 20–29.

13. Wolff K, Johnson RA, Saavedra AP. *Fitzpatrick's Color Atlas and Synopsis of Clinical Dermatology.* 7th ed. New York, NY: McGraw-Hill Education; 2013.

14. Tully A, Studdiford JS. *USMLE Images for the Boards: A Comprehensive Image-Based Review.* Philadelphia, PA: Elsevier Saunders; 2013.

15. Rhoads J, Petersen SW. *Advanced Health Assessment and Diagnostic Reasoning.* 2nd ed. Burlington, MA: Jones & Bartlett Learning; 2013.

16. Bristow I, Turner R. Dermatological assessment. In: Yates B, ed. *Merriman's Assessment of the Lower Limb.* 3rd ed. Philadelphia, PA: Elsevier Churchill Livingstone; 2012: 164–200.

17. Derrer DT. Cysts, lumps, bumps, and your skin. WebMD Web site. http://www.webmd.com/skin-problems-and-treatments/guide/cysts-lumps-bumps?page=5. Updated September 21, 2014. Accessed April 27, 2015.

18. Williams G, Katcher M. Primary care dermatology: Nomenclature of skin lesions. The University of Wisconsin Department of Pediatrics Web site. http://www.pediatrics.wisc.edu/education/derm/. Accessed April 27, 2015.

19. Sharma A, Lambert PJ, Maghari A, Lambert WC. Arcuate, annular, and polycyclic inflammatory and infectious lesions. *Clin Dermatol.* 2011; 29(2): 140–150.

20. Greydanus DE. The acnes: Acne vulgaris, acne rosacea, and acne excoriée. In: Tareen RS, Greydanus DE, Jafferany M, Patel DR, Merrick J, eds. *Pediatric Psychodermatology: A Manual of Child and Adolescent Psychocutaneous Disorders.* Boston, MA: Walter de Gruyter; 2013: 163–192.

21. Cole GW. Acne. In: Stöppler MC, ed. eMedicine Health. http://www.emedicinehealth.com/acne/page2_em.htm. Updated November 7, 2014. Accessed April 27, 2015.

22. Sylvia LM. Drug allergy, pseudoallergy, and cutaneous diseases. In: Tisdale JE, Miller DA, eds. *Drug-Induced Diseases: Prevention, Detection, and Management.* 2nd ed. Bethesda, MD: American Society of Health-System Pharmacists; 2010: 51–97.

23. Zouboulis CC, Abdel-Naser MB. Acne and its variants. In: Krieg T, Bickes DR, Miyachi Y, eds. *Therapy of Skin Diseases: A Worldwide Perspective on Therapeutic Approaches and Their Molecular Basis.* New York, NY: Springer; 2010: 359–375.

24. Fabbrocini G, Annunziata MC, D'Arco V, et al. Acne scars: Pathogenesis, classification and treatment. *Dermatol Res Pract.* 2010; 2010: 893080. http://www.ncbi.nlm.nih.gov/pmc/articles/PMC2958495/# Accessed May 1, 2015.

25. Bowers ES. How your period affects acne. WebMD Web site. http://www.webmd.com/skin-problems-and-treatments/acne/features/period. Updated April 11, 2011. Accessed May 1, 2015.

26. Bauer KA, Schlosser B, Mirowski GW. Acne vulgaris and steroid acne. In: Fife RS, Schrager SB, eds. *The APC Handbook of Women's Health*. Philadelphia, PA: ACP Press; 2009: 337–346.

27. Graber E. Treatment of acne vulgaris. In: Basow DS, ed. *UpToDate*. Waltham, MA: UpToDate; 2015. http://www.uptodate.com/contents/treatment-of-acne-vulgaris?detectedLanguage=en&source=search_result&search= acne+treatment&selected Title=1~150&provider=noProvider. Updated February 18, 2015. Accessed May 1, 2015.

28. Herrier RN. Dermatotherapy and drug-induced skin disorders. In: Alldredge BK, Corelli RL, Ernst ME, et al, eds. *Koda-Kimble and Young's Applied Therapeutics: The Clinical Use of Drugs*. 10th ed. Philadelphia, PA: Wolters Kluwer Health/Lippincott Williams & Wilkins; 2013: 925–946.

29. Kober MM, Bowe WP, Shalita AR. Topical therapies for acne. In: Zeichner JA, ed. *Acneiform Eruptions in Dermatology: A Differential Diagnosis*. New York, NY: Springer; 2014: 19–26.

30. Titus S, Hodge J. Diagnosis and treatment of acne. *Am Fam Physician*. 2012; 86(8): 734–740. http://www.aafp.org/afp/2004/0501/p2123.html. Accessed May 1, 2015.

31. Richardson MD, Warnock DW. *Fungal Infection: Diagnosis and Management*. 4th ed. Hoboken, NJ: Wiley-Blackwell; 2012.

32. Van der Vlugt TM. Regional dermatitis. In: Amieva-Wang NE, Shandro J, Fassl B, Sohoni A, eds. *A Practical Guide to Pediatric Emergency Medicine: Caring for Children in the Emergency Department*. New York, NY: Cambridge University Press; 2011: 147–150.

33. Robbins CM, Elewski BE. Tinea pedis. In: Elston DM, ed. Medscape. http://emedicine.medscape.com/article/1091684-overview. Updated December 10, 2014. Accessed May 4, 2015.

34. Cafardi JA. *The Manual of Dermatology*. New York, NY: Springer; 2012.

35. McKinney ES, James SR, Murray SS, Nelson K, Ashwill JW. *Maternal-Child Nursing*. 4thed. Philadelphia, PA: Elsevier Saunders; 2012.

36. Lescher JL Jr. Tinea corporis. In: Elston DM, ed. Medscape. http://emedicine.medscape.com/article/1091473-overview. Updated July 21, 2014. Accessed May 4, 2015.

37. Craft N, Fox LP, Goldsmith LA, Papier A, Birnbaum R, Mercurio MG. *VisualDx: Essential Adult Dermatology*. Philadelphia, PA: Wolters Kluwer Health/Lippincott Williams & Wilkins; 2011.

38. Burkhart CG, Burkhart CN. Tinea versicolor workup. In: Elston DM, ed. Medscape. http://emedicine.medscape.com/article/1091575-workup. Updated July 21, 2014. Accessed May 4, 2015.

39. Dourmishev LA. Pediatric tinea versicolor workup. In: Elston DM, ed. Medscape. http://emedicine.medscape.com/article/911138-workup. Updated November 4, 2014. Accessed May 4, 2015.

40. Rakel RE, Rakel DP. *Textbook of Family Medicine*. 9th ed. Philadelphia, PA: Elsevier Saunders; 2015.

41. Michaels BD, Del Rosso JQ. Tinea capitis in infants: Recognition, evaluation, and management suggestions. *J Clin Aesthet Dermatol*. 2012; 5(2): 49–59.

42. McQueen L, Lio P. Pediatric dermatologic conditions. In: Aghababian RV, ed. *Essentials of Emergency Medicine*. 2nd ed. Sudbury, MA: Jones & Bartlett Learning; 2011: 551–561.

43. Phillips RM, Rosen T. Topical antifungal agents. In: Wolverton SE, ed. *Comprehensive Dermatologic Drug Therapy*. 3rd ed. Philadelphia, PA: Elsevier Saunders; 2013: 460–472.

44. Berger TG. Dermatologic disorders. In: Papadakis MA, McPhee SJ, Rabow MW, eds. *Current Medical Diagnosis & Treatment*. 53rd ed. New York, NY: McGraw-Hill; 2014: 90–158.

45. Weber DJ, Rutala WA. Prevention and control of varicella-zoster virus in hospitals. In: Basow DS, ed. *UpToDate*. Waltham, MA: UpToDate; 2015. http://www.uptodate.com/contents/prevention-and-control-of-varicella-zoster-virus-in-hospitals. Updated September 20, 2013. Accessed May 5, 2015.

46. Albrecht MA. Clinical features of varicella-zoster virus infection: Chickenpox. In: Basow DS, ed. *UpToDate*. Waltham, MA: UpToDate; 2015. http://www.uptodate.com/contents/clinical-features-of-varicella-zoster-virus-infection-chickenpox?source=-search_result&search=chickenpox&selectedTitle=1~150. Updated June 30, 2014. Accessed May 5, 2015.

47. Mersch J. Chickenpox. In: Stöppler MC, ed. eMedicineHealth. http://www.emedicinehealth.com/chickenpox/article_em.htm. Reviewed June 18, 2015. Accessed June 19, 2015.

48. Papadopoulos J, Janniger CK, and Schwartz RA. Chickenpox clinical presentation. In: Elston DM, ed. Medscape. http://emedicine.medscape.com/article/1131785-clinical. Updated February 10, 2015. Accessed May 5, 2015.

49. Albrecht M. Diagnosis of varicella-zoster virus infection. In: Basow DS, ed. *UpToDate*. Waltham, MA: UpToDate; 2015. http://www.uptodate.com/contents/diagnosis-of-varicella-zoster-virus-infection. Updated October 8, 2013. Accessed May 5, 2015.

50. United States Department of Health and Human Services, Centers for Disease Control and Prevention. Chickenpox VIS. http://www.cdc.gov/vaccines/hcp/vis/vis-statements/varicella.html. Updated June 18, 2013. Accessed May 5, 2015.

51. Acyclovir (oral route, intravenous route). Mayo Clinic Web site. http://www.mayoclinic.org/drugs-supplements/acyclovir-oral-route-intravenous-route/proper-use/drg-20068393. Updated April 1, 2015. Accessed May 5, 2015.

52. Marks JG Jr, Miller JJ. *Lookingbill and Marks' Principles of Dermatology*. 5th ed. Philadelphia, PA: Elsevier Saunders; 2013.

53. United States Department of Health and Human Services, Centers for Disease Control and Prevention. Chickenpox (varicella): Prevention & treatment. http://www.cdc.gov/chickenpox/about/prevention-treatment.html. Updated November 16, 2011. Accessed May 5, 2015.

54. United States Department of Health and Human Services, Centers for Disease Control and Prevention. Molluscum (molluscum contagiosum). http://www.cdc.gov/ncidod/dvrd/molluscum/faq/everyone.htm#whatis. Updated January 13, 2011. Accessed May 5, 2015.

55. Saavedra A, Rosmarin D. Tropical dermatology. In: Magill AJ, Ryan ET, Hill D, Solomon T, eds. *Hunter's Tropical Medicine and Emerging Infectious Diseases*. 9th ed. Philadelphia: Elsevier Saunders; 2012: 68–76.

56. Eckert LO, Lentz GM. Infections of the lower and upper genital tracts: Vulva, vagina, cervix, toxic shock syndrome, endometritis, and salpingitis. In: Lentz GM, Lobo RA, Gershenson DM, Katz VL, eds. *Comprehensive Gynecology*. 6th ed. Philadelphia, PA: Elsevier Mosby; 2012: 519–560.

57. Isaacs, SN. Patient information: Molluscum contagiosum (beyond the basics). In: Basow DS, ed. *UpToDate*. Waltham, MA: UpToDate; 2015. http://www.uptodate.com/contents/molluscum-contagiosum-beyond-the-basics. Updated October 17, 2013. Accessed May 5, 2015.

58. Warrell DA. Molluscum contagiosum. In: Warrell DA, Cox TM, Firth JD, Török E, eds. *Oxford Textbook of Medicine: Infection*. Oxford, UK: Oxford University Press; 2012: 264–266.

59. Brice SL. Viral diseases of the skin. In: Bope ET, Kellerman RD, eds. *Conn's Current Therapy 2013*. 65th ed. Philadelphia, PA: Elsevier Saunders; 2013: 288–293.

60. Medically prescribed treatments for molluscum contagiosum. Natural Molluscum Web site. http://www.naturalmolluscum.com/treatments. Accessed May 5, 2015.

61. Bhatia AC. Molluscum contagiosum treatment & management. In: Elston DM, ed. http://emedicine.medscape.com/article/910570-treatment#aw2aab6b6b2. Updated November 4, 2014. Accessed May 5, 2015.

62. Mathes EFD, Frieden IJ. Treatment of molluscum contagiosum with cantharidin: A practical approach. *Pediatr Ann*. 2010; 39(3): 124–128.

63. Berk DR. Tutorial: Dermatologic medications and dermatologic diagnostics. In: Amieva-Wang NE, Shandro J, Sohoni A, Fassl B, eds. *A Practical Guide to Pediatric Emergency Medicine: Caring for Children in the Emergency Department*. New York: Cambridge University Press; 2011: 176-183.

64. United States Department of Health and Human Services, National Institutes of Health, National Institute of Arthritis and Musculoskeletal and Skin Diseases. Handout on health: Atopic dermatitis (a type of eczema). http://www.niams.nih.gov/health_info/atopic_dermatitis/#d. Published May 2013. Accessed May 6, 2015.

65. Weston WL, Howe W. Epidemiology, clinical manifestations, and diagnosis of atopic dermatitis (eczema). In: Basow DS, ed. *UpToDate*. Waltham, MA: UpToDate; 2015. http://www.uptodate.com/contents/epidemiology-clinical-manifestations-and-diagnosis-of-atopic-dermatitis-eczema?source=search_result&search=atopic+dermatitis&selectedTitle= 2~150. Updated April 29, 2015. Accessed May 6, 2015.

66. Honig PJ, Castelo-Soccio L, Yan AC. Dermatologic urgencies and emergencies. In: Fleisher GR, Ludwig S, eds. *Textbook of Pediatric Emergency Medicine*. Philadelphia, PA: Lippincott Williams & Wilkins; 2010: 730–757.

67. Nagaraju K. *Manual of Pediatric Allergy*. London and New Dehli: JP Medical; 2014.

68. Barkley TW Jr. *Family Nurse Practitioner Certification Review / Clinical Update Continuing Education Course*. West Hollywood, CA: Barkley and Associates; 2015.

69. Topical corticosteroids. National Eczema Association Web site. http://nationaleczema.org/eczema/treatment/topical-corticosteroids/. Accessed May 6, 2015.

70. Basics of topical corticosteroids. National Eczema Association Web site. http://nationaleczema.org/eczema/treatment/topical-corticosteroids/basics-of-topical-corticosteroids/. Accessed May 6, 2015.

71. Winland-Brown JE, Porter BO, Allen S. Skin problems. In: Dunphy LM, Winland-Brown JE, Porter BO, Thomas DJ, eds. *Primary Care: The Art and Science of Advanced Practice Nursing*. 3rd ed. Philadelphia, PA: F. A. Davis Company; 2011: 145–244.

72. Ratini M. Contact dermatitis: Facts about skin rashes. WebMD web site. http://www.webmd.com/skin-problems-and-treatments/contact-dermatitis?page=2. Accessed May 6, 2015.

73. Hogan DJ. Allergic contact dermatitis. In: James WD, ed. Medscape. http://emedicine.medscape.com/article/1049216-overview. Updated April 23, 2015. Accessed May 6, 2015.

74. Usatine RP, Riojas M. Diagnosis and management of contact dermatitis. *Am Fam Physician*. 2010; 82(3): 249–255.

75. Singh AK, Loscalzo J. *The Brigham Intensive Review of Internal Medicine*. 2nd ed. New York, NY: Oxford University Press; 2014.

76. Horii KA, Prossick TA. Overview of diaper dermatitis in infants and children. In: Basow DS, ed. *UpToDate*. Waltham, MA: UpToDate; 2015. http://www.uptodate.com/contents/overview-of-diaper-dermatitis-in-infants-and-children?source=search_result&search=irritant+diaper+dermatitis&selectedTitle=1~150. Updated July 9, 2013. Accessed May 7, 2015.

77. Findlay JS. Dermatologic conditions. In: Silbert-Flagg J, Sloand E, eds. *Pediatric Nurse Practitioner Certification Review Guide*. 5th ed. Sudbury, MA: Jones and Bartlett Publishing; 2011: 153–192.

78. Cadeliña R. Diaper rash: Clinical considerations and evaluation. The University of British Columbia Web site. http://learnpediatrics.com/body-systems/neonate/diaper-rash-clinical-considerations-and-evaluation/. Updated February 9, 2011. Accessed May 7, 2015.

79. Dib R, Kazzi AA. Diaper rash treatment & management. In: Bachur RG, ed. Medscape. http://emedicine.medscape.com/article/801222-treatment. Updated September 16, 2014. Accessed May 7, 2015.

80. Schalock PC. Topical therapy. In: Schalock PC, Hsu JTS, Arndt KA. *Lippincott's Primary Care Dermatology*. Philadelphia: Lippincott Williams & Wilkins; 2011: 12–19.

81. Meffert J. Psoriasis. In: James WD, ed. Medscape. http://emedicine.medscape.com/article/1943419-overview#showall . Updated January 22, 2015. Accessed May 8, 2015.

82. Cane EM. Psoriasis condition. Psoriasis Free Life Web site. http://www.psoriasisfreelife.net/psoriasis-condition.html. Published 2012. Accessed May 8, 2015.

83. White L, Duncan G, Baumle W. *Medical-Surgical Nursing: An Integrated Approach*. 3rd ed. Clifton Park, NY: Cengage Learning; 2013.

84. Schalock PC. Psoriasis. In: Porter RS, Kaplan JL, eds. The Merck Manual Online. http://www.merckmanuals.com/professional/dermatologic-disorders/psoriasis-and-scaling-diseases/psoriasis. Updated November 2014. Accessed May 8, 2015.

85. Ko HC, Jwa SW, Song M, Kim MB, Kwon KS. Clinical course of guttate psoriasis: Long-term follow-up study. *J Dermatol*. 2010; 37(10): 894–899.

86. Tidy C. Psoriatic nail disease. Patient.co.uk Web site. http://www.patient.co.uk/doctor/psoriatic-nail-disease. Updated November 20, 2012. Accessed May 8, 2015.

87. Knee NW, Blair G. Psoriasis. In: Buttaro TM, Trybulski J, Bailey PP, Sandberg-Cook J, eds. *Primary Care: A Collaborative Practice*. 4th ed. St. Louis, MO: Elsevier Mosby; 2013: 62–63.

88. Psoriasis: Tests and diagnosis. Mayo Clinic Web site. http://www.mayoclinic.org/diseases-conditions/psoriasis/basics/tests-diagnosis/con-20030838. Published April 11, 2014. Accessed May 5, 2015.

89. Topical treatment for psoriasis. National Psoriasis Foundation Web site. https://www.psoriasis.org/document.doc?id=164. Published September, 2013. Accessed May 11, 2015.

90. Kupetsky EA, Keller M. Psoriasis vulgaris: An evidence-based guide for primary care. *J Am Board Fam Med*. 2013; 26(6): 787–801.

91. Mild psoriasis: Non-steroidal prescription topical treatments. National Psoriasis Foundation Web site. https://www.psoriasis.org/about-psoriasis/treatments/topicals/non-steroid. Accessed May 11, 2015.

92. Phototherapy. National Psoriasis Foundation Web site. https://www.psoriasis.org/phototherapy. Accessed May 11, 2015.

93. Gruskin KD. Rash-maculopapular. In: Fleisher GR, Ludwig S, eds. *Textbook of Pediatric Emergency Medicine*. 6th ed. Philadelphia, PA: Wolters Kluwer Health/Lippincott Williams & Wilkins; 2010: 509–520.

94. Fletcher ST, Chaney SE. Dermatological disorders. In: Miller SK, ed. *Adult Nurse Practitioner Certification Review Guide*. 5th ed. Burlington, MA: Jones & Bartlett; 2012: 29–44.

95. Tidy C. Pityriasis rosea. Patient.co.uk Web site. http://www.patient.co.uk/doctor/pityriasis-rosea. Updated February 8, 2013. Accessed May 11, 2015.

96. Goldstein AO, Goldstein BG. Pityriasis rosea. In: Basow DS, ed. *UpToDate*. Waltham, MA: UpToDate; 2015. http://www.uptodate.com/contents/pityriasis-rosea?source=search_result&search=pityriasis+rosea&selectedTitle=1~18. Updated November 25, 2014. Accessed May 11, 2015.

97. Pityriasis rosea – Treatment. National Health Service Web site. http://www.nhs.uk/Conditions/pityriasis-rosea/Pages/Treatment.aspx. Updated March 23, 2015. Accessed May 14, 2015.

98. Perman MJ, Lucky AW, Marino BS. Dermatology. In: Marino BS, Fine KS, eds. *Blueprint Pediatrics*. 6th ed. Philadelphia, PA: Wolters Kluwer Health/Lippincott Williams & Wilkins; 2013: 74–85.

99. Pityriasis rosea. MedlinePlus Web site. http://www.nlm.nih.gov/medlineplus/ency/article/000871.htm. Updated October 14, 2012. Accessed May 14, 2015.

100. Baddour LM. Impetigo. In: Basow DS, ed. *UpToDate*. Waltham, MA: UpToDate; 2015. http://www.uptodate.com/contents/impetigo?source=search_result&search=impetigo&selectedTitle=1~62. Updated February 26, 2015. Accessed May 14, 2015.

101. Lewis LS. Impetigo. In: Steele RW, ed. Medscape. http://emedicine.medscape.com/article/965254-overview. Updated September 10, 2014. Accessed May 15, 2015.

102. Santiago TMG, Cardona JMO. Cutaneous disorders in the intensive care unit. In: Sánchez NP, ed. *Atlas of Dermatology in Internal Medicine*. New York, NY: Springer; 2011: 129–142.

103. Woo TM. Drugs used in treating infectious diseases. In: Woo TM, Wynne AL, eds. *Pharmacotherapeutics for Nurse Practitioner Prescribers*. 3rd ed. Philadelphia, PA: F. A. Davis Company; 2011: 741–868.

104. Gutierrez K. Infectious diseases. In: Bernstein D, Shelov S. *Pediatrics for Medical Students*. 3rd ed. Philadelphia, PA: Wolters Kluwer Health/Lippincott Williams & Wilkins; 2012: 160–223.

105. Kyle T, Carman S. *Essentials of Pediatric Nursing*. 2nd ed. Philadelphia, PA: Lippincott Williams & Wilkins; 2013.

106. Bose SK. Skin diseases. In: Srivastava RN, Kabra SK, eds. *Pediatrics: A Concise Text*. New Delhi, India: Elsevier India; 2011: 263–268.

107. Albakri L, Goldman RD. Permethrin for scabies in children. *Can Fam Physician*. 2010; 56(10): 1005–1006.

108. McCord S. Health problems of middle childhood. In: Hockenberry MJ, Wilson D, eds. *Wong's Nursing Care of Infants and Children Multimedia Enhanced Version*. 9th ed. St. Louis, MO: Elsevier Mosby; 2011: 684–737.

109. Workowski KA, Berman S. Sexually transmitted diseases treatment guidelines. *MMWR Morb Mortal Wkly Rep*. 2010; 59(RR-12): 1–110. http://origin.glb.cdc.gov/mmwr/pdf/rr/rr5912.pdf.

110. Beard CB. Epidemiology of Lyme disease. In: Basow DS, ed. *UpToDate*. Waltham, MA: UpToDate; 2015. http://www.uptodate.com/contents/epidemiology-of-lyme-disease?source=search_result&search=lyme+disease&selectedTitle=6~150. Accessed May 26, 2015.

111. United States Department of Health and Human Services, Centers for Disease Control and Prevention. Lifecycle of blacklegged ticks. Retrieved from http://www.cdc.gov/lyme/transmission/blacklegged.html. Updated November 15, 2011. Accessed May 26, 2015.

112. Misinformation about Lyme disease. American Lyme Disease Foundation Web site. http://aldf.com/lyme-disease/. Updated February 21, 2015. Accessed May 26, 2015.

113. Meyerhoff JO, Steele RW, Zaidman GW. Lyme disease clinical presentation. In: Diamond HS, ed. Medscape. http://emedicine.medscape.com/article/330178-clinical. Updated January 22, 2015. Accessed May 26, 2015.

114. Shapiro ED. Lyme disease: Clinical manifestations in children. In: Basow DS, ed. *UpToDate*. Waltham, MA: UpToDate; 2015. http://www.uptodate.com/contents/lyme-disease-clinical-manifestations-in-children?source=search_result&search=lyme+disease+children&selectedTitle=4~150#H3. Updated January 30, 2014. Accessed May 26, 2015.

115. Philip SS. Spirochetal infections. In: Papadakis MA, Mcphee SJ, Rabow MJ, eds. *Current Medical Diagnosis & Treatment*. 53rd ed. New York, NY: McGraw-Hill Education; 2014: 1417–1435.

116. Hu, L. Diagnosis of Lyme disease. In: Basow DS, ed. *UpToDate*. Waltham, MA: UpToDate; 2015. http://www.uptodate.com/contents/diagnosis-of-lyme-disease?source=search_result&search=lyme+disease& selectedTitle=3~150#H9. Updated March 20, 2015. Accessed May 26, 2015.

117. Measles. World Health Organization Web site. http://www.who.int/mediacentre/factsheets/fs286/en/. Updated February, 2015. Accessed May 26, 2015.

118. Fiebelkorn AP, Goodson JL. Measles (rubeola). In: Brunette GW, ed. *CDC Health Information for International Travel 2014: The Yellow Book*. New York, NY: Oxford University Press; 2013: 249–253.

119. Roig IL, Shandera WX. Viral and Rickettsial infection. In: Papadakis MA, McPhee SJ, Rabow MW, eds. *Current Medical Diagnosis & Treatment*. 53rd ed. New York, NY: McGraw-Hill Education; 2014: 1305–1370.

120. Barinaga JL, Skolnik PR. Clinical presentation and diagnosis of measles. In: Basow DS, ed. *UpToDate*. Waltham, MA: UpToDate; 2015. http://www.uptodate.com/contents/clinical-manifestations-and-diagnosis-of-measles. Updated February 12, 2015. Accessed May 26, 2015.

121. Pillitteri A. *Maternal & Child Health Nursing: Care of the Childbearing & Childrearing Family*. 7th ed. Philadelphia, PA: Wolters Kluwer Health/Lippincott Williams & Wilkins; 2013.

122. United States Department of Health and Human Services, Centers for Disease Control and Prevention. Rubella (German measles, three-day measles). http://www.cdc.gov/rubella/about/index.html. Updated December 17, 2014. Accessed May 26, 2015.

123. McLean H, Redd S, Abernathy E, Icenogle J, Wallace G. Congenital rubella syndrome. In: Roush SW, McIntyre L, Baldy LM, eds. *Centers for Disease Control and Prevention, Manual for the Surveillance of Vaccine-Preventable Diseases*. 5th ed. Atlanta, GA: Centers for Disease Control and Prevention; 2012. http://www.cdc.gov/vaccines/pubs/surv-manual/chpt15-crs.pdf. Accessed May 26, 2015.

124. Ezike E, Ang JY. Pediatric rubella clinical presentation. In: Steele RW, ed. Medscape. http://emedicine.medscape.com/article/968523-clinical#showall. Updated December 18, 2014. Accessed May 26, 2015.

125. Dijkmans AC, de Jong EP, Dijkmans BA, et al. Parvovirus B19 in pregnancy: prenatal diagnosis and management of fetal complications. *Curr Opin Obstet Gynecol*. 2012; 24(2): 95–101. doi: 10.1097/GCO.0b013e3283505a9d

126. Zellman GL. (2014). Erythema infectiosum. In: Elston DM, ed. Medscape. http://emedicine.medscape.com/article/1132078-overview#showall. Updated September 15, 2014. Accessed May 26, 2015.

127. Jordan JA. Clinical manifestations and pathogenesis of human parvovirus B19 infection. In: Basow DS, ed. *UpToDate*. Waltham, MA: UpToDate; 2015. http://www.uptodate.com/contents/clinical-manifestations-and-pathogenesis-of-human-parvovirus-b19-infection?source=search_result&search=erythema+infectiosum&selectedTitle=1~30. Updated December 15, 2014. Accessed May 26, 2015.

128. Pagana KD. *Mosby's Manual of Diagnostic and Laboratory Tests.* 5th ed. Philadelphia, PA: Elsevier Mosby; 2014.

129. Porth C. *Essentials of Pathophysiology: Concepts of Altered Health States.* 3rd ed. Philadelphia, PA: Wolters Kluwer Health/ Lippincott Williams & Wilkins; 2011.

130. Tremblay C, Brady MT. Human herpesvirus 6 infection in children: Clinical manifestations; diagnosis; and treatment. In: Basow DS, ed. *UpToDate*. Waltham, MA: UpToDate; 2015. http://www.uptodate.com/contents/human-herpesvirus-6-infection-in-children-clinical-manifestations-diagnosis-and-treatment?source=search_result&search=roseola+infantum+children&selectedTitle=2~150#H11. Updated January 7, 2015. Accessed May 26, 2015.

131. Gorman CR. Roseola infantum: Treatment & management. In: James WD, ed. Medscape. http://emedicine.medscape.com/article/1133023-treatment#showall. Updated October 13, 2014. Accessed May 26, 2015.

132. Davis CP. Coxsackie virus. In: Shiel WC Jr, ed. eMedicine Health. http://www.medicinenet.com/coxsackie_virus/article.htm. Updated July 11, 2014. Accessed May 26, 2015.

133. United States Department of Health and Human Services, Centers for Disease Control and Prevention. About hand, foot, and mouth disease (HFMD). http://www.cdc.gov/hand-foot-mouth/about/index.html. Updated July 7, 2014. Accessed May 26, 2015.

134. Romero JR. Hand, foot, and mouth disease and herpangina: An overview. In: Basow DS, ed. *UpToDate*. Waltham, MA: UpToDate; 2015. http://www.uptodate.com/contents/hand-foot-and-mouth-disease-and-herpangina-an-overview?source=-search_result&search=coxsackievirus&selectedTitle=2~70#H456270554. Updated December 2, 2014. Accessed May 26, 2015.

135. Hand-foot-mouth disease. A.D.A.M. Medical Encyclopedia Web site. http://www.nlm.nih.gov/medlineplus/ency/article/000965.htm. Updated August 18, 2013. Accessed May 26, 2015.

136. Modlin JF. Clinical manifestations and diagnosis of enterovirus and parechovirus infections. In: Basow DS, ed. *UpToDate*. Waltham, MA: UpToDate; 2015. http://www.uptodate.com/contents/clinical-manifestations-and-diagnosis-of-enterovirus-and-parechovirus-infections?-source=search_result&search=coxsackievirus&selectedTitle=1~70#H5882578. Updated October 7, 2014. Accessed May 26, 2015.

137. Nervi SJ, Schwartz RA, Kapila R. Hand-foot-and-mouth disease. In: Bronze MS, ed. Medscape. http://emedicine.medscape.com/article/218402-overview#showall. Updated June 10, 2014. Accessed May 26, 2015.

138. Balentine JR. Encephalitis and meningitis. In: Shiel WC Jr, ed. eMedicine Health. http://www.medicinenet.com/encephalitis_and_meningitis/article.htm. Updated February 10, 2015. Accessed May 26, 2015.

Chapter 12

Eye, Ear, Nose, and Throat Disorders

QUESTIONS

1. A 2-year-old is brought to your clinic presenting with red, irritated eyes. The mother says the symptoms manifested after they had visited a public swimming pool the day prior. Upon examination, you see no discharge. The child does not indicate any pain, only an itching sensation. You tell the mother that the condition is self-limiting, and you proceed with a normal saline flush on the patient's eyes. Which is the most likely diagnosis?

   a. Bacterial conjunctivitis

   b. Hordeolum

   c. Chemical conjunctivitis

   d. Viral conjunctivitis

2. Which of the following is most likely to be caused by *Chlamydia trachomatis*?

   a. Pharyngitis

   b. Croup

   c. Infectious mononucleosis

   d. Epiglottitis

3. Which of the following statements is most true regarding sinusitis in young children?

   a. Sinusitis occurs in children beginning at 6 years of age or older.

   b. Sinusitis is distinguished from acute otitis media by its typical pathogens.

   c. Radiological studies are the most common method of confirming a diagnosis.

   d. The paranasal sinuses are the most commonly affected sinuses.

4. A patient reports to your clinic with intense fatigue and a fever. Suspecting infectious mononucleosis, you begin a physical exam. Which of the following signs is <u>not</u> consistent with the common presentation of this condition?

   a. White exudate on the tonsils

   b. Generalized lymphadenopathy

   c. Discolored nasal discharge

   d. Petechial rash

5. Of the following, which eye disorder is characterized by an abrupt or sudden onset with painful swelling on the lid margin?

   a. Hordeolum

   b. Strabismus

   c. Conjunctivitis

   d. Chalazion

6. All of the following are viral causes of pharyngitis and tonsillitis <u>except</u>:

   a. Mumps virus

   b. Respiratory syncytial virus

   c. Influenza A and B

   d. Epstein-Barr virus

7. Which of the following conditions does <u>not</u> have a bacterial etiology?

   a. Epiglottitis

   b. Infectious mononucleosis

   c. Acute otitis media

   d. Conjunctivitis

8. Which of the following pathogens is most commonly responsible for epiglottitis?

   a. *Neisseria gonorrhoeae*

   b. *Streptococcus pneumoniae*

   c. *Moraxella catarrhalis*

   d. *Haemophilus influenzae*

9. Which of the following best distinguishes epiglottitis from croup?

   a. Epiglottitis presents with fever, whereas croup does not.

   b. Epiglottitis targets children between 3 months and 6 years of age, whereas croup usually presents in children 6–10 years of age.

   c. An x-ray for epiglottitis will show a thumb sign, whereas an x-ray for croup will show a steeple sign.

   d. Epiglottitis is entirely bacterial in nature, whereas croup is entirely viral.

10. Of the following, which form of conjunctivitis most often presents with watery discharge?

    a. Bacterial

    b. Viral

    c. Gonococcal

    d. Allergic

RATIONALES

1. c

Because the patient was treated with a normal saline flush and no discharge was present at the site, the most likely diagnosis is chemical conjunctivitis. Bacterial conjunctivitis, as well as viral conjunctivitis, can be self-limiting as well; however, purulent discharge accompanies bacterial conjunctivitis, and watery discharge typically accompanies viral conjunctivitis. The child's findings do not indicate a hordeolum, which presents with an abscess and is typically accompanied by pain, edema, and abrupt onset of symptoms.

2. a

Of the four choices, pharyngitis, or tonsillitis, is most likely caused by *Chlamydia trachomatis*. Common pathogens for epiglottitis include *Streptococci*, *Pneumococci*, and *Haemophilus influenzae*, but not *C. trachomatis*. Croup and infectious mononucleosis are both primarily caused by viral infections, rather than bacterial infections. Croup is mostly caused by parainfluenza, whereas infectious mononucleosis is caused by the Epstein-Barr virus.

3. d

In young children, the two sinuses most commonly affected by sinusitis are two of the paranasal sinuses: the maxillary and ethmoid sinuses. Sinusitis can occur in children younger than 6 years of age because the ethmoid and maxillary sinuses are present at birth. Sinusitis cannot be distinguished from acute otitis media (AOM) by its typical pathogens, as sinusitis shares the same typical pathogens with AOM, such as *Streptococcus pneumoniae*, *Haemophilus influenzae*, and *Moraxella catarrhalis*. Radiological studies are not commonly used to confirm a diagnosis in uncomplicated presentations of sinusitis, which is often diagnosed on clinical presentation. When imaging is required, CT scans are favored over standard x-rays, as a CT scan is more sensitive and equal in price.

4. c

Discolored nasal discharge is a presentation of sinusitis, not infectious mononucleosis. A petechial or maculopapular rash, white exudate on the tonsils, and generalized lymphadenopathy are all physical findings of infectious mononucleosis.

5. a

Of the choices, hordeolum is the only eye disorder that presents abruptly with painful swelling. Symptoms associated with strabismus, conjunctivitis, and cataracts develop over time. Strabismus is an ocular misalignment and does not normally cause painful swelling. Conjunctivitis has various types according to etiology; some types, such as allergic and bacterial conjunctivitis, can appear abruptly, but swelling is not typically painful with conjunctivitis as it is with hordeolum. Lastly, chalazia are typically not painful and usually occur inside the eyelid, rather than on the lid margin.

6. a

Although the mumps virus belongs to the same family as parainfluenza, which can produce pharyngitis and tonsillitis, it produces neither condition; the virus affects the salivary glands, genitals, and nervous system, rather than the throat and pharynx. The respiratory syncytial virus, Epstein-Barr virus, and influenza A and B are all viral causes of pharyngitis and tonsillitis.

7. b

Infectious mononucleosis is caused by the Epstein-Barr virus; thus, it does not have a bacterial etiology. Epiglottitis can be caused by a bacterial infection, with the most common pathogens being *Haemophilus influenzae* and members of the *Streptococci* and *Pneumococci* genera. *Streptococcus pneumoniae* and *H. influenzae* are the pathogens most commonly responsible for acute otitis media. Chlamydial and gonococcal pathogens can cause conjunctivitis.

8. d

Epiglottitis is most often caused by *Haemophilus influenzae* infection; as such, the number of cases has dropped in recent years due to widespread implementation of the *H. influenza* type B vaccine. *Moraxella catarrhalis* can be a bacterial cause of epiglottitis; however, the pathogen is more commonly associated with sinusitis. *Neisseria gonorrhoeae* is more likely to cause pharyngitis. *Streptococcus pneumoniae* does not typically produce epiglottitis but may produce conjunctivitis and sinusitis.

9. c

X-rays may be used to distinguish epiglottitis from croup; the former condition manifests as a thumb sign, whereas the latter condition manifests as a steeple sign upon x-ray. Both conditions can present with fever, and although patients with croup are typically afebrile, there are some manifestations of the condition, such as laryngotracheitis, that tend to produce fever. Epiglottitis produces high-grade fever in over half of all cases. Although croup is most commonly a viral infection, it may also be caused by bacteria, which results in bacterial tracheitis. Further, epiglottitis may be caused by bacterial or viral etiologies. Epiglottitis most often affects children 6–10 years of age, whereas croup affects children between 3 months and 6 years of age.

10. b

Of the choices, viral conjunctivitis most often presents with watery discharge. Bacterial conjunctivitis, along with gonococcal conjunctivitis, can present with purulent, not watery, discharge. With allergic conjunctivitis, patients may experience increased tearing, but the discharge is stringy, not watery.

DISCUSSION

Hordeolum (Stye)

Overview

Hordeolum, or stye, is a common type of staphylococcal abscess that presents on the upper or lower eyelid.[1]

Presentation

Styes typically have an abrupt onset with localized pain and edema. The eyelid is often extremely tender, and the amount of pain is usually proportional to the amount of edema.[2]

Workup

Differential diagnoses for a stye include conjunctivitis, chalazion, blepharitis, or dacryocystitis.[3] Before diagnosing a stye, the health care practitioner should closely examine the pediatric patient's general health to ensure that no other health conditions are complicating the diagnosis.[4] Generally, a diagnosis can be made by examining the patient's eyelid.

Treatment

Styes can be managed with warm compresses and antibiotics, such as topical bacitracin or erythromycin ophthalmic ointment. For severe cases, the nurse practitioner (NP) may refer the pediatric patient to an ophthalmologist for possible incision and drainage.[5]

Chalazion

Overview

A chalazion is a granulomatous nodule that slowly develops, blocks the oil gland in the eyelid, and causes swelling. This condition develops from an infection or retention cyst of the meibomian gland.[3]

Chalazia are more common in adults but may occur in children as well.[6] Sometimes chalazia appear due to an internal hordeolum that does not drain or resolve.[3] Unlike styes, chalazia are usually painless.

Presentation

Although often asymptomatic, signs and symptoms of a chalazion may include red conjunctiva, eyelid swelling, light sensitivity, itching, visual distortion, and increased tearing. If the chalazion pushes against the eye, the patient may also experience blurred vision due to pressure exerted on the cornea.[7]

Workup

Chalazia may be quite small and initially confused with styes. Other eye conditions may resemble a chalazion, including conjunctivitis, blepharitis, or dacryocystitis.[3] In order to diagnose a stye, the health care practitioner should closely examine the pediatric patient's eyelid, noting the lid structure, skin texture, and eyelash appearance. A patient history should also be conducted.[8]

Treatment

Chalazia can be treated with a warm compress.[3] A pediatric patient with a persistent chalazion should be referred to an ophthalmologist for possible surgical removal.

Conjunctivitis

Overview

Conjunctivitis (i.e., pink eye) is the most common eye disorder. Conjunctivitis is an inflammation of the conjunctiva. It may result from a variety of causes, such as allergies, chemical irritation, or bacterial or viral infection.[9]

Presentation

Signs and symptoms of conjunctivitis include inflammation, redness, irritation, itching, burning, increased tears, blurred vision, eyelid swelling, foreign body sensation, and discharge. The type of discharge that presents can often aid in distinguishing between variants of conjunctivitis. Both bacterial and gonococcal conjunctivitis may present with purulent discharge, but the discharge is typically more copious in cases of gonococcal infection. Watery discharge may indicate viral conjunctivitis, whereas stringy discharge and increased tearing may indicate allergic conjunctivitis.[10]

Workup

Because conjunctivitis has a variety of causes, a health care practitioner must identify the etiology in order to appropriately treat the condition. Viral conjunctivitis is often diagnosed based on clinical features alone. Severe cases may warrant culture and smear. Gram stains help to identify bacterial characteristics, whereas Giemsa stains help identify chlamydial bodies.[11,12] Bacterial cultures on blood and chocolate agar, along with a Gram stain and polymerase chain reaction assay, are indicated in neonatal cases.[13]

Treatment

As previously indicated, the proper identification of etiology of conjunctivitis is vital for appropriate management. See table 12.1 for treatment considerations for each type of conjunctivitis infection.

Cataracts

Overview

Cataracts are an abnormal, uniform, progressive opacity of the eye. Children with this condition most likely have comorbidities such as Down syndrome, diabetes mellitus, Marfan syndrome, or atopic dermatitis.[14] Cataracts may be congenital as a result of prolonged steroid use, trauma, undernutrition, or radiation.[15]

Presentation

Cataracts are painless, and pediatric patients typically present with decreased visual acuity; cloudy, blurred, dim vision; white reflex; poor visual fixation; and photophobia.[16]

Table 12.1 Treatment Considerations for Conjunctivitis

Type	Discharge	Treatment Considerations
Bacterial	Purulent; thick; white, yellow, or green; mostly at lid margins and corners of eyes[14]	1) Erythromycin ophthalmic ointment 2) Bacitracin ointment 3) Sulfacetamide ointment 4) Bacitracin-polymyxin B ointment[14]
Gonococcal (ophthalmic emergency)	Purulent; profuse exudate; swollen eyelids[15]	1) Hospitalization 2) Ceftriaxone, 25–50 mg/kg IV or IM, or 3) Cefotaxime, 100 mg/kg IV or IM (preferred if hyperbilirubinemia is present) 4) Frequent saline irrigation[15]
Chlamydial	Mild swelling of eyelids with mucopurulent, watery discharge; marked swelling of eyelids with thick, red conjunctivae[16]	1) Oral erythromycin, 50 mg/kg/day for 14 days, or 2) Oral azithromycin, 20 mg/kg/day for 3 days[16]
Allergic	Bilateral redness; watery; itchy; may have morning crusting[14]	1) Topical antihistamines with mast cell stabilizers 2) Topical antihistamine/vasoconstrictors 3) Refer to allergist/ophthalmologist in refractory cases[17]
Viral	Watery; may have morning crusting; occasional scants of mucous throughout the day; burning, sandy feeling in one eye[14]	1) Symptomatic: 2) Nonantibiotic lubricating agents 3) Topical antihistamine/decongestants[14]

Used with permission from Barkley TW Jr. Eyes, ears, nose, and throat issues and disorders. In: *Pediatric Primary Care Nurse Practitioner Certification Review/Clinical Update Continuing Education Course*. West Hollywood, CA: Barkley and Associates; 2015: 109–124.

Workup

In order to diagnose an infant or child with cataracts, the NP must consider the patient's medical history and ascertain if the patient has any systemic diseases that may cause cataracts. Laboratory and diagnostic tests may be unnecessary. If cataracts are indicated, the health care practitioner should refer the pediatric patient to an ophthalmologist.[15]

Treatment

Some cataracts that occur in infants do not need to be removed because the pediatric patient's vision will eventually develop normally. However, cataracts that continue to interfere with a child's vision must be surgically removed by an ophthalmologist.[17]

Strabismus

Overview

Strabismus is an ocular misalignment that results from uncoordinated ocular muscles. If strabismus is acquired after 6 months of age, the condition is usually related to underlying problems such as cerebral palsy, Down syndrome, hydrocephalus, or brain tumors.[16]

Presentation

Signs and symptoms of strabismus may include squinting; decreased visual acuity; head tilt; face-turning; inward deviation of the eyes (i.e., esotropia); outward deviation of the eyes (i.e., exotropia); upward deviation of the eyes (i.e., hypertropia); downward deviation of the eyes (i.e., hypotropia); and an unequal Hirschberg papillary light reflex.[18]

Workup

If a pediatric patient presents with strabismus, an NP should conduct a thorough examination of the eyes. Indications for referral to an ophthalmologist include strabismus that is fixed or continuous at 6 months of age or later; hypertropia or hypotropia; or signs that an underlying condition is the cause of strabismus.[19]

Treatment

Treatment for strabismus may include contact lenses, eyeglasses, or eye exercises. Patching may be required if amblyopia is also present. In some cases, surgical alignment of the eyes may be necessary.[19]

Otitis Externa (Swimmer's Ear)

Overview

Otitis externa is an inflammation of the external auditory canal or auricle. Though this condition is usually caused by a bacterial infection, the origin may also be viral or fungal. This condition occurs in all age groups, though children's narrow ear canals put them at increased risk. Recent water exposure is another risk factor because the retained water prevents not only drying, but removal of cerumen from the ear. Other causes of otitis externa include mechanical trauma, a foreign body in the ear, or excess cerumen.[20,21]

Presentation

Signs and symptoms of otitis externa include otalgia, pruritus, and purulent discharge.[20] Ear canal erythema, edema, purulent exudate, or pain upon manipulation of the auricle may also occur.

Workup

Diagnosis is based on a history and physical exam. Cultures should be obtained only in severe or recalcitrant cases of otitis externa.[22]

Treatment

In treating otitis externa, NSAIDs or corticosteroid ear drops may be administered to remedy inflammation. For otitis externa limited to the ear canal and not extending to adjacent tissues, topical antibiotics—or antifungals, if warranted—are the standard of care. In severe cases of malignant otitis externa, hospitalization is required; intravenous antibiotics are commonly administered, and surgery may be indicated. It is recommended that the patient keep the ear dry for 7-10 days, substitute showers for baths, and refrain from using earplugs or hearing aids until healed.[21]

Acute Otitis Media (AOM)

Overview

Acute otitis media (AOM) is a bacterial infection of the middle ear.[23] Although AOM may occur at any age, it is most prevalent in infants and young children. Between 60% –80% of all infants experience AOM in their first year, with 80%–90% experiencing it in their first 3 years. Risk factors include family history, lack of breastfeeding, exposure to tobacco smoke and air pollution, and pacifier use. Though viral infection is possible, AOM is more commonly caused by the bacteria *Streptococcus pneumoniae*, *Haemophilus influenzae*, or *Moraxella catarrhalis*.[24]

Presentation

Signs and symptoms of AOM include decreased hearing, otalgia, fever, aural pressure, vertigo, and nausea or vomiting. Other physical findings may include an erythematous and edematous tympanic membrane, purulent exudate from the ear, and the appearance of a bulging tympanic membrane. Impaired mobility of the tympanic membrane is another common indicator for AOM.[24]

Workup

In order to test for AOM, an NP should conduct a physical exam and diagnostic tests. A pneumatic otoscopy or a tympanometry test should be conducted to assess the status of the tympanic membrane; these measures will also help to confirm AOM and differentiate it from otitis media with effusion.[23]

Treatment

Pediatric patients may be administered acetaminophen to manage the pain associated with AOM. Benzocaine otic drops can be used for pain relief if the tympanic membrane has not perforated. These drops should only be used for 24–48 hours, as the pain should be decreased by then, and prolonged use can mask progressing symptoms. Otherwise, healthy children with the disorder should be observed. If the condition persists, amoxicillin can be administered orally at 80–90 mg/kg/day, twice daily. Cephalosporins may be administered to children with a delayed response penicillin allergy, whereas macrolides and lincosamides may be administered to children with an immediate responding penicillin allergy.[25]

AOM may be prevented by the *H. influenzae* type B and pneumococcal conjugate vaccines, as well as by annual flu vaccinations. Parents should also ensure that their children are not exposed to second-hand smoke, as there is an association between increased AOM and smoke exposure.[26]

Otitis Media with Effusion (OME)/ Serous Otitis Media

Overview

Otitis media with effusion (OME), or serous otitis media, is the buildup of fluid in the middle ears without infection. The fluid may build up as a result of allergies or respiratory infection. Although this condition can occur at any age, it is most common in children younger than 3 years of age due to their increased incidence of upper respiratory tract infections. Additionally, eustachian tubes are smaller and more horizontally aligned in children than in adults, making drainage more difficult. OME is most prevalent during the winter.[27]

Presentation

Unlike AOM, OME is mostly asymptomatic, although children may experience mild hearing loss, a popping sensation when pressure is altered, or a feeling of fullness in the ear.[28]

Workup

When a pediatric patient presents with symptoms of OME, a health care practitioner should conduct a physical exam. OME will typically present with opacity, impaired mobility of the tympanic membrane, bubbles, or an air fluid level. Furthermore, acute signs or symptoms should be absent, as these symptoms would more traditionally indicate AOM.[28] For prolonged cases of OME, especially in young children developing language abilities, audiometry to check for hearing loss would be indicated for lack of resolution after about four to six weeks.[29]

Treatment

Pediatric patients with OME should be monitored for 3 months. If fluid has not resolved by 3 months, pneumoeustacian tubes will typically be inserted to allow the fluid to drain, optimize normal hearing, and consequently improve verbal acquisition skills. Pediatric patients with OME should be re-evaluated 6 months after the first evaluation.[30]

Hearing Loss

Overview

Hearing loss is any degree of impairment in the ability to perceive sound, and may be conductive, sensorineural, or central.[31,32] Conductive hearing loss is characterized by the decreased ability to conduct sound from the external ear to inner ear. The most common causes of conductive hearing loss are cerumen impaction and middle ear fluid. Sensorineural hearing loss is characterized by problems of the inner ear, usually occurring at the cochlea, eighth cranial nerve, internal auditory canal, or the brain. Central hearing loss is the misperception of auditory information due to flaws in the central auditory nervous system or auditory nerve.[32]

Presentation

Pediatric patients with hearing loss should undergo both the Weber test and Rinne test (see table 12.1). The Weber test assesses if a pediatric patient hears sound equally in both ears and not laterally, whereas the Rinne test evaluates whether the patient's air conduction (AC) of sound is greater than bone conduction (BC) of sound.[33] The Weber test indicates conductive hearing loss if sound lateralizes to the affected ear; if the sound lateralizes to the unaffected ear, sensorineural hearing loss is indicated instead. A Rinne test presents normal results in the affected ear in cases of sensorineural hearing loss; in conductive hearing loss, however, the results of the Rinne test are abnormal in the affected ear, indicating that AC may be less than BC. [33]

Workup

An NP can administer a variety of diagnostic tests and labs to determine if hearing loss is present and possibly even determine the etiology. An otoscopic exam can be conducted to evaluate mobility of the tympanic membrane. Diminished mobility may indicate fluid or a mass in the middle ear cavity. Increased mobility may indicate ossicular chain disruption. Audiometric testing determines the softest decibel threshold a patient can hear. The test can be performed in an office but may fail to detect mild hearing loss. A complete neurological exam should be conducted to test for neurologic deficits. If a neurologic condition is suspected, a computerized tomography (CT) scan of the temporal bone and internal auditory meatus should be obtained. Finally, serum blood tests and tests for congenital infection should be obtained as warranted.[33]

Treatment

Treatment for hearing loss depends on etiology. Some causes of hearing loss are surgically correctable, such as hearing loss due to benign growths or malignant tumors. Amplification devices, such as hearing aids, are helpful for many people. Patients may benefit from hearing aids that either selectively amplify high frequencies or perform simple amplification. In those cases where traditional hearing aids are ineffective, bone conduction hearing aids and cochlear implants may be used. Children with permanent hearing loss should be managed by a multidisciplinary team of experts.[34]

Common Cold

Overview

The common cold occurs in the upper respiratory tract and is characterized as a self-limiting viral infection. Rhinoviruses are responsible for up to 50% of all colds in adults and children. Respiratory syncytial, influenza, parainfluenza, and adenoviruses are other common causes of colds in preschool children.[35]

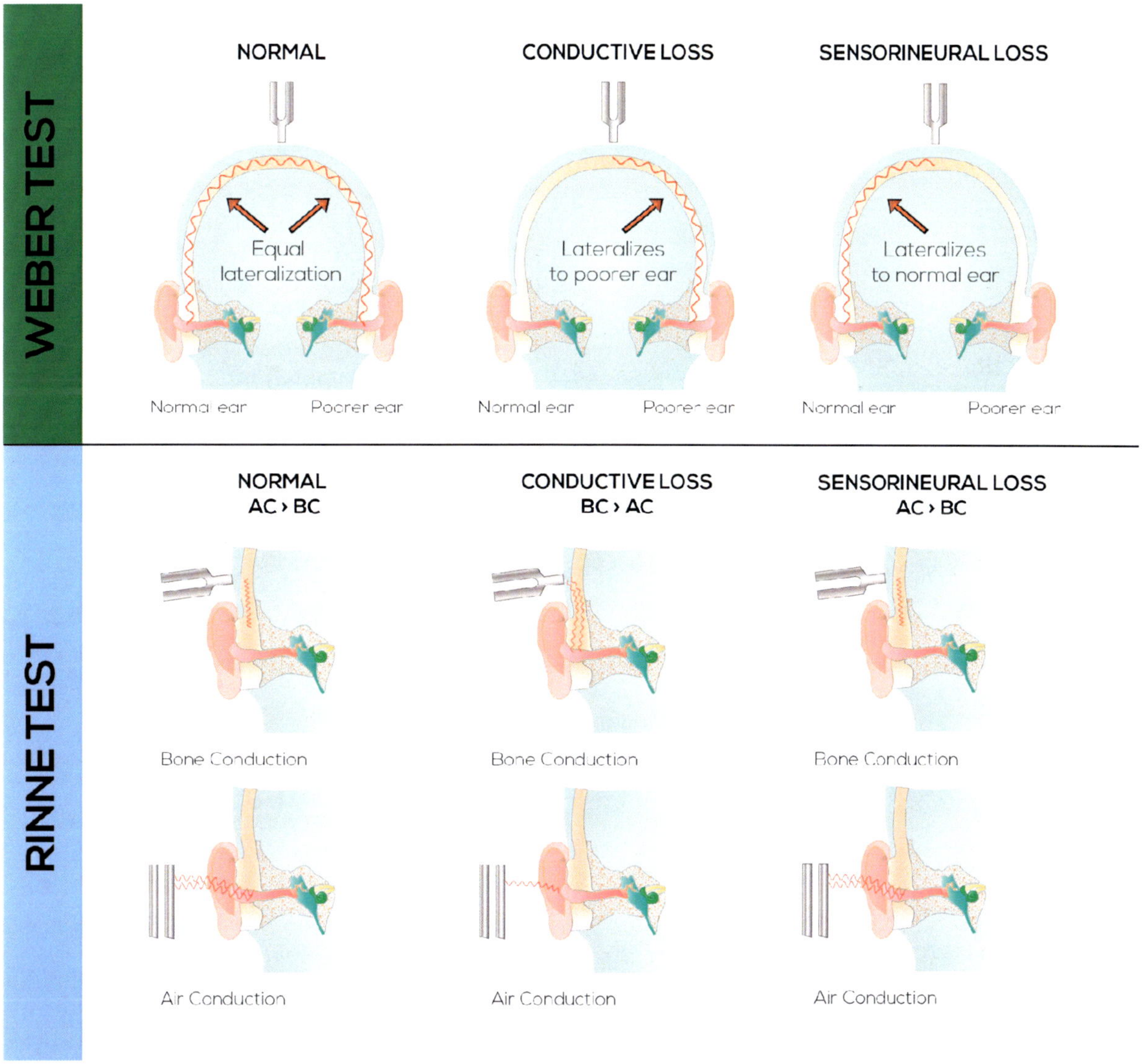

Figure 12.1. Weber and Rinne hearing loss tests.

Presentation

Symptoms of a common cold may include headache, rhinorrhea, sore throat, coughing, sneezing, and fever.[36]

Workup

To diagnose a common cold, a health care practitioner must conduct a physical exam focusing on the eyes, ears, nose, and throat, as well as determine the recent history of the patient. Based on physical exam findings, the health care practitioner can rule out other possible infections or illnesses that have similar symptoms to the common cold, such as influenza or sinusitis.[35]

Treatment

Treatment of the common cold is generally limited to supportive care. The NP should advise patients to rest and stay hydrated. Nasal saline drops and a humidifier can also provide some relief. Antibiotics should not be prescribed, and patients should be educated that time will alleviate the symptoms.[37]

Epistaxis (Nosebleed)

Overview

Epistaxis, commonly known as a nosebleed, involves bleeding from the inside of the nose.[38]

Presentation

Nosebleeds usually occur in one nostril.[38] Nosebleeds can result in an upset stomach due to drainage from the back of the throat into the stomach.

Workup

Nosebleeds are diagnosed by observation or evaluation of the pediatric patient's symptoms. Nosebleeds are typically caused from dryness, nose-picking, upper respiratory infections, or sinus complications. Frequent or prolonged nosebleeds may require an evaluation for a bleeding disorder.[38]

Treatment

In order to manage a nosebleed, the pediatric patient must sit upright, and the patient or parent must apply pressure for 10 minutes at Kiesselbach's triangle, which is the anterior inferior aspect of the nasal septum—the end of the bony ridge.[39] Ice should also be applied.[16] When compression is unsuccessful, cautery, matrix sealant, fibrin glue, or nasal packing may be used.

Pharyngitis/Tonsillitis

Overview

Pharyngitis is inflammation of the pharynx, whereas tonsillitis is inflammation of the tonsils. Pharyngitis and tonsillitis can occur at the same time or separately. Viruses such as respiratory syncytial virus, influenza A or B, or Epstein Barr virus are among the main causes of pharyngitis and tonsillitis. These conditions can also be caused by bacteria such as group A β-hemolytic *Streptococci* (GABHS), *Neisseria gonorrhoeae*, *Mycoplasma*, *Chlamydia trachomatis*, and *Corynebacterium*.[40]

Presentation

Pediatric patients with either condition typically present with the following symptoms: erythematous pharynx, dysphagia and cough, malaise, rhinorrhea, anterior cervical adenopathy, painful throat, and exudate. Fever may or may not be present.[41]

Workup

Diagnosing pharyngitis or tonsillitis does not typically require any routine testing. Numerous studies have shown that clinical judgment is not effective in determining if a sore throat is streptococcal pharyngitis or not. Consequently, a rapid strep test should be obtained. If the test is negative, a throat culture should be obtained and the patient should be treated appropriately.

Treatment

Treating pharyngitis or tonsillitis often requires supportive care measures, such as hydration, warm salt water gargles, and antipyretics. If a bacterial infection is present, antibiotics should be prescribed.[42] Penicillin VK, 250 mg orally, 3 times daily, for 10 days is the treatment of choice; however, this treatment tastes terrible, often making it a challenge to obtain compliance from pediatric patients. Amoxicillin, 45 mg/kg/day, is an acceptable alternative to prevent rheumatic complications of streptococcal A infection. For patients who are allergic to penicillin, erythromycin at 250 mg, 4 times daily, for 10 days is also commonly prescribed.[41]

Epiglottitis

Overview

Epiglottitis is a sudden and severe swelling of the epiglottis. The majority of pediatric cases are caused by *H. influenzae* type b, although *Streptococci* and *Staphylococcus aureus* may cause epiglottitis as well.[43]

Presentation

Pediatric patients with epiglottitis often present with a sudden onset of high fever, drooling, dysphagia, a restless and fearful state, and rapidly progressive signs of respiratory distress. Patients often prefer to sit, hyperextending their necks in an attempt to open the obstructed airway.[43]

Workup

Lab tests for epiglottitis include blood and tracheal cultures to determine the causative organism. A radiograph of the neck often shows a thumb-shaped patch, or "thumb sign."[44]

Treatment

Epiglottitis requires immediate hospitalization. Keeping the child calm is very important, and preparation for emergent intubation must be expedited in order to avoid cardiopulmonary arrest.[43,45] Intravenous third-generation cephalosporins should be started while waiting for culture verification of the offending pathogen.[46]

Croup

Overview

Croup is a parainfluenza viral infection of the larynx. The severity of this illness can range from mild to severe.[47] Croup affects males more often than females, with a peak incidence in pediatric patients occurring between the ages of 3 months and 6 years. Additionally, cases of croup are more common in the fall and winter.[48]

Presentation

Signs and symptoms of croup include a recent upper respiratory infection, a bark-like cough, a low-grade fever, dyspnea, and, in severe cases, stridor. Cyanosis may present late and is often indicative of impending respiratory failure.[49]

Workup

Croup is often diagnosed clinically, based on the physical examination and history of the patient. A pulse oximetry reading may be obtained to determine the child's oxygenation status, and x-rays may be obtained to differentiate croup from epiglottitis. However, neither of these measures confirms a diagnosis of croup.[50]

Treatment

The severity of croup must first be determined before treatment can begin. Corticosteroids or epinephrine may be used to reduce inflammation, though corticosteroids, such as dexamethasone, are preferred for more long-lasting effects.[49] Severe cases of croup require hospitalization and may require intubation.[51,52]

Infectious Mononucleosis

Overview

Infectious mononucleosis (mono) is an acute infectious disease that is caused by the Epstein-Barr virus and usually occurs in children older than the age of 10 years. Mono is transmitted via saliva and usually lasts about one month. The condition is usually self-limiting, but malaise and fatigue may endure for several months.[53]

Presentation

Fever, sore throat, swollen lymph nodes, and extreme fatigue are the typical presenting signs and symptoms of mono. A physical exam may reveal white tonsillar exudate and a maculopapular or petechial rash. Splenomegaly or hepatosplenomegaly, as well as jaundice, may also occur.[54]

Workup

Mono is often diagnosed clinically, based upon a physical examination that confirms the presence of the signs and symptoms listed above.[54] Lab tests should also be conducted to look for lymphocytic leukocytosis, neutropenia, an early rise in immunoglobulin M, and a permanent rise in immunoglobulin G. A positive heterophil antibody test or monospot test will also help to confirm a diagnosis.[53,55]

Treatment

Mono can be managed with supportive care, including NSAIDs and warm saline gargles.[56] Patients with strep throat should be prescribed penicillin or erythromycin instead of amoxicillin or ampicillin because amoxicillin and ampicillin often cause a rash in mono patients. In order to avoid splenic rupture, contact sports should be avoided for 3 weeks to several months, even in cases where splenomegaly is not clinically detectable.[57]

Sinusitis (Rhinosinusitis)

Overview

Sinusitis, also known as rhinosinusitis, occurs when one or more of the sinuses that drain into the nose become inflamed. The maxillary and ethmoid sinuses are the most commonly affected sinuses in patients with sinusitis. Sinusitis is most often caused by viral infections, such as the common cold.[58]

Presentation

Signs and symptoms of sinusitis include pain and pressure over the cheek, headache, and halitosis. Sinusitis also commonly presents with purulent postnasal drip and cough, usually occurring during the day and sometimes exacerbated at night. Additionally, patients may experience a dull, throbbing pain that worsens when the patient's head is in a dependent position.[59]

Workup

Diagnosis of sinusitis is often determined according to clinical presentation, especially when symptoms have lasted longer than 7–10 days. In some patients, the NP may need to order a CT scan to confirm the diagnosis.[59]

Treatment

Antibiotic therapy should be provided for children with a severe onset or worsening condition; amoxicillin with or without clavulanate is the typical first-line treatment.[60] For uncomplicated sinusitis with mild symptoms, pediatric patients should be treated as outpatients. Decongestants and antihistamines are not useful for acute sinusitis, but may be helpful for chronic sinusitis. The pain associated with sinusitis can be managed with acetaminophen. To reduce mucosal drying, nighttime humidification and supportive care can be used. In cases of chronic, refractory, or recurrent sinusitis, the patient should be referred to an otolaryngologist.[60]

Figures

Figure 12.1. Weber and Rinne hearing loss tests. Barkley & Associates, Inc. Published 2015.

References

1. Mayo Clinic Staff. Stye: definition. Mayo Clinic Web site. http://www.mayoclinic.com/health/sty/DS00257. Updated June 13, 2012. Accessed April 19, 2015.

2. Mayo Clinic Staff Sty: symptoms. Mayo Clinic Web site. http://www.mayoclinic.org/diseases-conditions/sty/basics/symptoms/con-20022698. Updated June 13, 2012. Accessed April 19, 2015.

3. Ghosh C, Ghosh T. Eyelid lesions. In: Basow DS, ed. *UpToDate*. Waltham, MA: UpToDate; 2015. http://www.uptodate.com/contents/eyelid-lesions. Last updated September 27, 2013. Accessed April 19, 2015.

4. Testing & diagnosis for stye (hordeolum) in children. Boston Children's Hospital Web site. http://www.childrenshospital.org/conditions-and-treatments/conditions/s/stye-hordeolum/testing-and-diagnosis. Accessed April 19, 2015.

5. Lindsley K, Nichols JJ, Dickersin K. Interventions for acute internal hordeolum. *Cochrane Database Syst Rev.* 2013; 4. doi: 10.1002/14651858.CD007742.pub3

6. Deschênes J, Fansler JL, Plouznikoff A. Chalazion. In: Roy H Sr, ed. Medscape. http://emedicine.medscape.com/article/1212709-overview#showall. Updated October 31, 2014. Accessed April 19, 2015.

7. Deschênes J, Fansler JL, Plouznikoff A. Chalazion clinical presentation. In: Roy H Sr, ed. Medscape. http://emedicine.medscape.com/article/1212709-clinical#showall. Updated October 31, 2014. Accessed April 19, 2015.

8. Chalazion. American Optometric Association Web site. http://www.aoa.org/patients-and-public/eye-and-vision-problems/glossary-of-eye-and-vision-conditions/chalazion?sso=y. Accessed April 19, 2015.

9. Azari AA, Barney NP. Conjunctivitis: A systematic review of diagnosis and treatment. *JAMA.* 2013; 310(16): 1721–1729. doi: 10.1001/jama.2013.280318

10. Conjunctivitis (pink eye). Centers for Disease Control and Prevention Web site. http://www.cdc.gov/conjunctivitis/about/symptoms.html. Last reviewed January 9, 2014. Accessed April 19, 2015.

11. Scott IU, Luu K. Viral conjunctivitis workup. In: Roy H Sr, ed. Medscape. http://emedicine.medscape.com/article/1191370-workup#showall. Updated May 2, 2014. Accessed April 19, 2015.

12. Yeung KK, Weissman BA, De Shazer ME. Bacterial conjunctivitis workup. In: Roy H Sr, ed. Medscape. http://emedicine.medscape.com/article/1191730-workup#showall. Updated March 27, 2014. Accessed April 19, 2015.

13. McCourt EA, Enzenauer RW, Jatla KK, Zhao F. Neonatal conjunctivitis workup. In: Roy H Sr, ed. Medscape. http://emedicine.medscape.com/article/1192190-workup#showall. Updated February 20, 2014. Accessed April 19, 2015.

14. McCreery KM. Cataract in children. In: Basow DS, ed. *UpToDate*. Waltham, MA: UpToDate; 2015. www.uptodate.com/contents/cataract-in-children. Last updated March 4, 2015. Accessed April 19, 2015.

15. Colby K. Cataract. In: Porter RS, Kaplan JL, eds. The Merck Manual Online. http://www.merckmanuals.com/professional/eye_disorders/cataract/cataract.html. Last reviewed July 2014. Accessed April 19, 2015.

16. Barkley TW Jr. Eyes, ears, nose, and throat issues and disorders. In: *Pediatric Primary Care Nurse Practitioner Certification Review/Clinical Update Continuing Education Course*. West Hollywood, CA: Barkley and Associates; 2015: 109–124.

17. Bashour M, Menassa J, Cerontis CC. Congenital cataract treatment & management: Surgical care. In: Roy H Sr, ed. Medscape. http://emedicine.medscape.com/article/1210837-treatment#a1128. Updated March 5, 2014. Accessed April 19, 2015.

18. Strabismus. A.D.A.M. Medical Encyclopedia. http://www.nlm.nih.gov/medlineplus/ency/article/001004.htm. Updated September 2, 2014. Accessed April 19, 2015.

19. Fecarotta C, Huang WW. Strabismus. In: Porter RS, Kaplan JL, eds. The Merck Manual Online. http://www.merckmanuals.com/professional/pediatrics/eye_defects_and_conditions_in_children/strabismus.html?qt=Strabismus&alt=sh#v7540269. Last reviewed December 2012. Accessed April 19, 2015.

20. Waitzman AA. Otitis externa. In: Elluru RG, ed. Medscape. http://emedicine.medscape.com/article/994550-overview#showall. Updated December 29, 2014. Accessed April 19, 2015.

21. McCarthy AA. Otitis externa. Surgical Center of South Jersey Web site. http://www.scasouthjersey.com/apps/healthgate/article.aspx?chunkiid=100689. Last reviewed August 2014. Accessed April 19, 2015.

22. Goguen LA. External otitis: Pathogenesis, clinical features, and diagnosis. In: Basow DS, ed. *UpToDate*. Waltham, MA: UpToDate; 2015. http://www.uptodate.com/contents/external-otitis-pathogenesis-clinical-features-and-diagnosis. Last updated September 19, 2014. Accessed April 19, 2015.

23. Wald ER. Acute otitis media in children: Diagnosis. In: Basow DS, ed. *UpToDate*. Waltham, MA: UpToDate; 2015. http://www.uptodate.com/contents/acute-otitis-media-in-children-diagnosis. Last updated October 21, 2014. Accessed April 19, 2015.

24. Klein JO, Pelton S. Acute otitis media in children: Epidemiology, microbiology, clinical manifestations, and complications. In: Basow DS, ed. *UpToDate*. Waltham, MA: UpToDate; 2015. http://www.uptodate.com/contents/acute-otitis-media-in-children-epidemiology-microbiology-clinical-manifestations-and-complications. Last reviewed November 11, 2014. Accessed April 19, 2015.

25. Klein JO, Pelton S. Acute otitis media in children: Treatment. In: Basow DS, ed. *UpToDate*. Waltham, MA: UpToDate; 2015. http://www.uptodate.com/contents/acute-otitis-media-in-children-treatment. Last updated January 31, 2014. Accessed April 19, 2015.

26. Vaccine recommendations of the ACIP. Centers for Disease Control and Prevention Web site. http://www.cdc.gov/vaccines/hcp/acip-recs/index.html. Last reviewed July 16, 2013. Last updated March 30, 2015. Accessed April 19, 2015.

27. Otitis media with effusion. Penn State Hershey Web site. http://pennstate-hershey.adam.com/content.aspx?productId=117&pid=1&gid=007010. Reviewed August 30, 2014. Accessed April 19, 2015.

28. Klein JO, Pelton S. Otitis media with effusion (serous otitis media) in children: Clinical features and diagnosis. In: Basow DS, ed. *UpToDate*. Waltham, MA: UpToDate; 2015. http://www.uptodate.com/contents/otitis-media-with-effusion-serous-otitis-media-in-children-clinical-features-and-diagnosis. Last updated May 28, 2013. Accessed April 19, 2015.

29. Higgins TS Jr. Otitis media with effusion. In: Meyers AD, ed. Medscape. http://emedicine.medscape.com/article/858990-overview. Updated February 20, 2015. Accessed April 19, 2015.

30. Lieberthal AS, Carrol AE, Chonmaitree T, et al. The diagnosis and management of acute otitis media. *Pediatrics*. 2013; 131(3): e964–e999. doi: 10.1542/peds.2012-3488

31. Hearing loss. A.D.A.M. Medical Encyclopedia. http://www.nlm.nih.gov/medlineplus/ency/article/003044.htm. Updated May 18, 2014. Accessed April 19, 2015.

32. Smith RJH, Gooi A. Hearing impairment in children: Etiology. In: Basow DS, ed. *UpToDate*. Waltham, MA: UpToDate; 2015. http://www.uptodate.com/contents/hearing-impairment-in-children-etiology. Last updated March 25, 2014. Accessed April 19, 2015.

33. Smith RJH, Gooi A. Hearing impairment in children: Evaluation. In: Basow DS, ed. *UpToDate*. Waltham, MA: UpToDate; 2015. http://www.uptodate.com/contents/hearing-impairment-in-children-evaluation. Last updated January 14, 2015. Accessed April 19, 2015.

34. Smith RJH, Gooi A. Hearing impairment in children: Treatment. In: Basow DS, ed. *UpToDate*. Waltham, MA: UpToDate; 2015. http://www.uptodate.com/contents/hearing-impairment-in-children-treatment. Last updated January 20, 2015. Accessed April 19, 2015.

35. Pappas DE, Hendley JO. The common cold in children: Clinical features and diagnosis. In: Basow DS, ed. *UpToDate*. Waltham, MA: UpToDate; 2015. http://www.uptodate.com/contents/the-common-cold-in-children-clinical-features-and-diagnosis. Last updated January 15, 2014. Accessed April 19, 2015.

36. Mayo Clinic Staff. Common cold. Mayo Clinic Web site. http://www.mayoclinic.org/diseases-conditions/common-cold/basics/symptoms/con-20019062. Updated April 17, 2013. Accessed April 19, 2015.

37. Pappas DE, Hendley JO. The common cold in children: Treatment and prevention. In: Basow DS, ed. *UpToDate*. Waltham, MA: UpToDate; 2015. http://www.uptodate.com/contents/the-common-cold-in-children-treatment-and-prevention. Last updated January 20, 2015. Accessed April 19, 2015.

38. Mayo Clinic Staff. Nosebleeds. Mayo Clinic Web site. http://www.mayoclinic.org/symptoms/nosebleeds/basics/definition/sym-20050914. Updated August 10, 2012. Accessed April 19, 2015.

39. Messner AH. Management of epistaxis in children. In: Basow DS, ed. *UpToDate*. Waltham, MA: UpToDate; 2015. http://www.uptodate.com/contents/management-of-epistaxis-in-children. Last updated September 10, 2014. Accessed April 19, 2015.

40. Pharyngitis and tonsillitis. Cincinnati's Children Hospital Web site. http://www.cincinnatichildrens.org/health/p/pharyngitis-tonsillitis. Last updated September 2013. Accessed April 19, 2015.

41. Drutz JE. Sore throat in children and adolescents: Symptomatic treatment. In: Basow DS, ed. *UpToDate*. Waltham, MA: UptoDate; 2015. http://www.uptodate.com/contents/sore-throat-in-children-and-adolescents-symptomatic-treatment. Last updated January 6, 2014. Accessed April 19, 2015.

42. Shah UK, Conrad DE, Grindle CR. Tonsillitis and pharyngitis organism–specific therapy. In: Bronze MS, ed. Medscape. http://emedicine.medscape.com/article/2011872-overview. Updated August 16, 2013. Accessed April 19, 2015.

43. Woods CR. Epiglottitis (supraglottitis): Clinical features and diagnosis. In: Basow DS, ed. *UpToDate*. Waltham, MA: UpToDate; 2015. http://www.uptodate.com/contents/epiglottitis-supraglottitis-clinical-features-and-diagnosis. Last updated October 2, 2013. Accessed April 19, 2015.

44. Abdallah C. Acute epiglottitis: Trends, diagnosis and management. *Saudi J Anaesth.* 2012; 6(3): 279–281. doi: 10.4103/1658-354X.101222

45. Epiglottitis. A.D.A.M. Medical Encyclopedia. http://www.nlm.nih.gov/medlineplus/ency/article/000605.htm. Updated February 25, 2014. Accessed April 19, 2015.

46. Gompf SG. Epiglottitis medication. In: Dyne PL, ed. Medscape. http://emedicine.medscape.com/article/763612-medication#2. Updated August 8, 2014. Accessed April 19, 2015.

47. Holmes A. Croup: What it is and how to treat it. *US Pharmacist.* 2013; 38(7): 47–50. http://www.medscape.com/viewarticle/809211

48. Woods CR. Croup: Clinical features, evaluation, and diagnosis. In: Basow DS, ed. *UpToDate*. Waltham, MA: UpToDate; 2015. http://www.uptodate.com/contents/croup-clinical-features-evaluation-and-diagnosis. Last updated February 18, 2015. Accessed April 19, 2015.

49. Defendi GL, Muñiz A, Molodow RE. Croup clinical presentation. In: Steele RW, ed. Medscape. http://emedicine.medscape.com/article/962972-clinical#showall. Updated April 15, 2014. Accessed April 19, 2015.

50. Perlstein D. Croup diagnosis. In: Davis CP, ed. eMedicineHealth. http://www.emedicinehealth.com/croup/page5_em.htm#croup_diagnosis. Reviewed June 20, 2014. Accessed April 19, 2015.

51. Perlstein D. Croup treatment. In: Davis CP, ed. eMedicineHealth. http://www.emedicinehealth.com/croup/page7_em.htm#croup_treatment. Reviewed June 20, 2014. Accessed April 19, 2015.

52. Mayo Clinic Staff. Croup. Mayo Clinic Web site. http://www.mayoclinic.org/diseases-conditions/croup/basics/treatment/con-20014673. Updated January 30, 2013. Accessed April 19, 2015.

53. Epstein-Barr virus and infectious mononucleosis. Centers for Disease Control and Prevention Web site. http://www.cdc.gov/epstein-barr/index.html. Last updated January 7, 2014. Accessed April 19, 2015.

54. Infectious mononucleosis symptoms & causes. Boston Children's Hospital Web site. http://www.childrenshospital.org/conditions-and-treatments/conditions/i/infectious-mononucleosis/symptoms-and-causes. Accessed April 19, 2015.

55. Mono test. Lab Tests Online Web site. http://labtestsonline.org/understanding/analytes/mono/tab/test. Last reviewed January 8, 2013. Accessed April 19, 2015.

56. Snellman L, Anderson G, Godfrey A, et al. Diagnosis and treatment of respiratory illness in children and adults. Institute for Clinical Systems Improvement Web site. https://www.icsi.org/_asset/1wp8x2/RespIllness.pdf. Published 2013. Accessed April 19, 2015.

57. Stöppler MC. Infectious mononucleosis. In: Shiel WC Jr. eMedicineHealth. http://www.medicinenet.com/infectious_mononucleosis/page5.htm#what_is_the_usual_course_and_treatment_of_mono. Reviewed February 3, 2015. Accessed April 19, 2015.

58. Ramadan H. Pediatric sinusitis. American Rhinologic Society Web site. http://care.american-rhinologic.org/pediatric_sinusitis. Revised February 17, 2015. Accessed April 19, 2015.

59. U.S. Department of Health and Human Services, National Institutes of Health, National Institute of Allergy and Infectious Diseases. Sinusitis. http://www.niaid.nih.gov/topics/sinusitis/Pages/Index.aspx. Last reviewed March 9, 2011. Last updated April 3, 2012. Accessed April 19, 2015.

60. Wald ER, Applegate KE, Bordley C, et al. Clinical practice guideline for the diagnosis and management of acute bacterial sinusitis in children aged 1 to 18 years. *Pediatrics*. 2013; 132(1): e262–e280. doi: 10.1542/peds.2013–1071

Chapter 13

Respiratory Disorders

QUESTIONS

1. In general, how frequently would a typical pediatric patient with mild persistent asthma use a rescue inhaler?

   a. Less than 2 days per week

   b. Several times per day

   c. More than 2 days per week

   d. Once per day

2. Which of the following regimens would best constitute Step 3 in the stepwise management of a patient with asthma, according to national recommendations?

   a. Preferred low-dose inhaled corticosteroid (ICS)

   b. Cromolyn or montelukast as required

   c. Preferred medium-dose ICS with considered oral systemic corticosteroid short course

   d. Preferred short-acting B2-agonist as required

3. In considering the need to refer a child to a specialist for cystic fibrosis, all of the following statements from the mother would typically support the decision <u>except</u>:

   a. "My child's stool is often bulky and foul smelling with an oily residue."

   b. "My child doesn't seem to be growing. Am I not breastfeeding her enough?"

   c. "My child always seems to be coughing and has a running nose that won't quit."

   d. "My child wets his diaper six times a day and nearly soaks it through each time."

4. A premature infant should typically be given palivizumab (Synagis) for the prevention of respiratory syncytial virus bronchiolitis if gestation is less than:

   a. 29 weeks

   b. 33 weeks

   c. 35 weeks

   d. 40 weeks

5. The practitioner would expect which of the following laboratory tests to be least useful in a workup for cystic fibrosis?
   a. Pilocarpine iontophoresis sweat test
   b. Pulmonary function tests
   c. White blood cell count
   d. Sputum culture
6. What is the most common etiology of pneumonia in children 1–3 years old?
   a. *Streptococcus pneumoniae*
   b. *Mycoplasma*
   c. Group B Streptococcus
   d. *Haemophilus influenzae*
7. A 7-year-old presents with symptoms indicative of asthma. His mother states that he typically experiences symptoms once per day. His mother adds that the symptoms also keep him out of some of the more active past times of his peers and cause him to wake 2–3 nights per week. How should you classify the patient's asthma?
   a. Intermittent
   b. Persistent mild
   c. Persistent moderate
   d. Persistent severe
8. Which of the following pathogens responsible for pneumonia does not typically demonstrate lobar consolidation as a radiographic characteristic?
   a. *Streptococcus pneumoniae*
   b. *Haemophilus influenzae*
   c. *Pneumocystis jiroveci*
   d. *Klebsiella pneumoniae*
9. Which two laboratory findings best characterizes the findings of restrictive disease in pulmonary function test results?
   a. Reduced airflow rates and lung volumes within normal range or larger
   b. Primarily reduced volumes and, to some extent, reduced expiratory flow rates
   c. Normal volumes and reduced expiratory flow rates
   d. Primarily reduced airflow rates and, to some extent, increased lung volumes
10. You are assessing for egophony in a young patient with suspected pneumonia. You ask the patient to produce a long "E" sound. What sound should you anticipate to auscultate when the patient has lung consolidation?
   a. A long "A," or "ay," sound
   b. A short "A," or "ah," sound
   c. A long "E," or "ee," sound
   d. A short "E," or "eh," sound

RATIONALES

1. c

Patients with mild persistent asthma commonly tend to use a rescue inhaler for symptom control more than 2 days per week. Use of a rescue inhaler less than 2 days per week, on the other hand, more often indicates intermittent asthma. Daily use of a rescue inhaler is typically indicated for moderate persistent asthma but not for lesser degrees of severity. Using a rescue inhaler several times per day is mostly seen in cases of severe persistent asthma.

2. c

Step 3 in managing a patient with moderate to severe asthma would commonly involve administering a medium-dose inhaled corticosteroid (ICS) and considering a short course of oral systemic corticosteroids. A low-dose ICS is often the preferred course in Step 2 of asthma management, with cromolyn and montelukast suggested as alternatives. Lastly, short-acting B2-agonists are the common preferred course in Step 1 of managing a patient with asthma.

3. d

Urinary frequency and polyuria are not signs and symptoms typically associated with cystic fibrosis. In infants and young children, cystic fibrosis is more likely to present with steatorrhea, or greasy, foul-smelling stool produced as a result of non-absorption of dietary fats. Other common signs and symptoms of cystic fibrosis may include failure to thrive, chronic cough, and rhinorrhea.

4. a

A premature infant born under 29 weeks gestation should be given palivizumab as prophylaxis for potential respiratory syncytial virus (RSV) infection. A premature infant born under 32 weeks gestation would qualify for prophylaxis if he or she required oxygenation for the first 28 days after birth, but not commonly on the basis of gestation. Earlier standards for RSV prophylaxis had qualifiers for children born at 32–35 weeks gestation, but these standards have since been modified. There is no common requirement for RSV prophylaxis in children born under 40 weeks gestation.

5. c

A white blood cell count is not a common diagnostic for cystic fibrosis. The pilocarpine iontophoresis sweat test is often considered the hallmark diagnostic for cystic fibrosis, with elevated salt levels serving as a bedrock for diagnosis. Pulmonary function tests see use to determine the possibility of airway obstruction, but may not be as reliable in patients under the age of 5. Sputum culture may likewise see use to find the presence of confirmatory pathogens for cystic fibrosis such as *Pseudomonas aeruginosa.*

6. a

The most common bacterial etiology for pediatric pneumonia in children 1–3 years old is by *Streptococcus pneumoniae*. The preferred outpatient oral antibiotic treatment for community-acquired pneumonia in this age group is amoxicillin, 90 mg/kg/day, dosed twice a day. The most common source of pediatric pneumonia is viral, which does not typically need any treatment other than supportive care.

7. c

A patient between the ages of 5 and 11 years who presents with daily asthma symptoms, some limitation of activity, and nighttime awakening more than once per week should be classified as experiencing persistent moderate asthma. Intermittent asthma typically presents with no limitation of activity, symptoms less than 2 days per week, and nighttime awakenings less than 2 nights per month. Mild persistent asthma commonly presents with minor activity limitation, as well as symptoms more than 2 days per week, but not daily and nighttime awakenings more than 3–4 times per month. Severe persistent asthma presents with nighttime awakenings more than once per week, but also presents with asthma symptoms throughout the day and extreme activity limitation.

8. c

Radiographic characteristics of pneumonia stemming from *Pneumocystis jiroveci* commonly include diffuse interstitial, alveolar, apical, or upper lobe infiltrates, but not lobar consolidation. Lobar consolidation is, however, a common shared radiographic characteristic of pneumonia stemming from *Haemophilus influenzae, Streptococcus pneumoniae*, and *Klebsiella pneumoniae*.

9. b

Restrictive disease in pulmonary function test results is primarily characterized by reduced volumes and, to some extent, expiratory flow rates. Primarily, reduced airflow rates and expiratory flow rates accompanied by lung volumes within the normal range or larger are, to some extent, more indicative of obstructive disease, not restrictive disease.

10. a

The technique to check for egophony requires listening to the lungs with a stethoscope as the patient says the letter "E"; when lung consolidation is present, the sound will typically be transmitted as the long "A," or "ay," sound. When the lungs are normal, the long "E," or "ee," sound can commonly be heard through the stethoscope. Short "A" ("ah") and short "E" ("eh") sounds are not typical findings of this technique, regardless of the state of the lungs. This assessment can be performed in conjunction with percussion to validate findings by assessment of resonance versus dullness for consolidation.

DISCUSSION

Respiratory Assessment

Overview

A respiratory assessment evaluates the type and location of a patient's breath sounds and consists of four components: inspection, palpation, percussion, and auscultation.[1] The nurse practitioner (NP) should inspect the thorax, vertebral column, and chest wall. The palpation component consists of palpating the trachea for mobility and any deviation from the midline. The lymph nodes of the head and neck should also be palpated. Percussion can be used to determine if the regions of the chest are hyper-resonant, dull, or flat. The NP should auscultate each lobe of both lungs, and should be able to recognize any abnormal breath sounds on either inspiration or expiration.[2] Egophony, which is a change in timbre from "E" to "A" that can be heard while auscultating, indicates lung consolidation and compression.[3] In cases of respiratory complications and if indicated, pulmonary function tests should also be included in a respiratory assessment if the patient is older than 5 years of age and is cooperative.[4]

Presentation

When a respiratory assessment detects abnormalities that derive from recurring respiratory complications, the patient's pulmonary condition can be classified as an obstructive or restrictive disease. Obstructive diseases are characterized by reduced airflow rates and lung volumes either within the normal range or higher. These findings are typical of conditions such as asthma, chronic bronchitis, and cystic fibrosis. Restrictive diseases, such as pneumonia, are characterized by reduced expiratory flow rates and volumes.[5]

Bronchiolitis

Overview

Bronchiolitis is a viral illness that affects the lower respiratory tract and produces inflammation, which then leads to blockage of the small respiratory airways. Most cases of bronchiolitis are caused by the respiratory syncytial virus (RSV) or the parainfluenza 3 virus.[6] Bronchiolitis usually affects children younger than 2 years of age and often occurs in epidemics.[6] Although bronchiolitis may occur at any age, severe symptoms of the condition usually appear only in young infants.[7]

Presentation

Bronchiolitis usually begins with a mild upper respiratory infection lasting for several days. After a few days, the patient presents with a moderate fever and signs of respiratory distress, (e.g., a wheezy or hacking cough, retractions, tachypnea).[6,8] More severe cases may present with additional signs of distress, such as cyanosis and nasal flaring.[7] Restlessness and changes in mental status may also accompany respiratory distress.[3] The patient's liver and spleen may be palpable due to hyperinflated lungs.[9]

Workup

A diagnosis of bronchiolitis is confirmed by a number of factors, such as seasonal occurrence, the patient's age, presentation, and physical examination findings.[7] A chest x-ray, usually reserved for if the patient exhibits severe symptoms or has a pre-existing condition, typically shows hyperinflated lungs and may show scattered areas of consolidation.[3,6] Other diagnostic tests that may be done include a nasal fluid culture, which helps to determine the causative virus, and arterial blood gas analysis.[10] Additionally, an immunofluorescence foci assay (IFA) may detect RSV in a mucus culture or nasal washing.[11]

Treatment

Outpatient treatment and supportive care are common options for infants with mild distress. RSV prophylaxis with a palivizumab (Synagis) injection is indicated in high-risk infants and helps decrease the risk of hospitalization.[6] Palivizumab should be administered every month during RSV season (maximum five doses) to premature infants (i.e., infants born before 29 weeks gestation) under 1 year of age, as well as premature infants born before 32 weeks gestation who present with chronic lung disease.[3,12] Infants may likewise be considered for palivizumab if they present with hemodynamically significant heart disease or would be immunocompromised during RSV season.[12,13]

Asthma

Overview

Asthma is a respiratory disease that is characterized by widespread narrowing of the airways and is distinguished by an increased responsiveness of the bronchi and trachea to a variety of stimuli. These stimuli trigger diffuse airway inflammation, which results in bronchoconstriction.[14] Severity of asthma may decrease either spontaneously or due to direct treatment.[3]

The pathophysiology of asthma involves acute inflammation and plugging of the airways by thick, viscous mucus. The airways are likewise narrowed by hypertrophy of smooth muscle and remodeled via thickening of the epithelial basement membrane.[3,14] Other pathophysiological features of asthma include mucosal edema and hyperemia.[15]

The most common asthma allergens are encountered indoors and include dust mites, indoor molds, respiratory infections, stress, cold air, pets, cockroaches, and smoke. Asthma may be triggered by exercise, especially in environments that are cold or dry.[14] Certain medications, such as aspirin and other NSAIDs, may also cause asthma.[16] Other contributing factors include airway irritants, such as cigarettes, air pollution, wood smoke, perfumes, aerosol sprays, paints or sealants, and cleaning agents.[17]

Presentation

Asthma is characterized by a pattern of respiratory symptoms that occur when the patient is exposed to triggers of the condition.[18] These symptoms may include coughing, wheezing, chest tightness, and respiratory distress; the patient may also experience difficulty speaking in sentences and may present with diaphoresis and hyperresonance.[19]

More ominous signs of asthma include absent breath sounds, cyanosis, and inability to maintain recumbency. Another ominous sign is pulsus paradoxus, which is indicated by a change in systolic blood pressure amplitude greater than 10 mmHg in between inspiration and expiration.[20]

Workup

When a diagnosis of asthma is suspected, the patient should undergo a pulmonary function test to assess for abnormalities typical of obstructive dysfunction.[14] Hospitalization is recommended if the peak flow is under 60 L/min initially or if there is no improvement in ventilation after aerosol treatment. Laboratory findings, such as slight white blood cell elevation with eosinophilia, are helpful in excluding other diagnoses. A chest x-ray is usually unnecessary but may be used to rule out other conditions.[3,21]

The severity of a patient's asthma can be classified according to table 13.1.[3]

Treatment (see table 13.2)

According to the 2007 National Heart, Lung, and Blood Institute/National Asthma

Table 13.1 Asthma Severity Classification

Classification	Intermittent	Mild Persistent	Moderate Persistent	Severe Persistent
Symptoms	≤ 2 days/week	> 2 days/week	Daily	Throughout the day
Nighttime awakenings	≤ 2/month	3 to 4/month	More than once per week but not nightly	Nightly
Rescue inhaler use	≤ 2 days/week	> 2 days/week but not daily	Daily	Several times per day
Interference with normal activity	None	Minor limitation	Some limitation	Extremely limited
Lung function	FEV1 > 80% predicted and normal between exacerbations	FEV1 > 80% predicted	FEV1 60% to 80% predicted	FEV1 less than 60% predicted

Used with permission from Barkley TW Jr. Pediatric Primary Care Nurse Practitioner Certification Review/Clinical Update Continuing Education Course. West Hollywood, CA: Barkley and Associates; 2015.

Table 13.2 Assessing Asthma Control and Adjusting Therapy in Children

Components of control			Well controlled		Not well controlled		Very poorly controlled	
			Ages 0–4	Ages 5–11	Ages 0–4	Ages 5–11	Ages 0-4	Ages 5–11
Impairment	Symptoms		2 days/week or less, but not more than once a day		More than 2 days/week or multiple times on 2 days/week or more		Throughout the day	
	Nighttime awakenings		1x/month or less		More than 1x/ month	2x/month or more	More than 1x/ week	2x/week or more
	Interference with normal activity		None		Some limitation		Extremely limited	
	SABA use for symptom control (not EIB prevention)		2 days/week or less		More than 2 days/week		Several times per day	
	Lung function	FEV_1	N/A	> 80%	N/A	60%–80%	N/A	< 60%
		FEV_1/FVC		> 80%		75%–80%		< 75%
Risk	Exacerbations requiring oral systemic corticosteroids		0–1x/year		2–3x/year	2x/year or more	>3x/year	2x/year or more
	Reduction in lung growth		N/A	Requires long-term followup	N/A	Requires long-term followup	N/A	Requires long-term followup
	Treatment-related adverse effects		Medication side effects can vary in intensity from none to very troublesome and worrisome. The level of intensity does not correlated to specific levels of control but should be considered in the overall assessment of risk.					
Recommended action for treatment			Maintain current step. Regular followup every 1–6 months. Consider step down if well controlled for at least 3 months		Step up 1 step.	Step up at least 1 step.	Consider short course of systemic corticosteroids. Step up 1–2 steps.	

Notes. 1. Before stepping up, review adherence to medication, inhaler technique, and environmental control. If alternative treatment was used, discontinue it and use preferred treatment for that step. 2. Re-evaluate the level of asthma control in 2–6 weeks to achieve control every 1–6 months to maintain control. Children 0–4 years old: If no clear benefit is observed in 4–6 weeks, consider alternative diagnoses or adjusting therapy. Children 5–11 years old: Adjust therapy accordingly. For side effects: consider alternative treatment options. EIB=exercise-induced bronchospasm; FEV_1=forced expiratory volume in 1 second; FVC_1=forced vital capacity; ICU=intensive care unit; N/A=not applicable. For more information on treatment, see "Stepwise approach for managing asthma for treatment steps" at http://www.nhlbi.nih.gov/files/docs/guidelines/asthsumm.pdf. Source: National Heart, Lung, and Blood Institute, National Institutes of Health. Assessing Asthma Control and Adjusting Therapy in Children. http://www.nhlbi.nih.gov/files/docs/guidelines/asthsumm.pdf. Published 2007. Retrieved April 2015. Reproduced with permission.

Education and Prevention Program Asthma Guidelines at a Glance, asthma treatment should focus on achieving and maintaining control of asthma symptoms.[22] In the treatment for persistent asthma, inhaled corticosteroids (ICS) commonly see use in all age groups.[22] Combination therapy is recommended when treatment needs to be stepped up; in patients over the age of 12 years, long-acting beta-2 adrenergic agonists are preferred for combination with ICS. Guidelines for asthma management are divided into three distinct age groups with consideration for current impairment and future risk. These age groups are 0–4 years of age, 5–11 years of age, and 12 years of age and older. More frequent monitoring should initially be conducted every 2–4 weeks until control is achieved. If the patient's asthma remains uncontrolled, the NP should move to the next step of treatment and check back with the patient at least every 2 weeks. If there is continued control for 3 months, however, the NP should step down therapy.[3,22]

Pneumonia

Overview

Pneumonia is a respiratory disorder characterized by inflammation of the lower respiratory tract. This condition typically produces when microorganisms gain access through aspiration, inhalation, or hematogenous dissemination. Although the majority of pneumonia cases are viral, the condition may be caused by a variety of other organisms, such as bacteria and fungi.[3,23] Additionally, the presentation of pneumonia typically differs depending on if the condition is acquired in the community or hospital.[24]

The most common bacterial cause of pneumonia includes group B *Streptococcus*, but can also include *Chlamydophila pneumoniae*, *Escherichia coli*, *Haemophilus influenzae*, and *Streptococcus pneumoniae*.[3,25] RSV also causes pneumonia, particularly in infants and children younger than 6 years of age.[26] Immunocompromised or malnourished patients are particularly susceptible to pneumonia caused by fungi or *Pneumocystis jiroveci*.[27]

Presentation

Signs and symptoms of pneumonia in pediatric patients vary based on age group. Fever and cough are common findings of pneumonia in all patients older than 1 month, but viral forms of pneumonia may present with low temperature or no fever at all. Toddlers and preschoolers commonly present with tachypnea and congestion, whereas older children and adolescents may experience constitutional symptoms such as headache and chest pain.[24,28] A physical exam may note lung consolidation, and pulse oximetry will show decreased oxygenation in the event of severe distress.[3]

Workup

If pneumonia is suspected, the NP may order diagnostic tests such as chest x-rays, pulse oximetry, and blood tests.[23] A sputum culture is warranted if the patient presents with a productive cough.[29]

Radiographic characteristics of pneumonia differ depending on the causative organism. For instance, lobar consolidation is indicative of *H. influenzae*, *S. pneumoniae*, and *Klebsiella pneumoniae*. Pneumocystis infections, on the other hand, are characterized by diffuse interstitial, alveolar, apical, or upper lobe infiltrates. Patchy infiltrates are characteristic of *E. coli*, *Staphylococcus aureus*, and *Pseudomonas aeruginosa*. *E. coli* infections may also be indicated by pleural effusion, whereas *P. aeruginosa* infections may also present with cavitation.[3,30]

Treatment

Viral pneumonia is treated by supportive measures such as hydration, antipyretics, humidified oxygen, chest physiotherapy, and bronchodilators, which help improve airway clearance. In viral cases, antibiotics only see use in the event of secondary bacterial infections.[31,32]

For patients with community-acquired pneumonia, pharmacological therapy is determined by the infecting organism. Penicillin is indicated for *S. pneumoniae* infections, whereas *Moraxella catarrhalis* infections are treated by macrolides such as azithromycin.[33,34] Amoxicillin and cephalosporin are indicated for *H. influenzae* infections.[35]

Cystic Fibrosis

Overview

Cystic fibrosis (CF) is the most common autosomal recessive disorder in the Caucasian population.[36] The condition is caused by a chromosome 7 long arm mutation. The mutation causes a defect in epithelial chloride transport, resulting in dehydrated, thick secretions. As a result of mucus buildup, patients may experience digestion problems and life-threatening lung infections.[37] Nearly all exogenic glands are affected by CF, including the respiratory, hepatobiliary, gastroenterology, and reproductive tracts.[3,37] CF is also characterized by progressive obstructive pulmonary disease, recurrent endobronchial infections, and pancreatic insufficiency with intestinal malabsorption. The median survival age of CF is 36.9 years, with males typically living longer than females.[38]

Presentation

Newborns with CF may present with meconium ileus, failure to thrive, or salty-tasting skin.[36,39] CF also presents with recurrent respiratory infections and chronic coughing, among other respiratory findings. Malabsorption causes large, liquid, bulky, and foul stool (i.e., steatorrhea). A nasal exam may reveal rhinorrhea, and gastrointestinal findings may include hepatosplenomegaly or fat-soluble vitamin deficiencies.[3,38] Delayed puberty is more common in CF patients than the general population. Infertility also frequently occurs in CF patients.[37]

Workup

Most cases are discovered during the universal newborn screening and confirmed through a pilocarpine iontophoresis sweat test.[36] Pulmonary function tests reveal an obstructive pattern, and a chest radiograph may detect cystic lesions and atelectasis.[3] Lastly, blood gas and serum electrolyte levels may detect chronic alkalosis.[37]

Treatment

CF patients should be referred to a CF center for care. Although there is no cure for CF, a number of treatment options exist to help reduce symptoms and complications.[40] The main goals of CF treatment are to maintain normal lung function and ensure normal growth through nutritional therapy.[38] Pulmonary treatment is aimed at preventing airway obstruction and also includes prophylaxis against pulmonary infections.[36] Exercise and dietary modifications are also beneficial for CF patients.[39]

References

1. Bickley LS, Szilagyi PG. *Bates' Guide to Physical Examination and History Taking.* 11th ed. Philadelphia, PA: Lippincott, Williams & Wilkins; 2011.

2. Taylor C, Gfeller P, Ring T. Respiratory examination. Learn Pediatrics Web site. http://learnpediatrics.com/files/2011/01/Respiratory-video-script.pdf. Accessed May 19, 2015.

3. Barkley TW Jr. *Pediatric Primary Care Nurse Practitioner Certification Review/Clinical Update Continuing Education Course*. West Hollywood, CA: Barkley and Associates; 2015.

4. Sawicki G, Haver K. Asthma in children younger than 12 years: Initial evaluation and diagnosis. In: Basow DS, ed. *UpToDate*. Waltham, MA: UpToDate; 2015. http://www.uptodate.com/contents/asthma-in-children-younger-than-12-years-initial-evaluation-and-diagnosis. Last updated January 4, 2015. Accessed April 19, 2015.

5. Healthwise, Inc. Obstructive and restrictive lung disease. WebMD Web site. http://www.webmd.com/lung/obstructive-and-restrictive-lung-disease. Reviewed September 4, 2012. Accessed April 19, 2015.

6. Caserta MT. Respiratory syncytial virus (RSV) and human metapneumovirus infections. In: Porter RS, Kaplan JL, eds. The Merck Manual Online. http://www.merckmanuals.com/professional/pediatrics/miscellaneous-viral-infections-in-infants-and-children/respiratory-syncytial-virus-rsv-and-human-metapneumovirus-infections. Last reviewed November 2014. Accessed April 19, 2015.

7. DeNicola LK, Maraqa NF, Custodio HT, & Udeani J. Bronchiolitis. In: Steele RW, ed. Medscape. http://emedicine.medscape.com/article/961963-overview. Updated November 10, 2014. Accessed April 19, 2015.

8. Piedra PA, Stark AR. Bronchiolitis in infants and children: Clinical features and diagnosis. In: Basow DS, ed. *UpToDate*. Waltham, MA: UpToDate; 2015. http://www.uptodate.com/contents/bronchiolitis-in-infants-and-children-clinical-features-and-diagnosis. Last updated January 19, 2015. Accessed April 19, 2015.

9. Tidy C. Bronchiolitis. Patient.co.uk Web site. http://www.patient.co.uk/doctor/bronchiolitis-pro. Last reviewed June 28, 2013. Accessed April 19, 2015.

10. Bronchiolitis. A.D.A.M. Medical Encyclopedia. http://www.nlm.nih.gov/medlineplus/ency/article/000975.htm. Updated August 22, 2013. Accessed April 19, 2015.

11. Pankaj K. Methods for rapid virus identification and quantification. *Mater Methods.* 2013; 3: 207.

12. Committee on Infectious Diseases, Bronchiolitis Guidelines Committee. Updated guidance for palivizumab prophylaxis among infants and young children at increased risk of hospitalization for respiratory syncytial virus infection. *Pediatrics.* 2014; 134(2): 415–420. doi: 10.1542/peds.2014-1665

13. Bollani L, Pozzi M. The prevention of respiratory syncytial virus infection. *Ital J Pediatr.* 2014; 40 (Suppl 2): A35. doi: 10.1186/1824-7288-40-S2-A35

14. Miles MC, Peters SP. Asthma. In: Porter RS, Kaplan JL, eds. The Merck Manual Online. http://www.merckmanuals.com/professional/pulmonary-disorders/asthma-and-related-disorders/asthma. Last reviewed July 2014. Accessed April 19, 2015.

15. Ball DR, McGuire BE. Airway pharmacology. In: Hagberg C, ed. *Benumof and Hagberg's Airway Management.* 3rd ed. Philadelphia, PA: Elsevier Saunders; 2013: 159–183.

16. Asthma. A.D.A.M. Medical Encyclopedia. http://www.ncbi.nlm.nih.gov/pubmedhealth/PMH0062942. Last updated June 11, 2014. Accessed April 19, 2015.

17. United States Department of Health and Human Services, Centers for Disease Control and Prevention. Common asthma triggers. http://www.cdc.gov/asthma/triggers.html. Last reviewed December 14, 2010. Last updated August 20, 2012. Accessed April 19, 2015.

18. Fanta CH. Diagnosis of asthma in adolescents and adults. In: Basow DS, ed. *UpToDate*. Waltham, MA: UpToDate; 2015. http://www.uptodate.com/contents/diagnosis-of-asthma-in-adolescents-and-adults. Last updated March 7, 2014. Accessed April 19, 2015.

19. United States Department of Health and Human Services, National Institutes of Health (NIH), National Heart, Lung, and Blood Institute (NHLBI). What are the signs and symptoms of asthma? http://www.nhlbi.nih.gov/health/health-topics/topics/asthma/signs.html. Updated August 4, 2014. Accessed April 19, 2015.

20. Heuer AJ, Scanlan CL, Wilkins RL. *Wilkins' Clinical Assessment in Respiratory Care.* 7th ed. Maryland Heights, MO: Elsevier Mosby; 2014: 43–45.

21. Morris MJ. Asthma workup. In: Mosenifar Z, ed. Medscape. http://emedicine.medscape.com/article/296301-workup. Updated September 30, 2014. Accessed April 19, 2015.

22. United States Department of Health and Human Services, NIH, NHLBI. Asthma care quick reference: Diagnosing and managing asthma (NIH Publication No. 12-5075). http://www.nhlbi.nih.gov/guidelines/asthma/asthma_qrg.pdf. Revised September 2012. Accessed April 19, 2015.

23. Mayo Clinic Staff. Pneumonia. Mayo Clinic web site. http://www.mayoclinic.com/health/pneumonia/DS00135. Updated March 14, 2015. Accessed April 19, 2015.

24. Pneumonia. A.D.A.M. Medical Encyclopedia. http://www.ncbi.nlm.nih.gov/pubmedhealth/PMH0063028. Updated June 11, 2014. Accessed April 19, 2015.

25. Kamangar N, Harrington A. Bacterial pneumonia. In: Byrd RP Jr, ed. Medscape. http://emedicine.medscape.com/article/300157-overview#showall. Updated October 8, 2014. Accessed April 19, 2015.

26. Understanding RSV. American Lung Association Web site. http://www.lung.org/lung-disease/respiratory-syncytial-virus/understanding-rsv.html. Accessed April 19, 2015.

27. Bennett NJ, Gilroy SA. Overview of pneumocystis jiroveci pneumonia. In: Bronze MS, ed. Medscape. http://emedicine.medscape.com/article/225976-overview. Updated September 2, 2014. Accessed April 19, 2015.

28. Bennett NJ, Domachowske J. Pediatric pneumonia clinical presentation. In: Steele RW, ed. Medscape. http://emedicine.medscape.com/article/967822-clinical. Updated April 28, 2014.

29. Ibrahim M. Sputum culture. In: Staros EB, ed. Medscape. http://emedicine.medscape.com/article/2119232-overview. Updated May 7, 2014. Accessed April 19, 2015.

30. Amanullah S, Posner DH, Farhad M, Lessnau K-D. Typical bacterial pneumonia imaging. In: Garg K, ed. Medscape. http://emedicine.medscape.com/article/360090-overview#showall. Updated May 22, 2013. Accessed April 19, 2015.

31. Lee FE, Treanor J. Viral infections. In: Mason RJ, Broaddus VC, Martin T, et al, eds. *Murray and Nadel's Textbook of Respiratory Medicine.* 5th ed. Philadelphia, PA: Elsevier Saunders; 2010: 661–698.

32. Limper AH. Overview of pneumonia. In: Goldman L, Schafer AI, eds. *Goldman's Cecil Medicine.* 24th ed. Philadelphia, PA: Elsevier Saunders; 2011: 587–595.

33. Falcó V, Sánchez A, Pahissa A, Rello J. Emerging drugs for pneumococcal pneumonia. *Expert Opin Emerg Drugs.* 2011; 16(3): 459–477. doi: 10.1517/14728214.2011.576669

34. Parnham MJ, Erakovic Haber V, Giamarellos-Bourboulis EJ, Perletti G, Verleden GM, Vos R. Azithromycin: Mechanisms of action and their relevance for clinical applications. *Pharmacol Ther.* 2014; 143(2): 225–245. doi: 10.1016/j.pharmthera.2014.03.003

35. Paterson DL, Daveson K. Cefoxitin, cefotetan, and other cephamycins (cefmetazole and flomoxef). In: Grayson ML, Crowe SM, McCarthy JS, eds. *Kucers' The Use of Antibiotics.* 6th ed. Boca Raton, FL: CRC Press; 2010: 301–310.

36. Katkin JP. Cystic fibrosis: Clinical manifestations and diagnosis. In: Basow DS, ed. *UpToDate.* Waltham, MA: UpToDate; 2015. http://www.uptodate.com/contents/cystic-fibrosis-clinical-manifestations-and-diagnosis. Last updated June 25, 2014. Accessed April 19, 2015.

37. Rosenstein BJ. Cystic fibrosis. In: Porter RS, Kaplan JL, eds. The Merck Manual Online. http://www.merckmanuals.com/professional/pediatrics/cystic-fibrosis-cf/cystic-fibrosis. Last reviewed January 2014. Accessed April 19, 2015.

38. Sharma GD. Cystic fibrosis. In: Bye MR, ed. Medscape. http://emedicine.medscape.com/article/1001602-overview#aw2aab6b2b6aa. Updated March 19, 2015. Accessed April 19, 2015.

39. Cystic fibrosis. A.D.A.M. Medical Encyclopedia. http://www.ncbi.nlm.nih.gov/pubmedhealth/PMH0063023. Last updated June 11, 2014. Accessed April 19, 2015.

40. Mayo Clinic Staff. Cystic fibrosis. Mayo Clinic Web site. http://www.mayoclinic.com/health/cystic-fibrosis/DS00287/DSECTION=treatments-and-drugs. Updated June 13, 2012. Accessed April 19, 2015.

Chapter 14

Musculoskeletal Disorders

QUESTIONS

1. You are conducting an assessment for a 12-year-old whose feet point slightly inward, though he walks normally without a limp. His chief complaint is pain in the "front, bottom part" of his knee, pointing towards the tibial tubercle. He indicates that he began playing soccer year-round 7 months prior without any significant incident or injury. The pain began 3 weeks ago and has been constant since. Which of the following conditions is the patient most likely experiencing?

   a. Genu valgum

   b. Osgood-Schlatter disease

   c. Grade I knee sprain

   d. Legg-Calvé-Perthes disease

2. Which of these clinical tests would be most useful in evaluating the degree of a patient's scoliosis?

   a. Genetic testing

   b. Radiograph

   c. Ultrasound

   d. Joint fluid aspiration

3. A 6-month-old appears to have a shorter left leg, which turns outward slightly further than her right leg. Given this finding, which of the following signs would you <u>least</u> expect to present during the diagnostic assessment?

   a. Galeazzi sign

   b. Barlow sign

   c. Gower's sign

   d. Allis' sign

4. Your patient has significant edema and ecchymoses around the elbow. After ordering a radiograph, you notice a fat pad sign on the x-ray but no visible fracture. What would be the best course of action to take regarding treatment?

   a. Refer the patient to orthopedics

   b. Administer non-steroidal anti-inflammatory drugs

   c. Employ the RICE method

   d. Supinate the arm to correct subluxation

5. Which of the following is the most specific test for muscular dystrophy?

   a. Transaminase level

   b. Prolactin level

   c. Creatine kinase determination

   d. Polymerase chain reaction result

6. A 4-year-old presents with an awkward walk and run, without any pain and with full range of motion. The physical exam reveals that the distance between his ankles exceeds 3 inches. Which of these conditions would be the most likely diagnosis?

   a. Genu varum

   b. Muscular dystrophy

   c. Genu valgum

   d. Slipped capital femoral epiphysis

7. A 6-year-old male presents to your office with a limp and complains of pain in his groin. Upon further examination, you notice stiffness in the hip area on the affected side, as well as significant muscle loss in the upper thigh due to limited motion. Which of the following diagnostics would be most helpful in confirming Legg-Calvé-Perthes disease?

   a. Radiograph

   b. Ultrasound

   c. Muscle biopsy

   d. Electromyography

8. Which of these diagnostics is <u>not</u> routinely recommended for patients presenting with classic symptoms of slipped capital femoral epiphysis?

   a. Radiography

   b. Bone scans

   c. Endocrine studies

   d. Computed tomography

9. A 6-year-old patient arrives at your clinic with a painful limp that seemed to develop out of nowhere. While examining the patient, you discover that the internal rotation of the hip causes spasms. Suspecting toxic synovitis, you order a series of lab panels and imaging studies for confirmation. Which of these procedures would <u>not</u> typically be ordered?

   a. Ultrasonography

   b. Creatine kinase test

   c. Magnetic resonance imaging

   d. Erythrocyte sedimentation rate test

10. All of these statements are true of slipped capital femoral epiphysis <u>except</u>:

    a. The condition typically occurs in girls prior to menarche.

    b. The condition usually occurs without sudden severe force or trauma.

    c. There is an increased incidence of the condition amongst obese adolescents.

    d. The condition is more common in males and Caucasian adolescents.

RATIONALES

1. b

Pain at the tibial tubercle is commonly a strong indicator for Osgood-Schlatter disease. Though the patient appears to be pigeon-toed, this does not typically indicate that the knees point inward, as seen in genu valgum. A mild knee sprain is possible, but the patient did not indicate any injury; extraneous sports-related activity and pain isolated at the tibial tubercle would commonly make Osgood-Schlatter disease the more likely condition of the two. Although Legg-Calvé-Perthes disease may also indicate limp and knee pain, the patient's hip is not affected, as it commonly would be in cases of this condition.

2. b

Although scoliosis can be diagnosed with Adam's Forward Bend Test, radiographs are often recommended to determine the actual curvature of the spine. Genetic testing can be used to predict the development of scoliosis, but is more often used to diagnose muscular dystrophy. An ultrasound is more often used to diagnose developmental dysplasia of the hip. Lastly, joint fluid aspiration is commonly used to diagnose toxic synovitis.

3. c

Gower's sign, which is usually indicated when the hands are used to walk back towards the legs in order to attain a standing position due to weakness of the proximal muscles, is typically seen in patients with muscular dystrophy and would not likely present in this patient, who shows signs more indicative of developmental dysplasia of the hip (DDH). Signs of DDH would commonly produce positive results for the Galeazzi and Barlow test, though the latter would not typically present after 6 months of age. The Galeazzi sign is indicated by asymmetry in knee height while the infant lies supine with knees and hips flexed. The Barlow sign is indicated when the hip becomes dislocated upon pressure applied posteriorly by the nurse practitioner while the patient lies supine with knees flexed and hip adducted. Allis' sign is another name for the Galeazzi sign and would be present in the diagnostic assessment for a patient with DDH.

4. a

An elbow fracture may present with edema and ecchymosis, and is more often indicated with radiographs that show the presence of the fat pad sign, rather than the presence of any visible fracture; hence, you would refer the patient to orthopedics to be treated for fracture. Administering non-steroidal anti-inflammatory drugs and employing the RICE method are both appropriate steps for managing ankle sprains and other soft tissue injuries. Supinating the injured arm to correct subluxation is recommended for treatment of nursemaid elbow.

5. c

A creatine kinase determination aids in detecting the presence of inflammation or muscle damage stemming from muscular dystrophy (MD). Transaminase levels are used to detect disorders of the liver, whereas prolactin levels are used to measure erectile dysfunction in men and menstrual irregularities in women. A polymerase chain reaction test is used to diagnose viruses such as human papillomavirus and HIV, not genetic conditions such as MD.

6. c

Genu valgum, or knock-knees, typically manifests with abnormally close knees and increased ankle space; common signs and symptoms include no pain, full range of motion, and an awkward gait. The condition typically evolves to normal alignment by 7 years of age; if genu valgum persists past this age or unilaterally, further examination will often be necessary. Genu varum, or bowleg, is characterized by knees that remain apart while the feet and ankles are touching; these patients also typically have a full range of motion, and the condition is usually considered normal until 2 years of age. Muscular dystrophy may present with an awkward gait and posture, but patients may also experience pain and commonly exhibit limited range of motion. Common signs and symptoms of slipped capital femoral epiphysis include pain in the groin, the inability to properly flex the hip, and possible presentation of limb shortening.

7. a

The patient's limp, groin pain, stiffness of the hip, and muscle loss in the upper thigh most likely indicate Legg-Calvé-Perthes disease; radiograph studies would be most useful for both visualizing bone damage caused by this condition and confirming a diagnosis. Ultrasounds are more useful in the diagnosis of developmental dysplasia of the hip, and muscle biopsies and electromyography are often useful in the diagnosis and monitoring of muscular dystrophy.

8. c

Endocrine studies may be ordered in patients presenting with symptoms of slipped capital femoral epiphysis (SCFE) but are typically reserved for if the patient presents with atypical symptoms or has a medical history that would indicate a condition that may present with endocrine disorders. Radiography of the hips is typical in diagnosis of SCFE, with bone scans or magnetic resonance imaging serving to confirm the diagnosis.

9. b

Creatine kinase determination is used to detect inflammation of muscles, not joints, and would serve little use in confirming a diagnosis of toxic synovitis. The presence of inflammation stemming from toxic synovitis is usually detected through a complete blood count, an erythrocyte sedimentation rate test, or a C-reactive protein test. Ultrasonography is used to detect intracapsular effusion, whereas magnetic resonance imaging is used to rule out other potential causes of pain.

10. d

Slipped capital femoral epiphysis (SCFE) is most common in male and African American, not Caucasian, adolescents. Female adolescents are also likely to experience the condition during growth spurts and prior to menarche. SCFE also shows a higher incidence amongst children who are obese or who have sedentary lifestyles and often presents without sudden force or trauma.

DISCUSSION

Osgood-Schlatter Disease

Overview

Osgood-Schlatter disease is a common musculoskeletal condition among pediatric patients experiencing pubertal growth spurts. The disease is characterized by the growth of a painful lump due to inflammation at the tibial tubercle, just below the knee.[1] Incidence is usually seen in children between the ages of 11 and 14 and is especially prevalent in active children who play sports.[2]

Presentation

Patients often present with mild-to-severe swelling of the proximal tibia below one or both kneecaps. Patients may also complain of knee pain that is usually exacerbated by high-impact activities such as running, jumping, and climbing stairs.[3]

Workup

A clinical examination is usually all that is necessary to diagnose Osgood-Schlatter disease. X-rays are primarily ordered to rule out other possible conditions, such as neoplasms, osteomyelitis, and infection. Often, a radiograph will show a prominent, elevated tubercle with anterior soft-tissue swelling. A radiograph that shows ossicles separated from the tibial tuberosity indicates a more severe manifestation.[4,5]

Treatment

Because the disease is a self-limiting condition, pediatric patients should regulate their activity in order to control pain. To manage the condition, children and adolescents should practice the treatments that comprise the acronym R-I-C-E (Rest, Ice, Compress, and Elevate). However, complete activity restriction is not advised. Knee immobilizers may provide some relief, and non-steroidal anti-inflammatory drugs (NSAIDs) are often recommended for pain management.[6]

Toxic Synovitis

Overview

Toxic synovitis (i.e., transient synovitis) is a self-limiting inflammation of the hip that most often has a viral etiology.[7] This condition is most prevalent in children between 2 and 6 years of age but may also occur anywhere from ages 1 to 15. Toxic synovitis is more common in males than females and typically has an insidious onset.[1]

Presentation

Acute hip pain is the most common symptom of toxic synovitis. Pain may either be unilateral or present in both hips. Patients typically present with a painful limp, and additional findings may include spasms caused by internal rotation of the hip. There are usually no obvious signs of infection upon inspection or palpation.[1,8]

Workup

The diagnosis of toxic synovitis is a process of exclusion to rule out septic arthritis and osteomyelitis. Imaging studies may help to confirm toxic synovitis, with radiographs showing an increase in medial joint space and ultrasonography detecting intracapsular effusion. Patients with the condition will also typically show elevated white blood cells (WBC) on a complete blood count (CBC), as well as elevated erythrocyte sedimentation rate (ESR) and C-reactive protein levels.[7,9] Additional tests may be conducted to rule out other causes of pain, including a bone scan, magnetic resonance imaging (MRI), or aspiration of fluid from the hip joint.[7]

Treatment

Analgesics and bed rest should be given as needed. Full unrestricted activity can resume once the limp and pain have resolved. Hospitalization should be considered if the patient presents with a fever, limited range of motion (ROM), or other potential signs of septic arthritis.[7]

Legg-Calvé-Perthes Disease (LCPD)

Overview

Legg-Calvé-Perthes disease (LCPD) is a temporary pediatric condition caused by a lack of blood flow to the femoral head. The area often becomes inflamed and avascular necrosis of bone tissue can occur, which can cause the thigh bone to collapse. The stiffness in the hip joint that causes LCPD varies for each child, but most children with the condition present with a limp.[10] LCPD most commonly occurs in pediatric patients between 4 and 10 years of age who tend to be physically active. The condition also commonly occurs in children who are small for their age, but there is no known reason for this increased incidence.[11]

Presentation

Patients with LCPD usually present with an insidious onset of a limp accompanied by knee pain that may migrate to the groin and lateral hip area. Although the hip pain associated with LCPD is similar to transient synovitis and septic arthritis, LCPD pain is less acute than either condition. Patients with LCPD may be afebrile, which helps to distinguish the disease from osteomyelitis.[1,12]

Workup

Imaging tests, such as x-rays and an MRI, can be used to assess for LCPD. Although a CBC with measurement of ESR may be ordered to assess for inflammation, results may be normal.[12]

Treatment

Patients with LCPD should be referred to an orthopedic specialist. Restoring the patient's ROM while maintaining the femoral head within the acetabulum is the primary goal in treating LCPD. Measures to help alleviate pain include bed rest, limiting the amount of physical activity, and the use of anti-inflammatories. Treatment typically involves the use of orthotic devices. Surgical intervention may be necessary in severe cases. Observation and periodic x-rays are indicated for cases in which full ROM is preserved, the patient is younger than 6 years of age, and if less than half of the femoral head is involved.[1,13] Progress should be monitored through subsequent follow-ups.

Slipped Capital Femoral Epiphysis (SCFE)

Overview

Slipped capital femoral epiphysis (SCFE) is a condition of the adolescent hip characterized by spontaneous dislocation of the femoral head in both a downward and backward position relative to the femoral neck. As a result, the femoral head slips through the epiphyseal plate.[1]

Although etiology is unknown, SCFE may be precipitated by puberty-related hormone changes. The condition is not usually associated with injury but can occur with sudden or severe trauma to the area. The condition typically presents during the adolescent growth spurts or prior to menarche in girls.[1] Incidence is highest in obese adolescents with sedentary lifestyles.[14] The condition is rare, reported in 10.8 cases out of 100,000 adolescent patients. African-American adolescents have a higher incidence rate than adolescents of other races and ethnicities.[1]

Presentation

Patients typically present with pain in the hip that usually has an acute onset. Hip pain may be severe, and the patient may be unable to ambulate or move the hip. Pain may also be reported in the knee, thigh, or groin because the pain may be referred from the hip via the obturator nerve.[1,14]

Workup

The NP should assess both hips for passive and active ROM during the physical examination. The patient should be in the prone position with knees flexed at 90° for the assessment. In most cases of SCFE, internal rotation of the hip is decreased and often painful. Gentle passive hip flexion may result in external rotation and abduction of the lower extremity.[14]

Diagnostics include radiographs of the pelvis or bilateral hips.[15] Bone scans or an MRI may be used to confirm the diagnosis.[14] Laboratory tests should be ordered for patients who present with atypical presentations of endocrine disorders or other medical conditions, including Down syndrome and short stature.[14]

Treatment

Early diagnosis and treatment is paramount to a good outcome. The NP should refer the patient to an orthopedist, who will typically oversee a surgical course of correction for the condition. The NP should also monitor the patient's other hip for indications of SCFE.[1] NSAIDs may be prescribed to manage pain stemming from SCFE. Although most patients recover well, limb shortening may result from the proximal displacement of the metaphysis in more severe cases.[15]

Genu Varum (Bowleg)

Overview

Genu varum (i.e., bowleg) is a lateral bowing of the tibia that often occurs due to joint laxity. Bowleg is considered to be normal in toddlers younger than 2 years of age. By age 3, bowleg usually resolves and children should be able to stand with their ankles apart and their knees close together. Genu varum should be suspected in children older than age 3 if the knees remain wide apart while the child stands with feet and ankles close together.[1,16]

Presentation

Pediatric patients with bowleg present are unable to stand with their knees touching when the ankles are together. The condition is confirmed if the intercondylar distance is more than 2 inches.[17] Bowing is not typically a cause for concern in children younger than age 3, and if bowing does not increase after the child begins walking and the retains full ROM in the legs.

Workup

Diagnosis of genu varum can be determined by observation alone. Diagnostic tests or labs are often unnecessary. A radiograph may help to confirm an uncertain diagnosis. A genetic assessment may be required if an underlying syndrome is suspected.[1,16]

Treatment

No treatment is necessary for pediatric patients younger than age 2 if the condition appears as a normal variant. If genu varum persists after the age of 2, is unilateral, or becomes progressively worse after the first year, the patient should be referred to an orthopedist.[18]

Genu Valgum (Knock-Knee)

Overview

Genu valgum (i.e., knock-knee) is a condition characterized by a person's knees being abnormally close with the ankle space increased. Knock-knee most commonly presents during preschool age, but the condition typically resolves by age 7.[17]

Presentation

Patients with knock-knee present with knees touching while the legs are straightened. The ankles are spread apart and separated by a distance of more than 3 in. when the knees are together. Patients with knock-knee typically experience no pain and have full ROM. However, some patients may walk or run awkwardly. If the condition persists past 7 years of age, complications such as pain, dislocation, and meniscal tears may produce.[19]

Workup

The patient can be diagnosed through observation alone. Radiographs are only necessary if the patient is older than age 7 or if unilateral involvement is present.[1]

Treatment

In younger patients, knock-knee often requires no treatment.[1] Patients older than age 7 should be referred to orthopedics for potential surgical intervention.[1,19]

Scoliosis

Overview

Scoliosis is a lateral curvature of the spine that most commonly develops during adolescence. The condition is usually idiopathic but tends to run in families; approximately 70% of all cases of scoliosis are familial. Congenital and neuromuscular types of scoliosis are less common. Females are 8 times more likely than males to develop scoliosis.[1,20]

Presentation

Scoliosis patients often present with no distinctive symptoms. Characteristic indications include intense back pain with asymmetry of the shoulders, ribs, hips, and waistline.[21]

Workup

The Adam's Forward Bend Test is the standard physical exam to screen for scoliosis. Radiographs may be ordered for further evaluation.[22]

Treatment

Patients with mild scoliosis should be evaluated every 4 to 6 months for changes in pain. If no pain is present and if spine curvature is less than 25 °, the patient may be observed rather than treated. If the adolescent patient experiences pain or spine curvature that is more than 25 °, the patient should be referred to orthopedics.[1,23,24]

Developmental Dysplasia of the Hip (DDH)

Overview

Developmental dysplasia of the hip (DDH) is abnormal dislocation (i.e., luxation or subluxation) of the hip, which causes the femoral head to become either partially or completely displaced from the acetabulum.[25]

Presentation

Infants with DDH may present with Galeazzi's sign—asymmetrical knee height while the infant is supine and the hips and knees are flexed.[26] A positive Galeazzi test is not specific for DDH, though; other conditions may cause leg length discrepancy.[27] The combination of the Barlow and Ortolani maneuvers has a high specificity for DDH. The Barlow maneuver is performed with light posterior pressure applied to abducted hips, with a palpable dislocation indicating DDH.[27] The Ortolani maneuver is performed by flexing the infant's hips and knees to 90 °, then gently abducting the thighs. If a "clunk" sound is heard when the patient's hip shrinks into the acetabulum while the hip is abducted, DDH is indicated.[28]

Until age 1, DDH is painless. If not detected in infancy, the child may begin to walk with a limp. In older children, DDH may present with decreased hip abduction.[1,26]

Workup

Patients should be examined for DDH within the first few days of life and at every Well Child Check until the child begins to walk normally. Although the Ortolani and Barlow maneuvers are preferred because of the high specificity and absence of radiation, imaging studies may be used to diagnose the condition. Plain radiography relies on metrics such as the Hilgenreiner line to ensure the hips and femurs are properly aligned. Ultrasounds are used to assess for abnormal ranges in the alpha and beta angles.[29]

Treatment

Pediatric patients with DDH should be referred to orthopedics for treatment. Bracing measures, such as a Pavlik harness or abduction brace, may see use in patients younger than 6 months of age. Older pediatric patients typically require closed or open reduction.[29]

Muscular Dystrophy

Overview

Muscular dystrophy (MD) is a chronic progressive genetic disorder that commonly originates in the lower extremities and progresses to the upper extremities and torso. MD is the most commonly inherited neuromuscular disease in pediatric patients and affects 1 out of every 3,500 males.[1] Duchenne MD, which is the most common pediatric form of MD, affects males almost exclusively because it is an x-linked disease.[30] Duchenne MD usually presents between the ages of 3 and 5 and is caused by a lack of dystrophin, a protein that maintains muscle. MD varies in how it affects the muscular system, with some cases affecting the cardiac muscles. The age of onset and rate of progression also vary.[31]

Presentation

Pediatric patients with MD may present with a combination of symptoms, including abnormalities of gait and posture. Patients may also experience developmental clumsiness and have difficulty keeping up with their peers. Gower's maneuver, in which individuals push themselves up to a standing position by using their hands to "walk up" their own body, is a common sign of Duchenne MD.[32]

Calves may appear firm, large, and woody; this appearance indicates that the healthy muscle has been replaced by degenerative tissue. Patients often experience decreased proximal muscle strength[33]; up to 82% of all males age 10 to 14 with Duchenne or Becker MD require the use of a wheelchair.[34]

Workup

A creatine kinase (CK) lab detects inflammation or muscle damage. In males, CK is markedly elevated if MD is a cause of the muscle weakness; for example, CK would fall between 15,000–35,000 IU/L in a patient with MD.[1,35] An electromyography can be used to detect myopathic changes.[32,36] Because MD may cause cardiac issues, an electrocardiogram can be conducted to assess the rate and frequency of heartbeats.[37] Other tests for MD include a muscle biopsy to detect necrotic degenerating muscle fibers, and a DNA test for analysis of genes.[38]

Treatment

There is no cure for MD, but the condition can be managed to control symptoms, delay progression, and maintain strength, and mobility.

Ankle Sprain

Overview

Ankle sprains are the most common sports-related musculoskeletal injury. Ankle sprains are characterized by the stretching or tearing of the ligaments around the ankle. Usually, the lateral ligament complex is affected. Ankle sprain injuries are usually caused by actions or movement resulting in a forced inversion or eversion of the ankle.[1,39]

Presentation

Ankle sprains are graded by the severity of the patient's injury. A grade I ankle sprain occurs when there is stretching with no tearing of the ligaments around the ankle and no joint instability. This grade of ankle sprain is characterized by local tenderness and minimal edema, with the ability to bear weight on the ankle retained. Ecchymoses is typically insignificant or absent. The full ROM may remain, but the patient usually experiences discomfort.[40,41]

A grade II ankle sprain causes partial tearing of the ligaments with some joint instability but a definite endpoint to laxity. The pain after a grade II ankle sprain typically occurs immediately upon injury and is often significant with weight bearing. Edema and ecchymosis are typically localized with this type of sprain, and ROM is often limited.[40,41]

A grade III ankle sprain involves the complete tear of a ligament. Grade III ankle sprains result in severe pain immediately upon injury, with significant edema along the foot and ankle. As a result, the pediatric patient cannot bear weight upon the ankle and has significant loss of ROM.[40,41]

Workup

An ankle sprain can be diagnosed with a physical examination that confirms tenderness and swelling. For pediatric patients 5 years of age and older, Ottawa ankle rules for use of radiography should be followed when diagnosing ankle sprains. An ankle x-ray should be ordered if a patient exhibits pain in the malleolar zone and bone tenderness at (a) the posterior edge or tip of the lateral malleolus or (b) the posterior edge or tip of the medial malleolus. Additionally, an ankle x-ray should be ordered if the patient cannot bear weight immediately after the injury and in the examining room.

A foot x-ray should be ordered if the patient exhibits pain in the midfoot zone and bone tenderness at (a) the base of the fifth metatarsal or (b) the navicular. Additionally, an ankle x-ray should be ordered if the patient cannot bear weight immediately after the injury and in the examining room. If none of these symptoms are present, a physical examination may suffice in diagnosing the condition.[41]

Treatment

All grades of ankle sprains respond well to the R-I-C-E treatment standards. The ankle should be rested, especially during the first couple days. The patient can bear some weight as tolerated for daily activities, but sports should be curtailed. The compression bandage should be applied immediately after the injury to minimize swelling, and ice should be applied on top of the compression dressing as quickly as possible after the injury. Ice should be applied in alternating periods of 30 minutes at a time. The patient should also elevate the ankle for several days after injury in order to reduce pain and swelling and promote recovery. NSAIDs can be used for pain relief. In grade III ankle sprains, surgery may be required to repair the torn ligament.[41,42]

Elbow Fracture

Overview

Patients can experience a fracture in several places on and around the elbow, including the following: above the elbow (supracondylar), at the elbow knob (condylar), at the inside of the elbow tip (epicondylar), at the growth plate (physis), or on the forearm. The fracture may also manifest as a dislocation.[1,43]

Presentation

Even though an elbow fracture may occur in several places, signs and symptoms for most elbow injuries are the same and typically including pain, swelling, and limited ROM.[44]

Workup

Elbow fractures can be diagnosed with follow-up radiographs with an oblique view. If the radiograph cannot provide a clear indication of the fracture, elevation of the anterior and posterior fat pads will suggest the presence of an occult fracture.[45]

Treatment

Pediatric patients with elbow fractures should be referred to orthopedics for proper treatment and assessment for the possibility of neurovascular injury. NSAIDs may be administered to control pain.[45]

Nursemaid Elbow

Overview

Nursemaid elbow is a common injury in children between 1 and 4 years of age that results from swinging or pulling the child's arm, which causes radial head subluxation.[46]

Presentation

Common signs and symptoms of nursemaid elbow include the inability or refusal to use the affected arm and pain with supination. Patients may also hold their affected arm against the body, with the thumb and forearm turned inward.

Workup

Manipulation of the elbow can typically diagnose the condition without ordering any imaging studies. However, ultrasonography can assess for annular ligamentous injury and displacement of the radial head from the capitellum. An MRI may be used to confirm subluxation with a ligament tear.[48] Radiographs are not standard in diagnosis, as imaging results are often normal; however, if significant swelling and bruising are present, or attempts to correct subluxation are unsuccessful, radiographs may be ordered to check for fractures or to rule out other conditions.[1,47,48]

Treatment

If nursemaid elbow has been confirmed, the NP should manipulate the arm in order to return the elbow to its proper condition. This involves supporting the elbow with one hand while placing a thumb laterally over the radial head of the child's elbow, grasping the child's hand, and deliberately supinating and externally rotating the forearm while flexing the elbow. If the subluxation is corrected, the patient should feel immediate relief and be able to use the arm again in a matter of minutes. A splint may be recommended for the next few days in order to ensure comfort, especially if the injury persisted for hours before being corrected.[49] NSAIDs may also be recommended for supportive care.[1]

References

1. Barkley TW Jr. Musculoskeletal issues and disorders. In: Barkley TW Jr, ed. *Pediatric Primary Care Nurse Practitioner Certification Review/Clinical Update Continuing Education Course*. West Hollywood, CA: Barkley and Associates; 2015: 130–137.

2. Mayo Clinic Staff. Osgood-Schlatter disease. Mayo Clinic Web site. http://www.mayoclinic.com/health/osgood-schlatter-disease/DS00392. Updated February 28, 2014. Accessed April 20, 2015.

3. Mayo Clinic Staff. Osgood-Schlatter disease: Symptoms. Mayo Clinic Web site. http://www.mayoclinic.com/health/osgood-schlatter-disease/DS00392/DSECTION=symptoms. Updated February 28, 2014. Accessed April 20, 2015.

4. Weiler R, Ingram M, Wolman R. Osgood-Schlatter disease. *Praxis.* 2011; 100(22): 1369–1370. doi:10.1024/1661-8157/a000715

5. Sullivan JA. Osgood-Schlatter disease workup. In: Young CC, ed. Medscape. http://emedicine.medscape.com/article/1993268-workup#showall. Updated July 15, 2014. Accessed April 24, 2015.

6. Sullivan JA. Osgood-Schlatter disease treatment & management. In: Young CC, ed. Medscape. http://emedicine.medscape.com/article/1993268-treatment. Updated July 15, 2014. Accessed April 20, 2015.

7. Sankar WN, Horn BD, Wells L, Dormans JP. Transient monoarticular synovitis (toxic synovitis). In: Kliegman RM, Stanton BF, St. Geme JW III, Schor NF, Behrman RE, eds. *Nelson Textbook of Pediatrics.* 19th ed. Philadelphia, PA: Elsevier Saunders; 2011: 2360.

8. Whitelaw CC, Schikler KN. Transient synovitis. In: Jung LK, ed. Medscape. http://emedicine.medscape.com/article/1007186-overview#showall. Updated October 9, 2014. Accessed April 20, 2015.

9. Gutierrez K. Transient synovitis. In: Long SS, Pickering LK, Prober CG, eds. *Principles and Practice of Pediatric Infectious Diseases.* 4th ed. London, UK: Elsevier Churchill Livingstone; 2012: 485–486.

10. Legg-Calve-Perthes disease. A.D.A.M. Medical Encyclopedia. http://www.nlm.nih.gov/medlineplus/ency/article/001264.htm. Updated August 22, 2013. Accessed April 20, 2015.

11. Sankar WN, Horn BD, Wells L, Dormans JP. Legg-Calve-Perthes disease. In: Kliegman RM, Stanton BF, St. Geme JW III, Schor NF, Behrman RE, eds. *Nelson Textbook of Pediatrics.* 19th ed. Philadelphia, PA: Elsevier Saunders; 2011: 2361–2362.

12. McQuillen KK. Musculoskeletal disorders. In: Marx JA, Hockberger RS, Walls RM, et al., eds. *Rosen's Emergency Medicine: Concepts and Clinical Practice.* 8th ed. Philadelphia, PA: Elsevier Saunders; 2014: 2250–2270.

13. Kim HKW, Herring JA. Legg-Calvé-Perthes disease. In: Herring JA, ed. *Tachdijan's Pediatric Orthopaedics.* 5th ed. Philadelphia, PA: Elsevier Saunders; 2013: 580–629.

14. Walter KD, Lin DY, Schwartz E. Slipped capital femoral epiphysis. In: Young CC, ed. Medscape. http://emedicine.medscape.com/article/91596-overview#showall. Updated December 17, 2014. Accessed April 20, 2015.

15. Germann CA, Fix ML. Hip and femur injuries. In: Wolfson AB, Cloutier RL, Hendey GW, Ling LJ, Rosen CL, Schaider JJ, eds. *Harwood-Nuss' Clinical Practice of Emergency Medicine.* 6th ed. Philadelphia, PA: Wolters Kluwer Health/Lippincott Williams & Wilkins; 2015: 285–288.

16. Stevens PM. Pediatric genu varum. In: Grogan DP, ed. Medscape. http://emedicine.medscape.com/article/1355974-overview#showall. Updated August 29, 2013. Accessed April 24, 2015.

17. Wells L, Sehgal K. Coronal plane deformities. In: Kliegman RM, Stanton BF, St Geme JW III, Schor NF, Behrman RE, eds. *Nelson Textbook of Pediatrics.* 19th ed. Philadelphia, PA: Elsevier Saunders; 2011: 2348–2349.

18. Canale ST. Osteochondrosis or epiphysitis and other miscellaneous affections. In: Canale ST, Beatty JH, eds. *Campbell's Operative Orthopaedics.* 12th ed. Philadelphia, PA: Elsevier Mosby; 2012: 1133–1201.

19. Stevens PM, Holmstrom MC. Pediatric genu valgum. In: Grogan DP, ed. Medscape. http://emedicine.medscape.com/article/1259772-overview#a0112. Updated April 24, 2014. Accessed April 20, 2015.

20. Hresko MT. Clinical practice: Idiopathic scoliosis in adolescents. *N Engl J Med.* 2013; 368(9): 834–841. doi: 10.1056/NEJMcp1209063

21. Idiopathic scoliosis: Adolescents. Scoliosis Research Society Web site. http://www.srs.org/patient_and_family/scoliosis/idiopathic/adolescents. Accessed April 20, 2015.

22. Mayo Clinic Staff. Scoliosis. Mayo Clinic Web site. http://www.mayoclinic.com/health/scoliosis/DS00194. Updated February 3, 2012. Accessed April 20, 2015.

23. Scherl SA. Adolescent idiopathic scoliosis: Management and prognosis. In: Basow DS, ed. *UpToDate*. Waltham, MA: UpToDate; 2015. http://www.uptodate.com/contents/adolescent-idiopathic-scoliosis-treatment-and-prognosis. Last updated September 2, 2014. Accessed May 22, 2015.

24. Ullrich PF Jr. Scoliosis treatment. Spine-Health Web site. http://www.spine-health.com/conditions/scoliosis/scoliosis-treatment. Updated January 20, 2012. Accessed April 24, 2015.

25. Sankar WN, Horn BD, Wells L, Dormans JP. The hip. In: Kliegman RM, Stanton BF, St. Geme JW III, Schor NF, Behrman RE, eds. *Nelson Textbook of Pediatrics*. 19th ed. Philadelphia, PA: Elsevier Saunders; 2011: 2355–2364.

26. Tamai J, McCarthy JJ. Development dysplasia of the hip. In: Jaffe WL, ed. Medscape. http://emedicine.medscape.com/article/1248135-overview#showall. Updated March 31, 2014. Accessed April 20, 2015.

27. Rosenfeld SB. Developmental dysplasia of the hip: Clinical features and diagnosis. In: Basow DS, ed. *UpToDate*. Waltham, MA: UpToDate; 2015. http://www.uptodate.com/contents/developmental-dysplasia-of-the-hip-clinical-features-and-diagnosis. Last updated April 14, 2015. Accessed May 22, 2015.

28. Sewell MD, Eastwood DM. Screening and treatment in developmental dysplasia of the hip – where do we go from here? *Int Orthop*. 2011; 35(9): 1359–1367. doi: 10.1007/s00264-011-1257-z

29. Blanco JS, Doyle SM, Scher DM, Sink EL, Widmann RF. Developmental pediatric hip dysplasia – an overview. Hospital for Special Surgery Web site. http://www.hss.edu/conditions_developmental-pediatric-hip-dysplasia-overview.asp. Reviewed and updated December 18, 2012. Accessed May 22, 2015.

30. Duchenne muscular dystrophy: Causes/inheritance. Muscular Dystrophy Association Web site. http://www.mda.org/disease/duchenne-muscular-dystrophy/causes-inheritance. Accessed April 24, 2015.

31. U. S. Department of Health and Human Services, National Institutes of Health, National Institute of Neurological Disorders and Stroke, Office of Communications and Public Liaison. NINDS muscular dystrophy information page. http://www.ninds.nih.gov/disorders/md/md.htm. Last updated April 8, 2015. Accessed April 20, 2015.

32. Darras BT. Clinical features and diagnosis of Duchenne and Becker muscular dystrophy. In: Basow DS, ed. *UpToDate*. Waltham, MA: UpToDate; 2015. http://www.uptodate.com/contents/clinical-features-and-diagnosis-of-duchenne-and-becker-muscular-dystrophy?source=search_result&search=Duchenne+becker&selectedTitle=1~79. Last updated November 18, 2014. Accessed April 20, 2015.

33. Darras BT. Patient information: Overview of muscular dystrophies (beyond the basics). In: Basow DS, ed. *UpToDate*. Waltham, MA: UpToDate; 2015. http://www.uptodate.com/contents/overview-of-muscular-dystrophies-beyond-the-basics. Last updated October 2, 2013. Accessed April 20, 2015.

34. U.S. Department of Health and Human Services, Centers for Disease Control and Prevention, National Center on Birth Defects and Developmental Disabilities. http://www.cdc.gov/ncbddd/musculardystrophy/data.html. Last updated March 23, 2015. Accessed April 24, 2015.

35. American Association for Clinical Chemistry. CK: The test. Lab Tests Online Web site. http://labtestsonline.org/understanding/analytes/ck/tab/test. Last reviewed February 25, 2013. Last updated February 24, 2015. Accessed April 20, 2015.

36. Mayo Clinic Staff. Electromyography (EMG). Mayo Clinic Web site. http://www.mayoclinic.com/print/emg/MY00107/METHOD=print&DSECTION=all. Updated October 25, 2012. Accessed April 20, 2015.

37. Muscular dystrophy. A.D.A.M. Medical Encyclopedia. http://www.nlm.nih.gov/medlineplus/ency/article/001190.htm. Updated February 24, 2014. Accessed April 20, 2015.

38. Darras BT. Treatment of Duchenne and Becker muscular dystrophy. In: Basow DS, ed. *UpToDate.* Waltham, MA: UpToDate; 2015. http://www.uptodate.com/contents/treatment-of-duchenne-and-becker-muscular-dystrophy. Last updated October 15, 2014. Accessed April 20, 2015.

39. Mayo Clinic Staff. Sprained ankle. Mayo Clinic Web site. http://www.mayoclinic.com/health/sprained-ankle/DS01014. Updated August 21, 2014. Accessed April 20, 2015.

40. Maughan KL. Ankle sprain. In: Basow DS, ed. *UpToDate.* Waltham, MA: UpToDate; 2015. http://www.uptodate.com/contents/ankle-sprain. Last updated April 3, 2015. Accessed April 20, 2015.

41. Tiemstra JD. Update on acute ankle sprains. *Am Fam Physician.* 2012; 85(12): 1170–1176. http://www.aafp.org/afp/2012/0615/p1170.html.

42. Young CC. Ankle sprain. In: Ho SSW, ed. Medscape. http://emedicine.medscape.com/article/1907229-overview#showall. Updated December 16, 2014. Accessed April 20, 2015.

43. Nishijima DK, Goldman M. Elbow fracture. In: Kulkarni R, ed. Medscape. http://emedicine.medscape.com/article/824654-overview#showall. Updated February 26, 2014. Accessed April 20, 2015.

44. Bachman D, Santora S. Orthopedic trauma. In: Fleisher GR, Ludwig S, Bachur RG, Gorelick MH, Shaw KN, Ruddy RM, eds. *Textbook of Pediatric Emergency Medicine.* 6th ed. Philadelphia, PA: Wolters Kluwer Health/Lippincott Williams & Wilkins; 2010: 1335–1375.

45. Blanco JS, Doyle SM, Green DW, Scher DM, Sink EL, Widmann RF. Elbow fractures in children: An Overview. Hospital for Special Surgery Web site. http://www.hss.edu/conditions_elbow-fractures-children-overview.asp. Reviewed and updated December 12, 2012. Accessed May 22, 2015.

46. Wolfram W, Boss DN. Nursemaid elbow: Overview. In: Bachur RG, ed. Medscape. http://emedicine.medscape.com/article/803026-overview#a0104. Updated February 7, 2014. Accessed April 20, 2015.

47. Mayo Clinic Staff. Dislocated elbow. Mayo Clinic Web site. http://www.mayoclinic.com/health/dislocated-elbow/DS01165. Updated April 3, 2015. Accessed April 20, 2015.

48. Wolfram W, Boss DN. Nursemaid elbow workup. In: Bachur RG, ed. Medscape. http://emedicine.medscape.com/article/803026-workup. Updated February 7, 2014. Accessed April 24, 2015.

49. Sigman LJ. Procedures. In: Tschudy MM, Arcara KM, eds. *The Harriet Lane Handbook.* 19th ed. Philadelphia, PA: Elsevier Mosby; 2011: 57–88.

Chapter 15

Neurologic Disorders

QUESTIONS

1. In what area of the brain do childhood tumors predominately occur?

   a. Infratentorial region

   b. Supratentorial region

   c. Tentorium cerebelli

   d. Occipital lobes

2. Which cranial nerve controls hearing and equilibrium?

   a. CN II

   b. CN IV

   c. CN VI

   d. CN VIII

3. The practitioner knows that which of the following prophylactic drugs is not used in pediatric migraine management?

   a. Doxepin

   b. Bisoprolol

   c. Ibuprofen

   d. Amitriptyline

4. Which of the following characteristics is not typically associated with febrile seizures?

   a. Fever with rectal temperature of 102 °F or above

   b. Generally manifests in early infancy by 3 months of age

   c. There is usually a family history of febrile seizures

   d. There is typically a loss of consciousness with this type of seizure

5. Tension and psychogenic headaches are commonly associated with what mechanism of headache pain?

   a. Vascular dilation

   b. Traction

   c. Muscular contraction

   d. Inflammation

6. Jamie, a 4-year-old male, presents to the clinic in a sleepy, afebrile state. His mother mentions that, after his afternoon nap, he started screaming in their brightly-lit den and began vomiting. When she tried to talk to him, he spoke nonsense. When you talk to Jamie, he rouses, exhibits normal speech, and says he feels fine. What is the most likely source of Jamie's symptoms?

   a. Viral meningitis

   b. Brain tumor

   c. Neurofibromatosis

   d. Confusional migraine

7. A patient has been referred to your practice by an optometrist, who found Lisch nodules in the patient's irises. Which finding would best help to confirm the suspected diagnosis?

   a. Photophobia

   b. Failure to thrive

   c. Axillary freckling

   d. Aphasia

8. Which of the following best defines a simple partial seizure?

   a. Staring for 25 seconds prior to onset of minor autonomic symptoms

   b. Minor motor symptoms with no loss of consciousness

   c. Staring for 10 seconds with brief onset and termination

   d. Partial loss of consciousness with increased muscle tone

9. Which of these signs would indicate meningitis in a patient?

   a. Pain upon external rotation of the knee

   b. Pain upon extension of the leg when the hip is flexed 90 °

   c. Sciatic pain when both legs are elevated off the exam table

   d. Pain with internal rotation of the flexed right thigh

10. In a patient with tic disorders, all of the following presentations would typically be recognized as a simple tic <u>except</u>:

   a. Blinking for 30 seconds without interruption

   b. Extensive clearing of the throat

   c. Jerking the head back and forth

   d. Repeating a word another person said

RATIONALES

1. a

Seventy to 80% of childhood brain tumors occur in the infratentorial region of the brain. Despite ongoing research, the etiology of these tumors is unknown. The supratentorial region, tentorium cerebelli, and occipital lobes may develop tumors; however, these regions are not predominating areas of occurrence of brain tumors in children.

2. d

CN VIII is known as the acoustic nerve, which controls hearing and equilibrium. CN II, on the other hand, controls vision. CN IV controls downward and inward eye movement, whereas CN VI controls lateral eye movement.

3. a

Doxepin is a tricyclic antidepressant used to treat depression and anxiety disorders, but is not suitable for migraine prophylaxis and is not approved for pediatric patients. Although tricyclic antidepressants are generally not used in migraine management, amitriptyline may see use when the migraines are accompanied by chronic pain, insomnia, or depression. Bisoprolol and other beta-blockers are thought to interfere with arterial dilation, and thus are commonly considered a drug of choice for preventing chronic migraine. Lastly, ibuprofen belongs to the class of NSAIDs widely used in migraine treatment.

4. b

Febrile seizures do not generally manifest before 6 months of age; such an early manifestation should call for a referral to a pediatric neurologist. Febrile seizures generally develop between 6 months of age and 5 years of age, with peak incidence in the toddler years. A patient with a familial history of febrile seizures often stands a higher risk of developing the condition. Febrile seizures often present when rectal temperature exceeds 102 °F and generally cause a loss of consciousness.

5. c

Tension and psychogenic headaches are closely associated with muscular contraction. Vascular dilation, on the other hand, is a mechanism of pain associated with migraine headaches. Traction is associated with space-occupying lesions, such as hematomas and increased intracranial pressure. Lastly, inflammation is associated with infections of parts of the body, such as the meninges.

6. d

Confusional migraines may present with confusion, aphasia, vomiting, photophobia, and agitation; once these symptoms pass, the patient may fall into a deep sleep, only to wake up feeling well. Since confusional migraine is commonly a diagnosis of exclusion, it warrants a work-up to rule out organic causes. Brain tumors may also produce aphasia, vomiting, and photophobia, and sleepiness; in children, however, tumors typically also present with headache that is at its worst in the morning. Viral meningitis produces vomiting and photophobia as well, but also typically exhibits fever. Neurofibromatosis is characterized by seizures and multiple café au lait spots.

7. c

Lisch nodules in the irises and axillary freckling are part of the diagnostic criteria for neurofibromatosis type 1; inguinal freckling would also indicate the condition. Photophobia would more likely indicate bacterial meningitis or migraines, aphasia more commonly produces as a result of migraines or brain tumor, and failure to thrive more often arises from disease or dysfunction of multiple bodily systems.

8. b

A simple partial seizure presents with no loss of consciousness and minor motor, autonomic, or sensory symptoms. A complex partial seizure will present with the same symptoms, but is accompanied by an episode of staring longer than 20 seconds that presents before, during, or after the symptoms. An absence, or petit mal, seizure is characterized by a brief staring episode of 10–20 seconds with brief onset and termination. Partial or complete loss of consciousness accompanying increased muscle tone indicates a tonic seizure.

9. b

Kernig's sign, a hallmark indicator of meningitis, presents as pain when the leg is elevated 90 ° from the hip and extended. Pain upon external rotation of the knee is Lachman's test, an indicator of damage to the anterior or posterior cruciate ligament of the knee. The positive straight leg raise test, meant to diagnose lower back pain, presents as radiating or sciatic pain when both legs are elevated off the exam table. Pain with internal rotation of the flexed right thigh is the Obturator sign, an indicator of appendicitis.

10. d

Repetition of another person's words, or echolalia, is typically recognized as a complex tic, not a simple tic. In tic disorders, simple tics are those which involve a single muscle group or a simple sound. Such simple tics may include sustained blinking, jerking the head back and forth, or throat clearing.

DISCUSSION

Headache

Overview

Headaches consist of pain in any part of the head, which is caused by activation of specific pain-sensitive structures.[1] Headaches may present for a multitude of reasons and can be difficult to evaluate. Although headaches commonly occur, serious causes are rare.[2] Proper evaluation of the history of the patient's headache and its associated symptoms is essential to making an accurate diagnosis.

Presentation

There are four primary mechanisms of headache pain: vascular pain, muscle contraction, traction, and inflammation.[2] Vascular dilation, which occurs in migraine headaches, consists of cranial artery distension caused by dilation or swelling of the blood vessels.[3] Causes of vascular dilation include fever, vasodilator drugs, metabolic disturbance, and systemic infections.[4] Muscular contraction, which occurs in tension headaches, involves tension of the head and neck muscles.[5] Traction pain may be caused by increased intracranial pressure and space-occupying lesions such as brain tumors, mass lesions, abscesses, and hematomas.[4] Lastly, headaches related to inflammation are often caused by infections in the meninges, sinuses, and teeth.[6]

For assessment of headache symptoms, the nurse practitioner (NP) may use the OLD CART system. This mnemonic reminds NPs to evaluate headache based on onset, location of pain, duration of headache, distinctive characteristics, aggravating factors, remedial and alleviating factors, and effective methods of treatment.[4]

Headache Considerations

Overview

Headache considerations in febrile patients include meningitis, which may be bacterial, viral, tuberculous, or aseptic. Brain abscess or other intracranial infections, encephalitis, and hypoglycemia should also be considered in febrile patients, as well as dehydration and sinusitis. Headache patients may also present with associated infections such as strep throat, influenza, mononucleosis, or rubeola.[4]

Headache considerations for afebrile patients include subarachnoid and intraparenchymal hemorrhages, postictal headaches, cerebral ischemia, severe hypertension, acute dental disease, and acute glaucoma. Space-occupying conditions such as brain tumors and hydrocephalies may also be suspected.[4]

Meningitis

Overview

Meningitis is an inflammation of the meninges, which envelop the brain and spinal cord. Although meningitis may occur in patients of any age, infants are at a higher risk for developing the condition.[7]

Most cases of meningitis in the United States are caused by viruses.[8] Enteroviruses are the most common source of viral meningitis; these infections usually occur in the summer and early autumn but may develop in sporadic cases throughout the year.[9] Bacterial meningitis, on the other hand, makes up only a small percentage of meningitis cases; when it does occur, it is extremely serious and is considered a medical emergency.[10] The most common bacterial causes of meningitis in children are *Streptococcus pneumoniae* and *Neisseria meningitidis*, the latter of which can cause death within hours.[11] Other causative agents of bacterial meningitis include group B *Streptococcus*, *Haemophilus influenzae*, and *Escherichia coli*, among others.[7]

Presentation

Meningitis is often indicated by temperatures higher than 101.8 °F (38.8 °C).[4,12] The classic triad of meningitis symptoms consists of fever, headache, and nuchal rigidity; however, many meningitis patients do not present with this triad of symptoms.[13] For example, most signs and symptoms of meningitis in pediatric patients are behavioral responses such as tantrums and sleep disturbance.[4,12] Newborns and young infants may present with other signs and symptoms such as irritability, lethargy, poor feeding, and a bulging fontanel.[14] Older infants and children may also present with headaches and irritability. Other typical signs and symptoms of meningitis include nausea and vomiting, photophobia, confusion, hyperesthesia, cranial nerve palsy, and ataxia.[4,15] Back pain may also occur in cases of meningitis caused by *Staphylococcus aureus* and other bacteria.[11]

Furthermore, nuchal rigidity can be demonstrated by both Kernig's and Brudzinski's signs.[16] A positive Kernig's sign consists of pain on extension of the leg when the hip is flexed at 90 °. A positive Brudzinski's sign is indicated by involuntary flexion of the legs when the neck is flexed.[17,18]

Workup

When meningitis is suspected, patients should undergo a cerebrospinal fluid (CSF) analysis via lumbar puncture.[19] A confirmatory finding will appear cloudy and show white blood cells, increased protein, and decreased glucose.[4]

Treatment

Antibiotics are the mainstay of treatment for bacterial meningitis,[11] and the choice of antibiotic typically depends on the type of bacteria that causes the patient's condition. Ceftriaxone and cefotaxime often see use against gram-negative organisms, whereas vancomycin may see use if *S. pneumoniae* is believed to be the causative pathogen.[19] Most cases of viral meningitis resolve on their own, and patients can be treated with bed rest, fluids, and over-the-counter medications.[8]

Brain Tumors

Overview

Brain tumors form as masses of abnormal cells, which may be either benign or malignant.[20] Although the cause of brain tumors is unknown, these masses are a leading cause of cancer-related deaths, as well as the most common type of solid cancer in children younger than 15 years of age.[21] Infratentorial brainstem tumors comprise the majority of tumors in children.[22]

Presentation

Frequently, headaches are the worst symptom in brain tumor patients. Headaches commonly appear in older children with brain tumors; upon manifestation, these headaches usually increase in frequency, are typically followed by vomiting, and are worse in the morning. Seizures are also a common symptom of brain tumors in both adult and pediatric patients.[20] Certain signs and symptoms depend on the location of the tumor; for example, ataxia is often associated with brain tumors located in the cerebellum.[21] Moreover, the patient may present with other abnormal neurologic or ocular findings, such as hemiparesis, cranial nerve palsies, somnolence, and papilledema. Additional abnormal neurologic findings include a positive Babinski sign, behavioral changes, loss of fine motor control, and diabetes insipidus. Finally, certain signs and symptoms are found specifically in infants and may include the following: increased head circumference, irritability, head tilt, failure to thrive, the loss of developmental milestones, and a tense, bulging fontanel.[4]

Workup

In most cases of brain tumors, magnetic resonance imaging (MRI) is the only diagnostic test needed.[23] Brain tumors may also be diagnosed with other imaging tests such as a computerized axial tomography (CAT) scan and computed tomography (CT) scan. A lumbar puncture (LP) may be used, but this test should only be performed after a neurological examination, and the NP should approach an LP with caution due to technical considerations.[24]

Treatment

Treatment of brain tumors is determined by the location and grade of the tumor.[21] Tumors are graded numerically from 1 to 4 according to their microscopic appearance and abnormality. Grade 1 tumors appear close to normal, whereas higher grade tumors appear abnormal and spread more rapidly.[25] Surgical removal of the tumor is often possible, and radiation therapy and chemotherapy are procedures that may be used if removal is not possible.[26]

Migraine Headaches (Vascular Headaches)

Overview

Migraine headaches are vascular headaches that are caused by dilation and excessive pulsation of branches of the external carotid artery. Females are more often affected by migraine headaches than males, and often there is a family history of migraines.[27] A variety of "triggers" associated with migraines include emotional or physical stress, lack or excess sleep, missed meals, and nitrate-containing foods. Alcoholic beverages, menstruation, and use of oral contraceptives may trigger migraines in adolescents.[28]

Visual and sensory symptoms of migraine headaches are known collectively as an aura, and onset usually occurs before the patient experiences head pain.[29] The presence or absence of an aura helps distinguish between classic and common migraines, as an aura typically appears in classic migraines, not common migraines. Furthermore, common migraines are the most frequent type of migraine in childhood, whereas classic migraines occur less frequently in children.[28]

Presentation

Migraines present with a dull or throbbing headache that may occur on one or both sides of the patient's head, accompanied by focal neurologic disturbances such as field defects and luminous visual hallucinations.[27] A number of other prominent signs and symptoms occur along with the headache, including nausea and vomiting, photophobia, and phonophobia.[1] The patient may also present with aphasia, numbness, tingling, clumsiness, and weakness.[4]

Confusional migraines are a type of migraine that commonly occur in younger children, and typically consist of a period of confusion and disorientation that is followed by vomiting and deep sleep, after which the patient awakens feeling well. Pediatric patients may or may not report a headache.[4] Another childhood periodic syndrome is abdominal migraines, which present with episodic abdominal pain, not head pain, as well as nausea and vomiting.[30]

Workup

Migraine headaches are commonly diagnosed by a physical examination, which helps detect characteristic signs and symptoms.[1] Additional studies are indicated by the patient's history and physical exam findings, and may also help to rule out other diagnoses.[29] Blood chemistries, basic metabolic panel, complete blood count (CBC), and an erythrocyte sedimentation rate test should be considered to rule out infection. A Venereal Disease Research Laboratory test may be used to rule out syphilis, and a CT scan of the head may rule out tumors.[4]

Treatment

When managing migraine headaches, avoidance of trigger factors is very important, and the NP should advise the patient to keep a headache diary.[27] A balanced diet, aerobic exercise, and regular sleep are recommended to improve general health, and relaxation and stress management can also help to reduce headaches.[27,28,29] Moreover, the patient should eliminate monosodium glutamate (MSG) and nitrates, or nitrites, from his or her diet. It is also recommended that the patient either reduce or eliminate his or her caffeine intake.[4]

Prophylactic therapy should be considered if attacks occur more than 3 or 4 times per month or if migraines interfere with the patient's daily functioning.[29] Non-steroidal anti-inflammatory drugs (NSAIDs) may be given in chronic low doses daily. Other prophylactic agents include propranolol, amitriptyline, and topiramate.[31] Imipramine, an antidepressant with tumor-fighting properties, is given in doses of 10–150 mg daily, whereas verapamil, a calcium channel blocker that exhibits antiproliferative action, is prescribed in doses of 15–30 mg/kg by mouth twice a day.[4]

The NP may manage an acute migraine attack by prescribing antiemetics as well as having the patient rest in a dark, quiet room.[4] Additionally, a simple analgesic such as ibuprofen taken immediately may provide some relief.[32] The NP should prescribe ibuprofen in doses of 7.5–10 mg/kg in younger children; doses may be increased up to 800 mg in older teens.[4]

Triptans are recommended when over-the-counter analgesics are not effective.[33] These triptans may include almotriptan, which is approved for children 12 years and older and is administered in doses of 6.25 mg. Rizatriptan is given in 5 mg doses, and sumatriptan and zolmitriptan are both given nasally in 5 mg doses. Sumatriptan tablets are less expensive, but they may not work as well due to slower absorption. All triptans noted above have been found to have the greatest effect in adolescents, whereas triptans recommended for ages 6–11 years include rizatriptan (Maxalt) 5 mg and sumatriptan (Imitrex) nasal 5 mg. The patient may take triptans at the first sign of a headache, and then repeat in 2 hours if needed; however, triptans should be avoided in children who are at risk for heart disease.[4]

Seizure Disorder

Overview

Seizure disorders consist of transient disturbances of cerebral function due to an abnormal paroxysmal neuronal discharge in the brain. There are several types of seizures, each with different presentations, diagnostic findings, and treatments. The term epilepsy denotes any disorder characterized by recurrent seizures; however, many individuals who have a seizure never experience a second one.[34] Moreover, fevers can lower the seizure threshold and, thus, make it easier for patients to develop seizures.[35]

Seizures may be caused by congenital abnormalities. Perinatal injuries may result in seizures presenting in infancy and early childhood. Among adolescents, trauma is a major cause of seizures. Metabolic disorders have also been linked to seizures, including hypocalcaemia, hypoglycemia, pyridoxine deficiency, renal failure, and acidosis. Furthermore, seizures can be caused by infectious diseases such as bacterial meningitis, herpes encephalitis, and neurosyphilis. Lastly, seizures are common in patients with brain tumors.[36]

Presentation

Seizures may be either partial or generalized. Partial seizures are concentrated in a limited area of the brain and do not typically affect the patient's awareness or memory. However, there may be a variety of other motor, autonomic, and sensory symptoms, such as abnormal perceptions, hallucinations, or uncontrollable muscle contraction.[37] Complex partial seizures, on the other hand, commonly impair the patient's awareness and memory during, before, and after the seizure.[37]

There are a variety of types of generalized seizures, which are typically bilateral and involve both hemispheres. Distinguishing between different types of seizures can be difficult, though eyewitness accounts and recorded evidence of the seizure can aid in diagnosis.[38]

Absence, or petit mal, seizures almost always begin in childhood and consist of brief "staring" episodes that usually last only a few seconds.[39]

Tonic seizures, on the other hand, cause a sudden increase in muscle tone, producing a number of characteristic postures that may make it difficult for the patient to breathe.[40] During the onset of tonic seizures, consciousness is usually partially or completely lost; postictal alteration of consciousness is usually brief and may last several minutes.[4]

Tonic-clonic (i.e., grand mal) seizures often present with a sudden loss of consciousness and arrested respirations during the tonic phase; subsequently, the patient enters the clonic phase, which involves increased muscle tone followed by rhythmic jerks.[40] Moreover, urinary or fecal incontinence may occur in the clonic phase. The postictal state can last minutes to hours, and is characterized by deep sleep for up to an hour, headaches, disorientation, muscle discomfort, and nausea.[4]

Lastly, atonic seizures cause sudden loss of muscle tone and may result in the patient falling to the ground or dropping his or her head.[41]

Workup

When investigating the underlying cause of the patient's seizures, an electroencephalogram (EEG) is an essential component of the patient's evaluation.[42] Additional tests may help rule out suspected causes that may be indicated by the patient's age and history, such as a CT scan, an MRI scan, and an LP.[14,43] A CBC, glucose test, renal and liver function test, and serologic test for syphilis should also be performed to assess the patient's overall health and to detect underlying conditions that may be causing the patient's seizures, such as anemia and diabetes mellitus.[4,43]

Treatment

The initial management of seizures is supportive, as most seizures are self-limiting. The NP should maintain an open airway, protect the patient from injuries, and administer oxygen if the patient is cyanotic. It is important, however, not to force artificial airways or objects between the patient's teeth, as this may result in chips, cracks, or other dental injuries.[4] Parenteral anticonvulsants, including benzodiazepines such as lorazepam, are used to stop convulsive seizures.[44] The NP should consider a referral to neurology or the emergency room if the patient's seizures continue despite therapeutic monitoring through anticonvulsant levels, if there is a regression of cognitive function or developmental skills, or if the patient's side effect profile is unacceptable.[4]

Febrile Seizures

Overview

Febrile seizures occur during the course of, and as a result of, fevers. Although febrile seizures occur in only a small percentage of children, these seizures are the most common type of seizure in pediatric patients.[45] After the onset of a fever, most febrile seizures develop within 24 hours; conversely, if a seizure occurs more than 24 hours after onset of fever, it is likely due to an infection.[4,46] Some pediatric patients have a family history that puts them at risk for febrile seizures.[47] Other risk factors for febrile seizures include tobacco use by mothers during pregnancy, prematurity, neonatal hospitalization for more than 28 days, and frequent infections in the first year of age.[4]

Presentation

The majority of febrile seizures are either clonic or tonic-clonic, and episodes typically last less than 5 minutes.[4,46] The NP should perform a physical exam to rule out meningitis and other infectious causes of seizures such as chickenpox, tonsillitis, herpes simplex virus, and the flu.[48]

Workup

Although diagnostic testing is usually unnecessary for patients with febrile seizures, an LP is indicated in cases where meningitis is suspected.[49] EEGs, chemistries, and serologies are not indicated, as febrile seizure patients typically do not need a full seizure workup.[47]

Treatment

Febrile seizures should be treated if they continue for more than 5 minutes.[49] During treatment, the NP should protect the patient's airway and place him or her in a side-lying position. Cooling measures and acetaminophen are recommended to treat febrile seizures as well. Seizure prophylaxis in collaboration with a neurologist is indicated based on considerations such as a family history of seizures, a prior abnormal neurological exam, previous seizures, and more than one seizure in 24 hours. Furthermore, prophylaxis is also warranted if the patient experiences recurring seizures.[4]

Neurofibromatosis (von Recklinghausen Disease)

Overview

Neurofibromatosis (NF) is a neurocutaneous syndrome characterized by numerous café-au-lait spots (CLS) on the skin, as well as nerve tumors on the skin and in the body. The condition is usually diagnosed in childhood or early adulthood, and may either be inherited or caused by a mutation in the patient's genes.[50,51] NF does not affect the patient's intelligence, and the severity of the condition is highly variable.[4] There are two common types of NF: Type 1 NF, also known as von Recklinghausen disease, is the more prevalent of the two and presents with neurologic and cutaneous manifestations; type 2 NF, on the other hand, only accounts for a small percentage of NF cases and primarily manifests itself as acoustic neuromas.[52]

Presentation

NF commonly presents with multiple CLS, which are usually the earliest clinical findings in patients with the condition.[53] To confirm a diagnosis of NF, the patient's presentation must include at least two of the following criteria: six or more CLS that are either larger than 5 mm in diameter in prepubertal children or larger than 15 mm in postpubertal children; two or more cutaneous neurofibromas; axillary or inguinal freckling; two or more iris Lisch nodules; distinctive osseous lesions; and an autosomal dominant NF1 gene mutation present in a first-degree relative.[54]

Workup

NF is usually diagnosed based on the patient's physical examination and medical history.[55] If neurologic signs and symptoms are present, the patient should undergo an MRI, which is the preferred imaging study for diagnosis. A CT scan may also be used for imaging screening of NF. Both imaging studies may be used to detect the presence of optic gliomas or acoustic neuromas.[4,52,53]

Treatment

Treatment of NF depends on the type of tumor and complications that appear in the patient's presentation.[56] Surgery may be used to remove the patient's tumors, and nerve resection can be accomplished by most surgeons.[53] Radiation or chemotherapy may also be needed if the tumors are cancerous.[51] Furthermore, NF patients should be referred to a neurologist, and genetic counseling may be recommended.[52]

Tic Disorders

Overview

Tic disorders consist of brief, abrupt, non-purposeful movements or utterances. Movements usually involve the face, neck, or shoulders, and may sometimes involve muscles of the limbs or other parts of the body. The onset of tic disorders usually occurs during school age; etiology is unknown, although tic disorders may be genetically inherited.[22,57] Frequently, tic disorders are unrecognized as a movement disorder in children. Many cases of tic disorders either resolve by themselves or become less severe by the time patients reach adulthood.[58]

The most common tic disorder is Tourette syndrome, which onsets before adulthood and is characterized by motor and vocal tics lasting more than 1 year.[59,60] Tic disorders are often caused by other psychobehavioral problems such as attention deficit hyperactivity disorder (ADHD).[61] Moreover, tic disorders may be associated with medications such as methylphenidate, pemoline, and amphetamines.[4]

Presentation

Patients with tic disorders present with movements that can be classified as simple or complex tics. Simple motor tics may include movements such as blinking or grimacing, among other behaviors.[58] Complex motor tics, on the other hand, last longer and may appear intentional because they involve recognizable words and gestures.[60] These tics may include copropraxia (i.e., obscene gestures), coprographia (i.e., obscene writing), coprolalia (i.e., obscene speech), palilalia (i.e., repeating one's own words), and echolalia (i.e., repeating another's words). In addition to recognizable words, other vocal tics may consist of nonsense words or phrases, as well as oropharyngeal, nasopharyngeal, or laryngeal sounds, consonants, or syllables.[4]

Workup

A diagnosis of tic disorders is based on clinical features. Typically, no further workup is necessary after the NP finds indications of Tourette syndrome or other tic disorders but may be required if the patient's history indicates the tic disorder is an abnormal presentation.[59]

Treatment

Pharmacotherapy is recommended for treatment of tic disorders if the patient's tics are interfering with daily living.[62] Clonidine, an antihypertensive that serves to treat ADHD, may be effective in controlling tics. Antipsychotics may likewise help to manage tics. It is important to treat comorbidities as well.[60] Furthermore, treatment is administered in collaboration with neurology.

References

1. Silberstein SD. Migraine. In: Porter RS, Kaplan JL, eds. The Merck Manual Online. http://www.merckmanuals.com/professional/neurologic_disorders/headache/migraine.html?qt=migrainealt=sh. Last reviewed April 2014. Accessed April 20, 2015.

2. Headaches. Mayo Clinic web site. http://www.mayo.edu/research/departments-divisions/department-neurology/programs/headaches. Accessed April 20, 2015.

3. Vascular headache. MedicineNet web site. http://www.medicinenet.com/script/main/art.asp?articlekey=5962. Last reviewed August 28, 2013. Accessed April 20, 2015.

4. Barkley TW Jr. *Pediatric Primary Care Nurse Practitioner Certification Review/Clinical Update Continuing Education Course*. West Hollywood, CA: Barkley and Associates; 2015.

5. Tension headache. A.D.A.M. Medical Encyclopedia. http://www.nlm.nih.gov/medlineplus/ency/article/000797.htm. Updated October 29, 2013. Accessed April 20, 2015.

6. United States Department of Health and Human Services, National Institutes of Health (NIH), National Institute of Neurological Disorders and Stroke (NINDS), Office of Communications and Public Liaison. NINDS headache information page. http://www.ninds.nih.gov/disorders/headache/headache.htm. Last updated February 23, 2015. Accessed April 20, 2015.

7. United States Department of Health and Human Services, Centers for Disease Control and Prevention. Bacterial meningitis. http://www.cdc.gov/meningitis/bacterial.html. Last updated April 1, 2014. Accessed April 20, 2015.

8. Mayo Clinic Staff. Meningitis. Mayo Clinic web site. http://www.mayoclinic.org/diseases-conditions/meningitis/basics/definition/con-20019713. Updated March 19, 2013. Accessed April 20, 2015.

9. Greenlee JE. Viral meningitis. In: Porter RS, Kaplan JL, eds. The Merck Manual Online. http://www.merckmanuals.com/professional/neurologic_disorders/meningitis/viral_meningitis.html. Last reviewed February 2013. Accessed April 20, 2015.

10. Hasbun R. Meningitis. In: Bronze MS, ed. Medscape. http://emedicine.medscape.com/article/232915-overview#showallHeadache. Updated January 28, 2015. Accessed April 20, 2015.

11. Greenlee JE. Acute bacterial meningitis. In: Porter RS, Kaplan JL, eds. The Merck Manual Online. http://www.merckmanuals.com/home/brain_spinal_cord_and_nerve_disorders/meningitis/acute_bacterial_meningitis.html. Updated February 2013. Accessed April 20, 2015.

12. Garralda E, Als L. What are the behavioural, emotional and cognitive impacts of meningitis and septicaemia on children? Meningitis Research Foundation web site. http://www.meningitis.org/impact-in-children. Accessed April 20, 2015.

13. Fraimow HS, Reboli AC. Specific infections with critical care implications. In: Parrillo JE, Dellinger RP, eds. *Critical Care Medicine: Principles of Diagnosis and Management in the Adult.* 4th ed. Philadelphia, PA: Elsevier Saunders; 2013: 936–964.

14. Mayo Clinic Staff. Epilepsy. Mayo Clinic web site. http://www.mayoclinic.org/diseases-conditions/epilepsy/basics/tests-diagnosis/con-20033721. Updated November 22, 2014. Accessed April 20, 2015.

15. Green NA. Meningitis. http://kidshealth.org/parent/infections/lung/meningitis.html#. Reviewed April 2013. Accessed April 20, 2015.

16. Tunkel AR. Clinical features and diagnosis of acute bacterial meningitis in adults. In: Basow DS, ed. *UpToDate*. Waltham, MA: UpToDate; 2015. http://www.uptodate.com/contents/clinical-features-and-diagnosis-of-acute-bacterial-meningitis-in-adults. Last updated April 28, 2014. Accessed April 20, 2015.

17. Kernig's sign of meningitis. A.D.A.M. Medical Encyclopedia. http://www.nlm.nih.gov/medlineplus/ency/imagepages/19077.htm. Updated October 6, 2012. Accessed April 20, 2015.

18. Brudzinski's sign of meningitis. A.D.A.M. Medical Encyclopedia. http://www.nlm.nih.gov/medlineplus/ency/imagepages/19069.htm. Updated October 6, 2012. Accessed April 20, 2015.

19. Meningitis. A.D.A.M. Medical Encyclopedia. http://www.nlm.nih.gov/medlineplus/ency/article/000680.htm. Updated October 6, 2012. Accessed April 20, 2015.

20. Brain tumor – primary – adults. A.D.A.M. Medical Encyclopedia. http://www.nlm.nih.gov/medlineplus/ency/article/007222.htm. Updated October 30, 2013. Accessed April 20, 2015.

21. What is neuroblastoma? American Cancer Society web site. http://www.cancer.org/cancer/neuroblastoma/detailedguide/neuroblastoma-what-is-neuroblastoma. Last revised March 10, 2015. Accessed April 20, 2015.

22. Rull G, Tidy C. Brain tumors in children. Patient.co.uk web site. http://www.patient.co.uk/doctor/brain-tumours-in-children. Last updated June 22, 2011. Accessed April 21, 2015.

23. Wong ET, Wu JK. Clinical presentation and diagnosis of brain tumors. In: Basow DS, ed. *UpToDate*. Waltham, MA: UpToDate; 2015. http://www.uptodate.com/contents/clinical-presentation-and-diagnosis-of-brain-tumors. Last updated September 26, 2014. Accessed April 21, 2015.

24. Shlamovitz GZ, Shah NR. Lumbar puncture. In: Lutsep HL, ed. Medscape. \http://emedicine.medscape.com/article/80773-overview#showall. Updated December 2, 2014. Accessed April 21, 2015.

25. U.S. Department of Health and Human Services, NIH, National Cancer Institute. Tumor grade. http://www.cancer.gov/cancertopics/factsheet/detection/tumor-grade-fact-sheet. Reviewed May 3, 2013. Accessed April 21, 2015.

26. Childhood brain tumors. A.D.A.M. Medical Encyclopedia. http://www.nlm.nih.gov/medlineplus/childhoodbraintumors.html. Accessed April 21, 2015.

27. Mayo Clinic Staff. Migraine. Mayo Clinic web site. http://www.mayoclinic.org/diseases-conditions/migraine-headache/basics/definition/CON-20026358. Updated June 4, 2013. Accessed April 21, 2015.

28. Cleveland Clinic Staff. Migraines in children. Cleveland Clinic web site. http://my.clevelandclinic.org/disorders/pediatric_headache/ns_migraines.aspx. Accessed April 21, 2015.

29. Chawla J. Migraine headache. In: Lutsep HL, ed. Medscape. http://emedicine.medscape.com/article/1142556-overview. Updated September 15, 2014. Accessed April 21, 2015.

30. Draper R, Tidy C. Migraine in children. Patient.co.uk web site. http://www.patient.co.uk/doctor/Migraine-in-Children.htm. Last updated October 22, 2014. Accessed April 21, 2015.

31. Shahein R, Beiruti K. Preventive agents for migraine: Focus on the antiepileptic drugs. *J Cent Nerv Syst Dis.* 2012; 4: 37–49. doi:10.4137/JCNSD.S9049

32. Healthwise, Inc. Drugs for migraine and headache pain. WebMD web site. http://www.webmd.com/migraines-headaches/pain-relief-headaches. Reviewed April 18, 2015. Accessed April 21, 2015.

33. Kenny T, Tidy C. Triptans. Patient.co.uk web site. http://www.patient.co.uk/health/triptans. Last updated July 31, 2014. Accessed April 21, 2015.

34. Adamolekun B. Seizure disorders. In: Porter RS, Kaplan JL, eds. The Merck Manual Online. http://www.merckmanuals.com/professional/neurologic_disorders/seizure_disorders/seizure_disorders.html?qt=-seizures&alt=sh. Last reviewed May 2013. Accessed April 21, 2015.

35. Donner EJ. What causes seizures? About Kids' Health web site. http://www.aboutkidshealth.ca/en/resourcecentres/epilepsy/aboutepilepsy/anoverviewofepilepsy/pages/what-causes-seizures.aspx. Published February 4, 2010. Accessed April 21, 2015.

36. Seizures. American Brain Tumor Association web site. http://www.abta.org/brain-tumor-information/symptoms/seizures.html. Accessed April 21, 2015.

37. Partial (focal) seizure. A.D.A.M. Medical Encyclopedia. http://www.nlm.nih.gov/medlineplus/ency/article/000697.htm. Updated February 20, 2014. Accessed April 21, 2015.

38. Borton C, Tidy C. Managing epilepsy in primary care. Patient.co.uk web site. http://www.patient.co.uk/doctor/Managing-Epilepsy-in-Primary-Care.htm. Last updated March 14, 2012. Accessed April 21, 2015.

39. Absence seizure. A.D.A.M. Medical Encyclopedia. http://www.nlm.nih.gov/medlineplus/ency/article/000696.htm. Updated February 20, 2014. Accessed April 21, 2015.

40. Tonic and clonic seizures. Johns Hopkins Medicine web site. http://www.hopkinsmedicine.org/neurology_neurosurgery/specialty_areas/epilepsy/seizures/types/tonic-and-clonic-seizures.html. Accessed April 21, 2015.

41. Healthwise, Inc. Epilepsy: Atonic seizures – Topic overview. WebMD web site. http://www.webmd.com/epilepsy/atonic-seizures. Last updated March 12, 2014. Accessed April 21, 2015.

42. Sheth RD. EEG in common epilepsy syndromes. In: Benbadis SR, ed. Medscape. http://emedicine.medscape.com/article/1138154-overview#showall. Updated October 8, 2014. Accessed April 21, 2015.

43. Healthwise, Inc. Epilepsy health center – Diagnosis & tests. WebMD web site. http://www.webmd.com/epilepsy/guide/epilespy-diagnosis-tests. Accessed April 21, 2015.

44. Healthwise, Inc. Epilepsy – Medications. WebMD web site. http://www.webmd.com/epilepsy/tc/epilepsy-medications. Reviewed March 12, 2014. Accessed April 21, 2015.

45. Tejani NR. Febrile seizures. In: Bechtel KA, ed. Medscape. http://emedicine.medscape.com/article/801500-overview. Updated September 12, 2014. Accessed April 21, 2015.

46. McBride MC. Febrile seizures. In: Porter RS, Kaplan JL, eds. The Merck Manual Online. http://www.merckmanuals.com/professional/pediatrics/neurologic_disorders_in_children/febrile_seizures.html. Last reviewed August 2013. Accessed April 21, 2015.

47. Febrile seizures. A.D.A.M. Medical Encyclopedia. http://www.nlm.nih.gov/medlineplus/ency/article/000980.htm. Updated February 26, 2014. Accessed April 21, 2015.

48. National Health Service (UK). Febrile seizures – Causes. http://www.nhs.uk/Conditions/Febrile-convulsions/Pages/Causes.aspx. Last reviewed June 10, 2014. Accessed April 21, 2015.

49. Fishman MA. Patient information: Febrile seizures (Beyond the Basics). In: Basow DS, ed. *UpToDate*. Waltham, MA: UpToDate; 2015. http://www.uptodate.com/contents/febrile-seizures-beyond-the-basics. Last updated August 30, 2013. Accessed April 21, 2015.

50. Mayo Clinic Staff. Neurofibromatosis. Mayo Clinic web site. http://www.mayoclinic.org/diseases-conditions/neurofibromatosis/basics/definition/con-20027728. Updated January 3, 2013. Accessed April 21, 2015.

51. United States Department of Health and Human Services, NIH, NINDS, Office of Communications and Public Liaison. NINDS neurofibromatosis information page. http://www.ninds.nih.gov/disorders/neurofibromatosis/neurofibromatosis.htm. Last updated February 23, 2015. Accessed April 21, 2015.

52. McBride MC. Neurofibromatosis. In: Porter RS, Kaplan JL, eds. The Merck Manual Online. http://www.merckmanuals.com/professional/pediatrics/neurocutaneous_syndromes/neurofibromatosis.html?qt=neurofibromatosis&alt=sh. Last reviewed September 2013. Accessed April 21, 2015.

53. Hsieh DT, Rohena LO. Neurofibromatosis type 1. In: Kao A, ed. Medscape. http://emedicine.medscape.com/article/1177266-overview. Updated December 16, 2014. Accessed April 21, 2015.

54. Peltonen S, Pöyhönen M. Clinical diagnosis and atypical forms of NF1. In: Upadhyaya M, Cooper DN, eds. *Neurofibromatosis Type 1: Molecular and Cellular Biology*. Berlin: Springer; 2013: 17–30.

55. Mayo Clinic Staff. Meningitis. Mayo Clinic web site. http://www.mayoclinic.org/diseases-conditions/meningitis/basics/definition/con-20019713. Updated March 19, 2013. Accessed April 22, 2015.

56. Korf BR. Neurofibromatosis type 1 (NF1): Management and prognosis. In: Basow DS, ed. *UpToDate*. Waltham, MA: UpToDate; 2015. http://www.uptodate.com/contents/neurofibromatosis-type-1-nf1-management-and-prognosis. Last updated March 25, 2015. Accessed April 22, 2015.

57. United States Department of Health and Human Services, Centers for Disease Control and Prevention. Tourette syndrome (TS). http://www.cdc.gov/ncbddd/tourette/facts.html. Last updated August 8, 2014. Last reviewed March 9, 2015. Accessed April 22, 2015.

58. Jankovic J. Tourette syndrome. In: Basow DS, ed. *UpToDate*. Waltham, MA: UpToDate; 2015. http://www.uptodate.com/contents/tourette-syndrome. Last updated April 9, 2015. Accessed April 22, 2015.

59. Robertson WC Jr. Tourette syndrome and other tic disorders. In: Kao A, ed. Medscape. http://emedicine.medscape.com/article/1182258-overview. Updated April 30, 2014. Accessed April 22, 2015.

60. McBride MC. Tic disorders and Tourette syndrome in children and adolescents. In: Porter RS, Kaplan JL, eds. The Merck Manual Online. http://www.merckmanuals.com/professional/pediatrics/neurologic_disorders_in_children/tic_disorders_and_tourette_syndrome_in_children_and_adolescents.html?qt=tic%20disorders&alt=sh. Last reviewed August 2013. Accessed April 22, 2015.

61. Myers EF, Zinner SH. Attention deficit hyperactivity disorder and co-occurring tics. *Contemp Pediatr.* 2013; 30(4): 24. http://contemporarypediatrics.modernmedicine.com/contemporary-pediatrics/news/modernmedicine/welcome-modernmedicine/attention-deficit-hyperactivity-d?page=full

62. Roessner V, Schoenefeld K, Buse J, Bender S, Ehrlich S, Münchau A. Pharmacological treatment of tic disorders and Tourette syndrome. *Neuropharmacology*, 2013; 68: 143–149. doi:10.1016/j.neuropharm.2012.05.043

Chapter 16

Hematologic and Oncologic Disorders

QUESTIONS

1. A 6-year-old female who is new to this country presents with a racing heart, rapid breathing, and pale-colored skin. During the physical examination, you notice splenomegaly and a very bony facial structure. Based on the patient's findings, which of the following would be most likely to present?

   a. MCV: 82 fl; MCHC: 32%; reticulocyte count: 2%

   b. MCV: 72 fl; MCHC: 30%; reticulocyte count: 3%

   c. MCV: 70 fl; MCHC: 34%; reticulocyte count: 1%

   d. MCV: 88 fl; MCHC: 36%; reticulocyte count: 1%

2. Joey, an 11-month-old infant, is brought in by his mother because he's been sleeping more than usual. A physical examination indicates pallor, palpitations, and tachycardia. In discussing recent events with the mother, she says that she has been alternating between breast milk and formula for Joey; when pressed for time and lacking formula, she gives him whole milk instead. After he responded well to the taste, she replaced breast milk with whole cow's milk. Joey most likely has which of these dietary insufficiencies?

   a. Insufficient iron

   b. Insufficient folic acid

   c. Insufficient fiber

   d. Insufficient vitamin D

3. Which of the following is <u>least</u> likely to result in lead poisoning?

   a. A red wagon from the 1970s

   b. Mexican soft drinks

   c. Inner-city playgrounds near major highways

   d. Indian herbal remedies

4. A febrile 5-year-old patient with sickle cell anemia has continued bedwetting. You order a urinalysis. Which of the following findings would you expect?

   a. Proteinuria

   b. Red blood cells

   c. Leukocyte esterase

   d. Specific gravity of 1.008

5. Which form of leukemia accounts for about 20% of all childhood leukemias and occurs primarily in infants and adolescents?

   a. Chronic myelogenous leukemia

   b. Chronic lymphocytic leukemia

   c. Acute myelogenous leukemia

   d. Acute lymphocytic leukemia

6. A toddler who presents with iron-deficiency anemia is also at increased risk for lead poisoning due to pica. After moving to a house built in 1965, the mother brings the child in for venous blood level testing. While going over the results, you explain that chelation therapy is not recommended because the toddler's venous blood level concentrations do <u>not</u> reach which threshold?

   a. Level 35 µg/dl

   b. Level 45 µg/dl

   c. Level 65 µg/dl

   d. Level 75 µg/dl

7. A mother brings her adopted 6-year-old to see you after he bruised his elbow bumping it on the kitchen counter. She became concerned the day after the injury because he said his elbow was tingling. After finding a normal complete blood count, you order a coagulation panel because you are most concerned about which disorder?

   a. Hemophilia

   b. Platelet disorder

   c. Anemia

   d. Leukemia

8. An otherwise healthy 4-year-old presents with bruises that the parents cannot explain. The parents first noticed the bruises a few days ago. The complete blood count results show the platelet count is low, hemoglobin is 12 g/dl, hematocrit is 36%, and her white blood cell count is 7,000/mm^3. Which of the following is the most likely diagnosis?

   a. Suspected child abuse

   b. Iron deficiency anemia

   c. Immune thrombocytopenic purpura

   d. Leukemia

9. A toddler recently diagnosed as anemic is found to have a reticulocyte count of 0.3%. All of the following may explain these findings <u>except</u>:

   a. Iron deficiency anemia

   b. Hemolytic anemia

   c. Folic acid deficiency

   d. Bone marrow failure

10. A 5-year-old is brought to your clinic by his mother because she is concerned about the multiple bruises on his extremities and back. The boy's mother also states that he looks pale. During your physical examination, you detect scattered, enlarged lymph nodes. Which of the following actions are you most likely to do?

    a. Order a peripheral smear

    b. Refer the patient to a hematologist-oncologist

    c. Do a bone marrow aspiration and biopsy

    d. Consult a child protective agency

RATIONALES

1. b

Values of MCV=72 fl, MCHC=30%, and reticulocyte count=3%, respectively, are suggestive of thalassemia, which may present with tachypnea, tachycardia, pale skin, splenomegaly, and frontal bossing. Thalassemia is a microcytic, hypochromic anemia with a high reticulocyte count. Patients with MCVs of 82 fl and 88 fl fall within the normocytic range. The normal range for mean corpuscular hemoglobin concentration (MCHC) is 32%–36%, so patients with an MCHC of either 32% or 36% would be normochromic, not hypochromic. A reticulocyte count of 1%–2% is considered normal, not elevated.

2. a

Iron deficiency anemia often presents with palpitations, lethargy, and tachycardia. In infants, this condition may be caused by an intake of whole milk before the age of 9 months, which may produce a microhemorrhage in the gut. Folic acid deficiency would be more likely if the child was on a goat's milk diet. Fiber deficiency is more likely to lead to constipation, not tachycardia or lethargy. Vitamin D deficiency is very rare in infancy, but may present with muscle twitching, muscle weakness, and softening or thinning of the skull.

3. b

Although certain Mexican foods and candies have been flagged for high lead content, Mexican soda is not likely to cause lead poisoning. Other common sources of lead poisoning include contaminated soil, especially when near freeways; toys that may contain lead paint, such as toys from the 1970s or earlier; and ethnic folk remedies, such as Indian Ayurvedic preparations.

4. d

The urinalysis for a child with sickle cell anemia is usually hypoconcentrated, as indicated by a urine specific gravity of 1.008. Presence of white blood cells, leukocyte esterase, or red blood cells would not be expected in a urinalysis of a child with sickle cell anemia. Proteinuria may be found in adult patients with sickle cell anemia because of sickle cell nephropathy, but pediatric sickle cell disease patients typically have normal renal function.

5. c

Acute myelogenous leukemia is a form of leukemia that accounts for about 20% of all leukemias and occurs primarily in infants and adolescents. Acute lymphocytic leukemia accounts for about 75% of pediatric leukemia cases, rather than 20%, and peak incidence occurs in children younger than 5 years of age. Chronic myelogenous leukemia and chronic lymphocytic leukemia rarely occur in children.

6. a

Chelation therapy is recommended for venous blood level concentrations that meet or exceed 45 mcg/dl. At levels below 45 mcg/dl, removing lead sources from the child's environment is considered to be more effective than chelation therapy. At levels above 70 mcg/dl, hospitalization for chelation, hydration, and close observation is recommended.

7. a

Easy bruising and joint tingling, a symptom of joint bleeding, may be indicative of a coagulation disorder, such as hemophilia. Platelet disorders, anemia, and leukemia would not likely present with joint tingling. Immunoglobulin assays are often performed in pediatric patients when platelet disorders are suspected. A complete blood count (CBC) would not be normal in individuals with anemia or leukemia. A CBC would show low red blood cells in individuals with anemia, which may also indicate leukemia.

8. c

The most likely diagnosis is immune thrombocytopenic purpura since the platelet count alone is shown to be abnormal. The child is not anemic because the hemoglobin and hematocrit are normal. Leukemia is also possible but less likely because only one blood component is abnormal. Although unexplained bruising may indicate child abuse, the abnormal platelet count makes immune thrombocytopenia purpura more likely than child abuse.

9. b

In hemolytic anemia, the destruction of red blood cells causes the bone marrow to produce an elevated reticulocyte count. A reticulocyte count of 0.3% is below the normal range of 1%–2%. A low reticulocyte count may indicate iron deficiency anemia, folic acid deficiency, or bone marrow failure.

10. a

A peripheral smear should be ordered to detect malignant cells. If malignant cells are detected, the next step would be a referral to a hematologist-oncologist who would likely perform a bone marrow aspiration and biopsy. Although abuse must be considered, especially with bruises on the back, enlarged lymph nodes would not be expected in suspected cases of child abuse.

DISCUSSION

Anemias

Overview

Anemias are a group of disorders characterized by a pathological process in which either the hemoglobin (Hgb) concentration in red blood cells (RBCs) or RBC mass is abnormally low.[1]

Anemias encompass various disorders that affect the patient's RBC count, quality of Hgb, or volume of packed RBCs. These disorders are classified according to both RBC size, which is determined by mean corpuscular volume (MCV), and Hgb content, which is determined by mean corpuscular hemoglobin concentration (MCHC).[1] Anemias are considered normocytic if the patient has an MCV of 80–100 fl; MCV values under 80 fl are classified as microcytic, whereas values over 100 fl are classified as macrocytic. Likewise, an anemia that presents with an MCHC of 32%–36% is considered normochromic, whereas an MCHC under 32% is considered hypochromic. An anemia that presents with MCHC greater than 36% is considered hyperchromic; many texts do not recognize this classification, however, on the grounds that it is impossible for an RBC to be "too red."[2]

Microcytic, hypochromic anemias, such as iron deficiency anemia, thalassemia, and lead poisoning, are more prevalent among pediatric patients. Macrocytic, normochromic anemias, such as vitamin B12 deficiency and pernicious anemia, are more prevalent among adults. Normocytic, normochromic anemias include anemia of chronic disease, acute blood loss, and early iron deficiency anemia.[2]

Iron Deficiency Anemia

Overview

Iron deficiency anemia is a microcytic, hypochromic anemia characterized by a defect in Hgb synthesis that reduces the capacity of the blood to deliver oxygen to body cells and tissues.[3] Iron deficiency anemia is caused by an overall deficiency of iron due to decreased iron intake or blood loss.[2]

Iron deficiency anemia develops in three stages: iron depletion, iron-deficient erythropoiesis, and iron deficiency anemia. Complications associated with iron deficiency include impaired cognitive and psychomotor function, as well as decreased leukocyte and lymphocyte function.[3]

Iron deficiency in children and infants is frequently attributed to nutritional factors. The risk of developing iron deficiency increases in toddlers and infants who rely on whole milk diets. Whole milk does not supply enough iron to meet dietary intake needs and can cause gastrointestinal bleeding in very young infants.[2]

A common cause of iron deficiency among adolescents is increased iron requirements related to rapid growth during the pubertal development stages. In males, iron intake requirements peak during puberty because of expanding blood volume.[4] Adolescent females who have experienced menarche require higher dietary intake of iron to compensate for menstrual blood loss.[2,4,5]

Presentation

Signs and symptoms of iron deficiency anemia depend on severity. Most pediatric patients with mild to moderate cases appear asymptomatic.[3] However, patients appearing asymptomatic may exhibit pica, pagophagia, or signs of impaired cognitive, psychomotor, or mental development.[3]

Severe cases of iron deficiency anemia may include presentations of lethargy, irritability, pallor, and poor feeding. Cardiovascular symptoms may include tachypnea and tachycardia. Shortness of breath and heart palpitations may also indicate cardiomegaly.[3] Other presenting signs include weakness, headache, irritability, brittle hair, and pale, dry skin and mucous membranes.[2,4]

Workup

The most common, cost-efficient method to screen for iron deficiency is to measure Hgb and hematocrit (Hct) levels for anemia. A presumptive diagnosis can be determined with findings of low Hgb and Hct.[1]

When screening for iron deficiency anemia, it is important to consider that Hgb and Hct levels vary among adolescents according to age and gender. The threshold for defining anemia is two standard deviations below the mean for the age- and sex-specific reference population.[1]

Following a presumptive diagnosis, the patient should be administered iron therapy and then evaluated for a response. Iron therapy is usually administered in the form of oral ferrous sulfate and is primarily recommended for confirming a diagnosis of iron deficiency in infants up to 24 months of age.[3] A presumptive diagnosis is supported if Hgb levels improve after administration of iron therapy. Patients who do not respond to iron therapy after a month should be screened to rule out other conditions, such as sickle cell trait, parasitic infections, or other types of anemia.[3] For older patients and infants who do not respond to ferrous sulfate iron therapy, additional assessment tests include a complete blood count (CBC), a reticulocyte count, and a peripheral blood smear.[3]

Confirmatory diagnostic findings include low serum ferritin and low Hgb and Hct levels.[1,6] Additional diagnostic findings include low serum iron, low MCV, low MCHC, low RBCs, increased total iron binding capacity (TIBC), and increased red cell distribution width (RDW).[2]

Treatment

Treatment should focus on raising Hgb levels and replacing iron stores. Dietary modifications should be made to increase vitamin C and iron intake.[6] Treatment should include oral iron therapy until iron levels have reached the age-adjusted normal range and iron storage pools have been replaced.[2,6]

Depending on severity and the patient's age, the recommended dose for pediatric patients is 3–6 mg/kg of elemental iron once or twice daily until Hgb normalizes.[6] This dosage should be taken between meals and preferably with juice rich in vitamin C to improve iron absorption. Once a reticulocyte response is seen, which may take up to 72 hours in severe cases, treatment should be reduced to 2–3 mg/kg/day of oral iron therapy for several months until iron stores are replaced.[2,6]

Prevention of iron deficiency anemia is recommended for infants and toddlers. Infants should undergo a risk assessment for iron deficiency at 4, 18, and 24 months of age, and a universal laboratory screening between 9 and 12 months of age. Parents should ensure infants are breastfed exclusively for the first 4–6 months, and toddlers are fed iron-fortified foods and foods rich in vitamin C.[6]

Screening recommendations vary for adolescents. Menstruating females should be screened annually during adolescence, and males should be screened at least once during the peak growth period.[4]

Thalassemia

Overview

Thalassemia is a group of hereditary disorders characterized by a partial or complete deficiency of α- or β-globin chain synthesis. This deficiency impairs production of globin chains and causes a reduction in the amount of Hgb deposited into each RBC.[7] This reduction of Hgb leads to a microcytic, hypochromic anemia with presentations that vary according to the classification of thalassemia.

Thalassemia is the second most common cause of microcytic anemias.[2] Classification of thalassemia is determined by which globin chain is affected, resulting in either α thalassemia or β thalassemia, and is further sub-classified according to the severity of impairment to globin chain synthesis.[7,8] Incidence of thalassemia is highest among Mediterranean, Middle Eastern, Indian, and Southeast Asian populations, as well as groups from the tropic and subtropic regions of Africa.[8]

Presentation

Presenting signs of thalassemia depend on the classification of the disease and the patient's age. Thalassemia is usually suspected in patients presenting with a hypochromic, microcytic anemia who do not respond to oral iron therapy.[7] Most pediatric patients with mild cases are asymptomatic but may feel tired from mild anemia. In addition to symptoms of mild anemia, mild to moderate cases may present with slowed growth, delayed puberty, brittle bones, or an enlarged spleen.[7,9]

In severe thalassemia cases, symptoms usually occur within the first 2 years of life. Patients typically have severe anemia but may also present with dark urine, pallor, lethargy, and slowed growth.[1,9] Bone marrow expansion may lead to bone abnormalities, such as frontal bossing.[9] Patients may also present with abdominal swelling and an enlarged heart with hyperdynamic precordium.[2,7] Patients who are not receiving blood transfusion therapy may develop debilitating symptoms, such as neuropathy and paralysis.[7] In older children and adolescents, presentations may include growth retardation, delayed puberty, mild to moderately severe jaundice, and iron overload from multiple blood transfusions. Signs of iron overload include bleeding tendencies, frequent infections, and organ dysfunction.[2,7]

Workup

A CBC count and peripheral blood smear examination are usually performed in suspected cases. Initial laboratory findings include a low MCV and low MCHC.[7] Lab findings that help to differentiate thalassemia from other microcytic, hypochromic anemias include normal to increased levels of ferritin and serum iron, normal TIBC, decreased Hgb, and decreased α- or β-globin chains.[9]

Classifying the type of thalassemia involves a bone marrow examination or Hgb electrophoresis.[7] Additional tests may involve β-globin gene mapping or evaluating ferritin and total bilirubin levels.[2]

Treatment

Patients should be referred to a hematologist for treatment.[2] Mild cases generally do not require treatment. In moderate and severe cases, treatment usually involves chronic blood transfusions, but chronic transfusions can cause severe iron overload and result in severe organ failure.[10] Iron overload can also damage the hypothalamic pituitary axis, which can adversely affect pubertal growth and sexual development. To counter the effects of iron overload, chelation therapy is recommended. Patients should also receive annual endocrine evaluations, bone mass evaluation, and nutritional counseling.[8]

For pediatric patients in the first decade of life, normal growth and development can be achieved by maintaining near-normal pretransfusion Hgb levels of 9–10 grams/dl.[8] Dietary recommendations include a high intake of folic acid, small doses of vitamin C and vitamin E, and avoidance of iron.[7] In very rare cases, a splenectomy may be required, particularly if the patient's spleen becomes hyperactive. However, this procedure can lead to excessive destruction of RBCs and an increased need for frequent blood transfusions. Because the spleen is a store for nontoxic iron, early removal of the spleen may be harmful, and caution should be taken to avoid further complications. As such, this procedure is usually delayed until the patient is at least 4 or 5 years of age.[7]

Sickle Cell Anemia

Overview

Sickle cell diseases are blood disorders caused by an autosomal recessive condition in which the Hgb S gene develops instead of Hgb A.[11] Sickle cell anemia, the most common form of sickle cell disease, is a hereditary anemia that typically manifests in early childhood. The mutated Hgb causes RBCs to be crescent- or sickle-shaped. These sickle-shaped RBCs block blood flow in the blood vessels, resulting in a chronic, hemolytic anemia. In sickle cell anemia, abnormal sickle cells have a significantly shorter life span than normal RBCs, and the bone marrow is often unable to make new RBCs to adequately replace those that have died.[12]

Pain, progressive organ damage, and increased risk of infection are associated with sickle cell disease, as well as cerebrovascular disease and cognitive impairment.[12,13] Young children are at increased risk of bacterial infection, splenic sequestration, and stroke. Indications of end-organ damage may manifest in adolescents and adults.[9]

Patients who are sickle cell trait carriers are clinically asymptomatic.[11,14] Carriers have some resistance to malaria, which can be a benefit in regions where malaria is common.[11]

The incidence of sickle cell disease is highest among populations of African or African-American ancestry.[13] The sickle cell gene is carried in 8% of African Americans.[2]

Presentation

Signs and symptoms of sickle cell anemia vary depending on age but typically manifest within the first year of life as levels of fetal Hgb (Hgb F), which inhibit deoxy-Hb S polymerization in the red blood cells, begin to fall.[11]

All patients present with hemolytic anemia, but signs and symptoms vary and may include fatigue, anemia, cholelithiasis, and possible development of vasculopathy.[13] Vaso-occlusive crisis, characterized by sudden, excruciating pain occurring in the back, chest, abdomen, and long bones, is the most common clinical presentation among patients with sickle cell disease.[11] Patients also may present with a low-grade fever, infection, or blood loss. Other manifestations include jaundice, retinopathy, delayed puberty, hepatosplenomegaly, an enlarged heart with hyperdynamic precordium, and systolic murmur.[2] In rare cases, end-organ damage may occur. Signs of end-organ damage include pulmonary hypertension, renal disease, stroke, leg ulcers, and chronic pain syndromes.[15]

Carriers of the sickle cell trait usually present with no clinical symptoms. Patients may, however, experience painful acute symptoms under conditions leading to hypoxia and may present with isosthenuria and hematuria.[2,11,14]

Workup

A diagnosis of sickle cell disease is determined through an Hgb analysis, which typically detects the disease in newborns during mandatory screening programs.[13] An analysis is usually performed through a hemoglobin electrophoresis; findings that show the presence of Hgb SS can confirm sickle cell anemia, whereas findings that show the presence of Hgb S and Hgb A can confirm sickle cell trait.[11,13]

Laboratory findings include decreased Hgb (5–9 grams/dl), decreased Hct (17%–29%), and an elevated total leukocyte count (12,000–20,000 cells/mm^3) with a predominance of neutrophils.[11] Additional lab findings may include indirectly elevated bilirubin and platelets above 400,000/µl. The reticulocyte count is usually elevated between 10% and 25% but may vary depending on the extent of baseline hemolysis. Further diagnostic findings include a peripheral blood smear that demonstrates target cells, characteristic sickle-shaped erythrocytes, and cells that appear elongated.[2] RBCs containing nuclear remnants, known as Howell-Jolly bodies, indicate asplenic conditions in the patient.[11] Urinalysis is usually hypoconcentrated.

Antenatal testing for sickle cell disease can be conducted for parents who are at risk of having a baby with the disease. An antenatal diagnosis can be made in the first trimester through chorionic villus biopsy or in the second trimester through amniocentesis.[13]

Treatment

Patients diagnosed with sickle cell anemia should be referred to a pediatric hematologist for treatment and management, with a focus on preventing associated complications.[2]

Both acute and chronic complications must be treated when dealing with sickle cell anemia. Management of acute complications may include fluids for dehydration, analgesics for pain, and oxygen for hypoxemia.[2,12] Blood transfusions may also be used to manage acute and chronic complications by correcting anemia, decreasing the percentage of Hgb S, suppressing Hgb S synthesis, and reducing hemolysis.[13] Hydroxyurea at 35 mg/kg/day is recommended for patients experiencing frequent painful episodes, severe symptomatic anemia, and severe chronic pain that is unmanageable through other medications.[2] Hydroxyurea, which stimulates Hgb F, is recommended for patients with a history of acute chest syndrome, stroke or high risk of stroke, and other severe vaso-occlusive events.[11]

Antibiotics are recommended for cases of infection and are given prophylactically until at least 5 years of age.[11] Immunization with Pneumovax is recommended at 2 and 5 years of age.[2,16] Vaccines to immunize against *Haemophilus influenzae*, *Neisseria meningitidis*, hepatitis B, and influenza are also recommended.[17]

Hemophilia A (X-Linked Recessive)

Overview

Hemophilia A is an X-linked recessive disorder caused by a deficiency of functional factor VIII (FVIII), which is a trace plasma glycoprotein that is vital to normal blood coagulation. This condition results in bleeding in the joints and muscles, with severe forms occurring in about 48% of all cases.[2,18]

Hemophilia A occurs in about 1 out of every 7,000 males.[2] Males inherit a hemophilic gene from the mother and a male chromosome from the father.[19] The frequency of carrier females is about 1 in 3,500. Among those female carriers, each pregnancy carries a 25% risk of having an affected son, a 25% risk of having a carrier daughter, and a 50% chance of having a healthy, non-carrier child.[2]

Presentation

Patients with hemophilia A are generally phenotypically normal at birth but may display easy bruising patterns or inadequate clotting following a traumatic injury.[2] Characteristic signs and symptoms include spontaneous and provoked bleeding of the mucocutaneous, joint, muscle, gastrointestinal, and central nervous systems. If left untreated or undertreated, bleeds can lead to major morbidity and even mortality.[20] Pediatric patients experiencing musculoskeletal hemorrhaging may complain of tingling or cracking sensations in the joints and refuse to use the affected joint. Additionally, patients may complain of warmth, pain, or stiffness in the joints. Gastrointestinal signs include hematemesis, melena, and abdominal pain. Genitourinary symptoms include hematuria, renal colic, and post-circumcision bleeding.[21]

In severe cases, spontaneous hemorrhaging may occur after a traumatic injury. General signs of hemorrhage include weakness, orthostasis, tachycardia, and tachypnea.[21]

Workup

Diagnosis of hemophilia A includes a CBC, coagulation studies, and an assay of FVIII.[21] Mild cases can be determined with FVIII measuring greater than 0.05 IU/ml. Moderate cases are supported by FVIII levels measuring between 0.05 and 0.01 IU/ml. A severe case of hemophilia A is determined with a finding of FVIII measuring less than 0.01 IU/ml.[18,21] CBC findings may indicate normal to low levels of Hgb and Hct, as well as normal platelet count. Coagulation studies include normal bleeding and prothrombin times.[21]

Treatment

Patients with hemophilia A should be referred to a comprehensive hemophilia care center for treatment. Treatment should involve management of hemostasis and bleeding episodes, replacement of FVIII, and rehabilitation of patients with hemophilia synovitis.[21] For severe cases, the current standard of care for pediatric patients is primary prophylaxis to prevent joint destruction.[18]

Lead Poisoning

Overview

Lead poisoning is a preventable chronic disease of toxic levels of lead in the body resulting from prolonged exposure. Lead exposure is dangerous to the developing brain in children because lead is easily absorbed in the nervous system and gastrointestinal tract.[22] Consequently, children younger than 6 years of age, especially young children between 12 and 36 months of age, are highly susceptible to the toxic effects of lead.[23] Lead poisoning can affect nearly every system in the body, including the peripheral and central nervous systems, and can impair several areas of cognitive, behavioral, and physical development. In severe cases, brain damage, coma, and even death may occur.[22,24]

Lead can be ingested or inhaled through toxins in the environment. Lead can be found in contaminated soil, gasoline emissions, food, and drinking water. The prevalence of lead poisoning is highest in poor, inner-city areas where housing built prior to 1978 still contains lead-based paint. Additional sources of lead include overseas products, such as toys or other household items, and herbal folk remedies or spices of Asian, Mexican-American, or Indian origin.[2,25]

Presentation

Signs and symptoms of lead poisoning depend upon the degree of exposure and the age of the patient. Presentations are usually vague or nonspecific in mild cases, and even in some severe cases.[23] Regardless, symptoms of lead poisoning usually involve the gastrointestinal, neuromuscular, and neurological systems.[26]

Classic presentations of lead poisoning found in pediatric patients include irritability, loss of appetite, weight loss, and sluggishness.[23] Gastrointestinal symptoms include abdominal pain, constipation, vomiting, and anorexia. Additional signs include muscle weakness, pallor, peripheral palsies, papilledema, and iron deficiency anemia. Cognitive defects may also present, such as inattentiveness, impulsiveness, distractibility, and learning problems. Encephalopathy may also result, and may be accompanied by lethargy, headaches, convulsions, and coma.[2,23,26,27]

Lead lines, also known as Burtonian lines, are a characteristic sign that rarely manifest but most often are a result of severe and prolonged lead exposure. A Burtonian line is a bluish-black line along the gingival border resulting from circulating lead reacting with sulfur ions released by oral bacteria.[2,23,28]

Diagnosis is normally made through a lead screening program. Patients suspected of having lead poisoning should undergo a complete physical examination and a patient history. The physical exam should focus on the neurologic portion of the examination, as well as psychological and language development, to assess possible neurologic consequences of lead toxicity.[23]

The history portion should assess the patient's nutritional, environmental, medical, and developmental history. When assessing nutritional history, particular attention should be given to the patient's iron and calcium intake. An environmental history should focus on potential sources of lead exposure. Such sources could be the patient's residence, surrounding soil, outside play areas, and any indoor or outdoor dust and dirt. Medical and developmental history should determine if there is a family history of lead poisoning or a patient history of pica. The patient's developmental milestones should also be evaluated. An assessment should also include an evaluation of behaviors, occupations, and hobbies of immediate family members, as well as exposure to imported products.[2,23]

Workup

To confirm a diagnosis of lead poisoning, the patient's blood lead levels (BLL) should be evaluated through venous sampling and compared to family members or other children who live near or with the patient.[27] Venous blood level concentrations are evaluated to categorize the degree of lead poisoning according to the following indications[2]:

Class I	Less than or equal to 10 µg/dL
Class IIA	10–14 µg/dL
Class IIB	15–19 µg/dL
Class III	20–44 µg/dL
Class IV	45–69 µg/dL
Class V	Higher than 70 µg/dL

Treatment

Therapy mainly depends on BLL, but treatment should primarily focus on managing the toxicity level and preventing further exposure to lead.[27] General treatment options include decontamination, chelation, and supportive therapy.[26] Patients should also be closely observed for hemoglobinopathies, impaired renal function, and vitamin D deficiencies.[2]

Patients with class IIA lead poisoning and higher should be referred to a hematologist. Patients with class IV lead poisoning should be recommended for chelation therapy, which involves injections of chemicals that bind to lead and draw it out of the tissues so that it can be excreted.[29] The injections must be administered over several weeks and can prevent death, but do not prevent brain damage.[22] Patients with class V lead poisoning should be hospitalized for chelation and hydration.

Leukemias

Overview

Leukemia is a cancer that encompasses a group of malignant hematological diseases characterized by abnormal, poorly differentiated lymphocytes (i.e., blast cells) replacing normal bone marrow elements. These blast cells may either fail to develop into mature cells or fail to mature correctly. Leukemia can be either acute or chronic. Acute leukemias spread quickly as many undeveloped malignant blast cells replace normal cells in the blood and marrow. Chronic leukemias develop slowly and with more mature-looking cells.[30]

Acute lymphocytic leukemia (ALL) and acute myelogenous leukemia (AML) are the two most prevalent forms of leukemia among pediatric patients. ALL, also known as acute lymphoblastic leukemia, is the most common type of leukemia diagnosed in pediatric patients, accounting for approximately 75% of all pediatric cancer cases. ALL is more prevalent among Caucasians and occurs predominantly in males.[2] The peak age of incidence of ALL is between 2 and 5 years of age.[2,31]

The etiology for ALL is unknown, although a variety of genetic and environmental factors have been related to incidence.[31] ALL originates in the lymphoid cells in the bone marrow, where lymphoblasts proliferate, thus affecting production of normal blood cells. These lymphoblasts also proliferate in the liver, spleen, and lymph nodes, and can infiltrate the testes, tonsils, adenoids, and orbital tissues.[31,32]

AML—also known as acute myelocytic, myeloid, or myoblastic leukemia—replaces normal bone marrow cells with abnormal, primitive hematopoietic cells. AML can be classified into eight different subtypes, depending on which type of bone marrow cells—myoblasts, monoblasts, erythroblasts, and megakaryoblasts—are being affected. The long-term survival rate of AML is 60% among pediatric patients.[33]

Etiology of AML has been associated with several risk factors that include genetic disorders, physical and chemical exposures, radiation exposure, and prior chemotherapy.[33]

Presentation

Generally, leukemia patients do not exhibit any symptoms in the early stages. Some of the general signs and symptoms of leukemia are flu or cold symptoms, minor fever or history of frequent infections, fatigue and pallor associated with anemia, and bone and joint pain. Signs associated with thrombocytopenia and neutropenia are also general signs of leukemia.[2,31,32]

With ALL, clinical presentations are most often acute but can evolve insidiously over the course of several months. Fever, fatigue, lethargy, and bone and joint pain are the most common symptoms of ALL, as well as a bleeding diathesis related to thrombocytopenia. Additional findings of ALL include lymphadenopathy, anemia, neutropenia, and either leucopenia or leukocytosis.[31,32]

Signs and symptoms of AML depend on the type of AML the patient has. Cytopenia, anemia, hemorrhage, and fever are attributed to a deficiency of normally functioning cells. In leukemia patients whose AML is characterized by proliferation and infiltration of the abnormal leukemic cell mass and infiltrative disease, typical findings include extramedullary infiltration, mediastinal mass, abdominal masses, and gingival hyperplasia or central nervous system (CNS) infiltration.[33]

Workup

Patients suspected of having leukemia should undergo a CBC with differential WBC, platelet counts, and reticulocyte counts. Further diagnostic tests include a peripheral blood smear, which may indicate malignant cells, and a bone marrow aspiration, which may show the poorly differentiated blast cells that have been replacing healthy bone marrow tissue. Anemia is a common finding of leukemia, and thrombocytopenia is present in up to 85% of all cases.[2]

The most common diagnostic findings of ALL include anemia, thrombocytopenia, neutropenia, and either leucopenia or leukocytosis. Additional findings may include hyperleukocytosis, which is found in approximately 15% of all pediatric patients, and elevated levels of serum uric acid and lactate dehydrogenase (LDH).[31] ALL can be distinguished from other malignant lymphoid disorders by the immunophenotype of the cells, which is similar to B- or T-precursor cells.[32]

The hallmark sign of AML is the reduction or absence of normal hematopoietic elements; a bone marrow examination can establish a diagnosis. Typical diagnostic findings of AML include a normocytic anemia, a low reticulocyte count, and decreased Hgb. Findings also include elevated or decreased WBC count and elevated levels of serum acid, serum muramidase, and LDH. A peripheral blood smear may indicate primitive granulocyte or monocyte precursors.

Immunophenotyping, such as cytogenic testing and human leukocyte antigen (HLA) typing, is used to further characterize leukemic cells for different cell lineages and stages of development. Cytogenic tests confirm the diagnosis, and HLA typing identifies HLA-matched family donors if a bone marrow transplant is required. Imaging studies are not required to diagnose AML but are useful for managing possible complications, such as sinusitis.

Lastly, a lumbar puncture and cerebral spinal fluid examination may be required for diagnostic and therapeutic purposes.[33]

Treatment

Pediatric patients should be referred to an oncologist.[2] Chemotherapy and blood transfusions are the primary treatments for leukemia patients; however, some patients may undergo additional procedures that include radiation therapy and stem cell transplantation. For all leukemia patients, treatment intensity should be adjusted according to prognostic factors associated with the risk of recurrence.

Treatment of ALL varies according to the patient's presenting features, leukemia features, and response to early therapy. Treatment should focus on eliminating residual leukemia, preventing or eradicating CNS leukemia, and ensuring continuation of remission. Therapy should be adapted according to the level of risk for relapse, degree of supportive care, and optimization of chemotherapy drugs.[31]

Treatment is generally broken down into separate phases: the remission-induction phase, intensification and consolidation phase, and continuation therapy targeted at eliminating disease.[32]

In most treatment centers, ALL treatment involves short-term intensive chemotherapy with a combination of high-dose antineoplastic agents and corticosteroids.[31] Antineoplastic agents include methotrexate (Trexall) and cytarabine. Corticosteroids include dexamethasone (Baycadron, Maxidex, Ozurdex) and prednisone.[32] Antimicrobials and antifungals are used in conjunction with chemotherapy to prevent infection and to provide further supportive therapy. Antimetabolite therapy should be considered for patients with a low risk of relapse. High-risk patients and patients showing either induction failure or persistent minimal residual disease after the first 2 weeks of induction therapy should be considered for more aggressive therapy and for allogeneic hematopoietic stem-cell transplantation.[31] CNS or testicular leukemia requires aggressive treatment, as these systems are poorly penetrated by chemotherapeutic agents. Although radiation therapy may be warranted to treat these sites in adults, the procedure is not recommended for pediatric patients; rather, an aggressive, directed course of conventional chemotherapy is the best first option for treatment in children.[31] Additional supportive care for patients may include blood transfusions, or antibiotics to manage complications associated with ALL therapy.[32]

The goals of AML therapy are to quickly destroy leukemic cells and prevent the emergence of a resistance clone. Therefore, patients with AML are normally transferred to pediatric cancer centers and hospitalized for extended periods of time, with intensive chemotherapy as an essential component of treatment. Hospitalization is also beneficial because it allows the patient to receive supportive care, particularly during extended periods of pancytopenia, until the bone marrow achieves hematologic remission and is again producing normal hematopoietic cells. Blood transfusions are critical to correcting anemia, thrombocytopenia, and other coagulopathies.[33]

Radiation may be recommended in AML cases where chloromas and other masses are pressing on a vital structure. Chemotherapeutic agents, such as purine antimetabolite (e.g., cytarabine) and daunomycin (Cerubidine), are used to destroy myeloblasts. Other drugs included in AML therapy in conjunction with chemotherapeutic agents include antiemetics, such as ondansetron (Zofran), to prevent nausea and vomiting; prophylactic broad-spectrum antimicrobials, such as sulfamethoxazole and trimethoprim (Bactrim), to prevent infection; and prophylactic antifungals, such as fluconazole (Diflucan), to treat and decrease host colonization of candidiasis. The role of surgery is limited; however, some patients may be referred for allogeneic or autologous bone marrow transplant therapy following chemotherapy and radiation treatment.[33]

References

1. Sandoval C. Approach to the child with anemia. In: Basow DS, ed. *UpToDate*. Waltham, MA: UpToDate; 2015. http://www.uptodate.com/contents/approach-to-the-child-with-anemia?source=search_result&search=thalassemia&selectedTitle=28~150#H9. Last updated September 25, 2013. Accessed April 22, 2015.

2. Barkley TW Jr. Hematological issues and disorders. In: Barkley TW Jr, ed. *Pediatric Primary Care Nurse Practitioner Certification Review/Clinical Update Continuing Education Course*. West Hollywood, CA: Barkley & Associates; 2015: 148–155.

3. Mahoney DH Jr. Iron deficiency in infants and young children: Screening, prevention, clinical manifestations, and diagnosis. In: Basow DS, ed. *UpToDate*. Waltham, MA: UpToDate; 2015. http://www.uptodate.com/contents/iron-deficiency-in-infants-and-young-children-screening-prevention-clinical-manifestations-and-diagnosis?detectedLanguage=en&source=search_result&search=iron+deficiency+anemia&selectedTitle=1~150&provider=noProvider#H1. Last updated February 2, 2015. Accessed April 22, 2015.

4. Abrams SA. Iron requirements and iron deficiency in adolescents. In: Basow DS, ed. *UpToDate*. Waltham, MA: UpToDate; 2015. http://www.uptodate.com/contents/iron-requirements-and-iron-deficiency-in-adolescents?detectedLanguage=en&source=search_result&search=iron+deficiency+anemia&selectedTitle=3~150&provider=noProvider#H1. Last updated December 8, 2014. Accessed April 22, 2015.

5. United States Department of Health and Human Services, National Institutes of Health (NIH), Office of Dietary Supplements. Iron. http://ods.od.nih.gov/factsheets/Iron-HealthProfessional. Reviewed February 19, 2015. Accessed April 22, 2015.

6. Mahoney DH Jr. Iron deficiency in infants and young children: Treatment. In: Basow DS, ed. *UpToDate*. Waltham, MA: UpToDate; 2015. http://www.uptodate.com/contents/iron-deficiency-in-infants-and-young-children-treatment?source=search_result&search=iron+deficiency+anemia&selectedTitle=2~150. Last updated February 2, 2015. Accessed April 22, 2015.

7. Yaish HM. Pediatric thalassemia. In: Coppes MJ, ed. Medscape. http://emedicine.medscape.com/article/958850#showall. Updated April 24, 2013. Accessed April 22, 2015.

8. Rachmilewitz EA, Giardina PJ. How I treat thalassemia. *Blood*. 2011; 118(13): 3479–3488. doi:10.1182/blood-2010-08-300335

9. Benz EJ Jr. Clinical manifestation and diagnosis of the thalassemias. In: Basow DS, ed. *UpToDate*. Waltham, MA: UpToDate; 2015. http://www.uptodate.com/contents/clinical-manifestations-and-diagnosis-of-the-thalassemias?source=search_result&search=thalassemia&selectedTitle=1~150. Last updated December 17, 2014. Accessed April 22, 2015.

10. Disease & treatment. Thalassemia Foundation of Canada Web site. http://www.thalassemia.ca/disease-treatment. Accessed April 22, 2015.

11. Maakaron JE. Sickle cell anemia. In: Besa EC, ed. Medscape. http://emedicine.medscape.com/article/205926-overview#showall. Updated September 15, 2014. Accessed April 22, 2015.

12. United States Department of Health and Human Services, NIH, National Heart, Lung, and Blood Institute (NHLBI). What is sickle cell anemia? http://www.nhlbi.nih.gov/health/health-topics/topics/sca. Updated September 28, 2012. Accessed April 22, 2015.

13. Rees DC, Williams TN, Gladwin MT. Sickle-cell disease. *The Lancet*. 2010; 376(9757): 2018–2031. doi:10.1016/S0140-6736(10)61029-X

14. United States Department of Health and Human Services, NIH, NHLBI. What causes sickle cell anemia? http://www.nhlbi.nih.gov/health/health-topics/topics/sca/causes. Updated September 28, 2012. Accessed April 22, 2015.

15. United States Department of Health and Human Services, NIH, NHLBI. What are the signs and symptoms of sickle cell anemia? http://www.nhlbi.nih.gov/health/health-topics/topics/sca/signs. Updated September 28, 2012. Accessed April 22, 2015.

16. Quinn CT, Rogers ZR, McCavit TL, Buchanan GR. Improved survival of children and adolescents with sickle cell disease. *Blood.* 2010; 115(17): 3447–3452. doi:10.1182/blood-2009-07-233700

17. Booth C, Inusa B, Obaro SK. Infection in sickle cell disease: A review. *Int J Infect Dis.* 2010; 14(1): e2–e12. doi:10.1016/j.ijid.2009.03.010

18. Gouw SC, van der Bom JG, Ljung R, et al. Factor VIII products and inhibitor development in severe hemophilia A. *N Engl J Med.* 2013; 368(3): 231–239. doi:10.1056/NEJMoa1208024

19. United States Department of Health and Human Services, Centers for Disease Control and Prevention. Hemophilia. http://www.cdc.gov/ncbddd/hemophilia/facts.html. Last updated August 26, 2014. Accessed April 22, 2015.

20. Wong TE, Majumdar S, Adams E, et al. Overweight and obesity in hemophilia: A systematic review of the literature. *Am J Prev Med.* 2011; 41(6S4): S369–S375. doi:10.1016/j.amepre.2011.09.008

21. Zaiden RA. Hemophilia A. In: Dronen SC, ed. Medscape. http://emedicine.medscape.com/article/779322-overview#showall. Updated November 7, 2014. Accessed April 22, 2015.

22. Lead. American Cancer Society Web site. http://www.cancer.org/cancer/cancercauses/othercarcinogens/athome/lead. Last reviewed May 27, 2014. Accessed April 22, 2015.

23. Hurwitz RL, Lee DA. Childhood lead poisoning: Clinical manifestations and diagnosis. In: Basow DS, ed. *UpToDate.* Waltham, MA: UpToDate; 2015. http://www.uptodate.com/contents/childhood-lead-poisoning-clinical-manifestations-and-diagnosis?detectedLanguage=en&source=search_result&search=lead+poisoning&selectedTitle=2~102&provider=noProvider. Last updated July 15, 2014. Accessed April 22, 2015.

24. Tiwari S, Tiwari HL, Tripathi IP. Lead effects on health. *Int Res J Environment Sci.* 2013; 2(8): 83–87. http://www.isca.in/IJENS/Archive/v2/i8/14.ISCA-IRJEvS-2013-149.pdf

25. Minnesota Department of Health. Lead poisoning in children: Early detection, intervention and prevention. http://www.health.state.mn.us/divs/fh/mch/webcourse/lead. Accessed April 22, 2015.

26. Badawy MK. Pediatric lead toxicity clinical presentation. In: Conners GP, ed. Medscape. http://emedicine.medscape.com/article/1009587-clinical#showall. Updated June 26, 2013. Accessed April 22, 2015.

27. Hurwitz RL, Lee DA. Childhood lead poisoning: Management. In: Basow DS, ed. *UpToDate.* Waltham, MA: UpToDate; 2015. http://www.uptodate.com/contents/childhood-lead-poisoning-management. Last updated November 17, 2014. Accessed April 22, 2015.

28. Babu MS, Murthy KV, Sasidharan S. Burton's line. *Am J Med.* 2012; 125(10): 963–964. doi: 10.1016/j.amjmed.2012.04.004

29. United States Department of Health and Human Services, Centers for Disease Control and Prevention. Blood lead levels in children. http://www.cdc.gov/nceh/lead/acclpp/lead_levels_in_children_fact_sheet.pdf. Accessed April 22, 2015.

30. Leukemia. Cedars-Sinai Web site. http://www.cedars-sinai.edu/Patients/Health-Conditions/Leukemia.aspx?gclid=CP3rwPHxo7sCFYF7QgodAmEA0A. Accessed April 22, 2015.

31. United States Department of Health and Human Services, NIH, National Cancer Institute. Childhood acute lymphoblastic leukemia treatment (PDQ). http://www.cancer.gov/cancertopics/pdq/treatment/childALL/HealthProfessional/page1/AllPages. Updated April 8, 2015. Accessed April 22, 2015.

32. Kanwar VS. Pediatric acute lymphoblastic leukemia. In: Arceci RJ, ed. Medscape. http://emedicine.medscape.com/article/990113-overview#showall. Updated December 5, 2014. Accessed April 22, 2015.

33. Weinblatt ME. Pediatric acute myelocytic leukemia. In: Arceci RJ, ed. Medscape. http://emedicine.medscape.com/article/987228-overview#showall. Updated April 25, 2014. Accessed April 22, 2015.

Chapter 17

Endocrine Disorders

QUESTIONS

1. A 17-year-old obese female undergoes a diabetes screening every 2 years. Which set of risk factors related to the patient's heritage and medical history would best justify this screening?

   a. Pacific Islander with polycystic ovarian disease

   b. Caucasian with hypertension

   c. Hispanic with dysmenorrhea

   d. Native American with hypotension

2. A 5-year-old male presents with weakness, muscle fatigue, and arthralgias. A physical examination reveals dry skin, diminished heart sounds, and diminished deep tendon reflexes. Suspecting hypothyroidism, you order a series of lab studies. Which of the following findings would confirm a diagnosis of hypothyroidism?

   a. Low liver enzymes

   b. Low serum cholesterol

   c. Elevated serum T3

   d. Increased thyroid stimulating hormone

3. You are providing nutritional education to the parents of a 12-year-old male who has been newly diagnosed with type 1 diabetes mellitus. All of the following statements regarding proper nutrition would be appropriate <u>except</u>:

   a. Consume no less than 2,000 calories per day.

   b. Carbohydrates should make up the majority of the diet.

   c. Protein should account for roughly 20% of caloric intake.

   d. The diet should be high in fiber.

4. During routine screening, a 22-month-old patient shows signs of short stature. The medical history, which reveals poor weight gain and recurrent gastrointestinal symptoms that include vomiting and chronic diarrhea, lead you to suspect celiac disease. Which of the following findings would enable you to establish this diagnosis and determine the etiology of the patient's short stature?

   a. Human leukocyte antibodies

   b. Endomysial antibodies

   c. Serum antinuclear antibodies

   d. Growth hormone antibodies

5. Margaret, an 11-year-old female diagnosed with type 1 diabetes mellitus, is experiencing hypoglycemia at 3 a.m. and elevated blood sugar at 7 a.m. What is the proper treatment for her?

   a. Reduce or eliminate the dose of insulin before bed

   b. Increase the dose of metformin before bed

   c. Add or increase the dose of insulin before bed

   d. Advise a snack before bed

6. Metformin is <u>not</u> recommended as a first line therapy for type 2 diabetes mellitus patients presenting with which of the following?

   a. Children less than 10 years of age

   b. Hypoglycemia

   c. Polydipsia

   d. Renal failure

7. You are treating Cynthia, age 9, who has recently been diagnosed with hyperthyroidism. What two drugs should you recognize as typical first-line treatment?

   a. Tapazole and Synthroid

   b. Propranolol and Tapazole

   c. Levothyroxine and propranolol

   d. Insulin and propylthiouracil

8. Which of these laboratory values would most likely be decreased in a patient with hyperthyroidism?

   a. Free thyroxine index

   b. Serum antinuclear antibodies

   c. Thyroid-stimulating hormone

   d. Triiodothyronine

9. Which of the following best describes the state of the pancreatic islet cells at symptom presentation in pediatric patients with type 1 diabetes mellitus?

   a. Pancreatic islet cells have shrunken in numbers but grown in size.

   b. Most pancreatic islet cells have been destroyed.

   c. The number of pancreatic islet cells is near normal levels but shrinking rapidly.

   d. Pancreatic cells produce insulin at a lower rate but their number doesn't change.

10. You are treating an overweight 7-year-old Hispanic female diagnosed with hypertension. She has a family history of type 2 diabetes mellitus (DM). Which of the following is true regarding risk factors and screening for type 2 DM for this patient?

   a. The patient should not be screened until age 10 or onset of puberty.

   b. The patient should be screened as soon as possible due to her hypertension.

   c. The patient should have been screened before the age of 7.

   d. The patient should be screened as soon as possible due to risk factors related to her ethnicity.

RATIONALES

1. a

For individuals with obesity and at least two risk factors, screening for diabetes mellitus (DM) should typically be conducted every 2 years, beginning around the onset of puberty. One risk factor is being Asian/Pacific Islander, African American, Native American, or Hispanic. Signs of insulin resistance, evidenced by polycystic ovarian disease, acanthosis nigricans, hypertension, or dyslipidemia, are also risk factors. Caucasians are not generally at an increased risk of developing DM. Hypotension and dysmenorrhea are also not considered to be risk factors for DM.

2. d

The thyroid-stimulating hormone (TSH) test is the standard diagnostic procedure for hypothyroidism, which is characterized by high TSH levels. While an individual with hypothyroidism may also present with a low serum and low serum cholesterol, these findings are not typically used to confirm this condition. The T3 is generally elevated in thyrotoxicosis, not hypothyroidism. Patients with hypothyroidism may present with elevated liver enzymes rather than low liver enzymes.

3. a

The caloric intake of a child with type 1 diabetes mellitus (DM) is commonly determined by the child's weight and growth patterns. A 2,000 calorie diet may be appropriate for one child, but not for another. Carbohydrates are the main energy source and should make up the majority of daily calories. Protein, which delays the absorption of carbohydrates, should account for about 20% of daily calories. Individuals with type 1 DM should generally consume about 25 grams of fiber per 1,000 calories, which equates to a high-fiber diet. High-fiber diets may help to control blood sugar levels and A1C.

4. b

Serologic testing for endomysial antibodies is commonly used to diagnose celiac disease, which is a condition that often causes short stature and presents with gastrointestinal symptoms. Human leukocyte antibodies are more relevant in cases of diabetes mellitus, and serum antinuclear bodies are a diagnostic of hyperthyroid conditions such as Addison's disease. Growth hormone deficiency may be seen in patients with short stature but is not indicative of celiac disease.

5. a

Reducing or eliminating insulin before bed is a common method of treating the Somogyi effect, which occurs when nocturnal hypoglycemia stimulates a surge of counter regulatory hormones that raise blood sugar. To treat the dawn phenomenon, which occurs when blood sugar levels peak at around 7 a.m. because of progressively elevated glucose levels during the night, bedtime insulin should be increased or added to the patient's regimen. Metformin does not stimulate insulin action and would not be appropriate to treat the Somogyi effect.

6. d

Patients with hepatic or renal failure should not be prescribed metformin, which is commonly used to control high blood glucose and reduce gluconeogenesis in patients with type 2 diabetes mellitus (DM). Metformin is known to upset the gastrointestinal tract and exacerbate lactic acidosis. Metformin does not generally produce or exacerbate hypoglycemia in DM patients. Polydipsia may present as a symptom in type 1 or type 2 DM patients, but is not a contraindication for metformin.

7. b

Propranolol and thiourea drugs, such as Tapazole, are commonly used in managing hyperthyroidism. Propranolol blocks the beta adrenergic activity of hyperthyroid disease, such as palpitations and anxiety. Thiourea drugs, such as Tapazole, and propylthiouracil block the synthesis of the thyroid hormones. Levothyroxine, on the other hand, is often used when treating hypothyroidism, while insulin is typically used in the management of diabetes mellitus.

8. c

Levels of thyroid-stimulating hormone are typically decreased in patients with hyperthyroidism. Conversely, hyperthyroidism patients will likely present with elevated levels of triiodothyronine, free thyroxine index, and serum antinuclear antibodies.

9. b

By the time of symptom presentation of type 1 diabetes mellitus (DM), most of the pancreatic islet cells are destroyed due to production of islet cell autoantibodies. The reduction in number of islet cells would have typically occurred before type 1 DM symptoms present, when the number of cells may still approximate normal levels. The pancreatic cells do not regenerate.

10. a

Screening for type 2 diabetes mellitus (DM) does not need to be conducted until age 10 or the onset of puberty unless the child is overweight and has at least two risk factors for type 2 DM. For children who meet this criteria, screening should begin at age 10 or at the onset of puberty, whichever comes first. The patient in the scenario displays three risk factors for type 2 DM (i.e., hypertension, Hispanic ethnicity, and family history of type 2 DM) and is also overweight. Therefore, she should be screened for type 2 DM at either the age of 10 or the onset of puberty, whichever comes first.

DISCUSSION

Diabetes Mellitus

Overview

Diabetes mellitus (DM) is defined as inappropriate hyperglycemia and disordered metabolism arising from either a reduction in the biologic effectiveness of insulin or an absolute deficiency of its secretion.[1] Classifications for DM fall into type 1 and type 2.[2] Type 1 DM produces ketosis if left untreated, whereas type 2 DM usually does not.[1]

Type 1 Diabetes Mellitus

Overview

Type 1 DM was previously known as insulin-dependent, or juvenile, diabetes. The presence of certain human leukocyte antigens (HLAs), such as HLA-DR3 and HLA-DR4, is strongly associated with the development of type 1 DM. By the time of symptom onset, most of the pancreatic islet cells are destroyed, and islet cell antibodies are detected through the autoimmune process. Type 1 DM is believed to be the result of an infectious disease, toxic environmental insult, or autoimmune destruction of pancreatic B cells.[3]

Presentation

Polyuria, polydipsia, and polyphagia are classic symptoms of type 1 DM.[3] Other presentations typically include nocturnal enuresis, weight loss with increased hunger, fatigue, weakness, parasthesia, dehydration, and dysfunction of peripheral sensory nerves. The patient's consciousness levels may change, ranging from mild cases of irritability to a comatose state. Muscle wasting and loss of subcutaneous fat are suggestive of an insidious onset. In advanced stages, an ophthalmic exam may detect the presence of cotton wool spots or microaneurysms; diminished deep tendon reflexes (DTRs) and evidence of peripheral vascular insufficiency may also present.[3]

Workup

A serum fasting blood sugar test producing results greater than or equal to 126 mg/dL on two separate occasions is a diagnostic of type 1 DM; results ranging from 100 to 125 mg/dL indicate impaired glucose tolerance, or prediabetes.[4] Glucosuria and ketonuria, as well as the presence of plasma ketones, are other typical laboratory findings of type 1 DM. Serum blood urea nitrogen, creatinine, and hemoglobin A1C levels may all be elevated. The presence of polyuria, polydipsia, and weight loss, along with a random blood sugar level greater than or equal to 200 mg/dL, indicate the diagnosis should be confirmed with fasting tests.

Baseline studies must first be established before initiating treatment. A family history should be taken, and a full physical evaluation should include a neurologic exam, a foot exam, and an assessment of peripheral pulses. The age of disease onset should be noted, as well as the presence of cardiac risk factors such as obesity. An electrocardiogram, as well as cholesterol and triglyceride fasting tests, should also be ordered to screen for potential cardiovascular complications. Ketone and antibody levels should be assessed. Whether or not administration of insulin is required is often determined on the basis of blood glucose levels.[5]

Treatment

Dietary competency, preferably with the aid of a dietitian, is of paramount importance in the management of type 1 DM. Caloric intakes must be noted. Maintaining proper caloric intake is necessary in order to achieve, and retain, ideal body weight.[1] Carbohydrates should account for 50%–60% of all calories; fats should account for 25%–30% of all calories; protein should account for 10%–20% of all calories; and 25 grams of fiber should be consumed for every 1,000 calories. Self-testing for blood glucose will help the patient to better tailor the regimen to his or her needs, minimizing the risk of complications resulting from DM.[6] The patient and family should both be trained in the process of self-tests.

Initiation of insulin is a necessity for patients who present with ketones in the blood or urine, as this signals the potential development of diabetic ketoacidosis. The benchmark for starting a course of insulin is 0.5 units/kg/day, with two-thirds of the dose administered in the morning and the other one-third given in the evening.[5]

Somogyi Effect and the Dawn Phenomenon

There are two conditions that produce early morning hyperglycemia; however, these conditions have separate etiologies and different management strategies. One is the Somogyi effect, which results when increased insulin levels in the evening produce a decrease in blood sugar. This nocturnal hypoglycemic state then triggers a rush of counterregulatory hormones that raise blood sugar. The patient will typically be hypoglycemic at 3 a.m., and will rebound around 7 a.m. with a corresponding rise in blood sugar. The treatment is aimed at reducing or eliminating the bedtime dose of insulin.

The other condition is the Dawn phenomenon, which occurs when tissue becomes desensitized to insulin over the course of the night. Blood sugar subsequently increases throughout the night, and typically peaks at 7 a.m. The tissue desensitization is most likely due to a nocturnal rise and spike in growth hormone levels. Proper treatment calls for adding an insulin regimen at bedtime or increasing the dose in an already present regimen.[1]

Type 2 Diabetes Mellitus

Overview

Type 2 DM was previously referred to as non-insulin-dependent DM. It is not linked to the HLA system, and no islet cell antibodies are identified. Although it is more common in adults, the presence of obesity increases the risk of type 2 DM in children.[6] A family history of type 2 DM is also considered a major risk factor.

Presentation

In early disease, physical findings typically do not present; insidious onset of hyperglycemia may also be asymptomatic with type 2 DM. The first symptom of type 2 DM in women is typically recurrent vaginitis. As in type 1 DM, peripheral neuropathies and blurred vision may present, but these findings are more common in type 2. Chronic skin infections typically present with type 2 DM, as do generalized pruritus and acanthosis nigricans. Polydipsia, polyphagia, and polyuria may be present,[7] but these are less common in type 2 than type 1. In women, symptoms of type 2 DM may warrant screening for polycystic ovarian disease, as the condition leads to increased insulin resistance.[8]

Workup

The workup for type 2 DM is the same as type 1; however, the presence of ketones in blood and urine is not expected. Screening for type 2 DM must be considered if the patient is obese and presents with two of the following risk factors: family history of type 2 DM; Hispanic, Native American, African American, or Asian/Pacific Islander ethnicity; or signs associated with insulin resistance, such as acanthosis nigricans, hypertension, dyslipidemia, or polycystic ovarian disease. Screening should be initiated at age 10 or at the onset of puberty,[9] whichever occurs first, and should be repeated every 2 years.

Treatment

Baseline data, as outlined for type 1 DM, should first be obtained; establishing weight management should follow. Metformin (Glucophage), 500 mg three times a day or 850 mg twice a day, may be used for the management of type 2 DM.[1] The drug does not trigger insulin action, but instead works to reduce gluconeogenesis. Metformin may cause significant gastrointestinal upset and minor hypoglycemia, though the gastrointestinal upset is typically transient. Metformin should not be given to patients with hepatic or renal failure, or patients prone to hypoxia. Administration of metformin should cease 48 hours before surgeries or tests that use contrast dye.[10]

In cases of severe hyperglycemia or ketoacidosis, insulin therapy should be employed in addition to the metformin regimen. In moderate to severe cases of ketoacidosis, fluids should be administered in order to remedy dehydration.

Hyperthyroidism

Overview

Hyperthyroidism, sometimes referred to as thyrotoxicosis, covers a group of clinical disorders characterized by increased circulating levels of free thyroxine (T4) or triiodothyronine (T3). Graves' disease, which is the most common manifestation of overt hyperthyroidism in children, is associated with diffuse enlargement and hyperactivity of the thyroid gland, as well as the presence of antibodies acting against different portions of the gland.[11]

Hyperthyroidism is more common in females by an 8:1 ratio. The onset is typically from 12 to 14 years of age. Common causes of hyperthyroidism include toxic adenoma, thyroid-stimulating hormone (TSH)-secreting pituitary tumor, subacute thyroiditis, and high-dosage amiodarone therapy.

Presentation

Patients with hyperthyroidism may complain of nervousness, restlessness, muscle cramps, chest pains, and migraines in the basilar region. Patients may also present with fine hair and heart palpitations, and female adolescent patients may exhibit menstrual irregularities. Heat intolerance may result, leading to increased sweating and warm, moist skin. Weight changes may also manifest, commonly producing as weight loss.[12] Physical findings typically include atrial fibrillation, tachycardia, and thyroid goiter, often without bruit. Graves' ophthalmopathy and hyperactive DTRs may also be present.

Workup

Mandatory newborn screenings often detect congenital hyperthyroidism in young patients. The TSH test is the most sensitive diagnostic for hyperthyroidism; TSH levels will typically be decreased in patients with a positive diagnosis. Elevated T3 and T4 levels are also diagnostics of hyperthyroidism.[13] Moreover, serum antinuclear antibodies (ANAs) are usually elevated without evidence of lupus.

Treatment

The first step in treating hyperthyroidism is to refer the patient to pediatric endocrinology. Pharmacologic treatment includes propranolol for symptomatic relief; dosing should begin at 10 mg, and may be titrated to 80 mg four times daily. For patients with mild cases of hyperthyroidism, or with small goiters or fear of isotopes, thiourea drugs (e.g., propylthiouracil, methimazole) may be utilized. Other treatments may include radioactive iodine 131-I or thyroid surgery. Before thyroid surgery can be performed, however, the patient must achieve a euthyroid state through medication.[14] Additionally, patients should receive 2–3 drops of Lugol's solution once a day for 10 days to diminish the vascularity of the gland.

Hypothyroidism

Overview

Hypothyroidism is a condition resulting in a lack of circulating thyroid hormone. The condition may occur due to disease that directly affects the thyroid gland, or due to a deficiency of pituitary TSH or hypothalamic thyrotropin-releasing hormone (TRH). Most often, hypothyroidism occurs due to autoimmune thyroiditis; however, other causes typically include deficient pituitary, iodine deficiency, and destruction of the gland by external radiation, surgery, or trauma.[1]

Hypothyroidism may be congenital or juvenile acquired. Congenital hypothyroidism may affect the fetus in the first trimester, and can lead to absence or underdevelopment of the thyroid gland, inherent dysfunction in transportation or assimilation of iodine, or development of hypothalamic or pituitary disorder.[15] Congenital hypothyroidism occurs in 1:4,000 live births.[1] Patients with juvenile acquired hypothyroidism may develop Hashimoto's thyroiditis, pituitary deficiency of TSH, hypothalamic deficiency of TRH, iodide deficiency, or damage to the gland.

Presentation

Signs and symptoms of hypothyroidism in neonates and infants are not obvious in the first month of life. However, signs that may appear after the first month include lethargy and poor feeding. Prolonged bilirubin elevation, growth deceleration, large fontanels, bradycardia, and hypotonia are other common findings in neonates and infants with hypothyroidism.

Older children with hypothyroidism may feel weak and achy, and can present with muscle fatigue, arthralgia, cramps, and lethargy. Constipation and weight gain are also common findings. Hypothyroidism may cause delayed bone age resulting in poor bone growth; dry skin, thinning hair, and brittle nails may also present. Various forms of swelling often occur; macroglossia and edema in the hands and face are typically found. Other manifestations of hypothyroidism in older children may include ascites, slowed DTRs, diminished heart sounds, and poor motor.[16]

Workup

Hypothyroidism screening for newborns is mandatory. Elevated TSH and serum cholesterol levels are indicative of hypothyroidism, as is an increase in liver enzymes. T4 and free T4 levels will typically be decreased in patients with hypothyroidism.[17] Lab findings indicating hyponatremia, hypoglycemia, and anemia are also typically present in cases of hypothyroidism.

Treatment

Treatment for hypothyroidism requires referral to a pediatric endocrinologist. Hormone replacement therapy with Synthroid[17]—as opposed to generic levothyroxine—is preferred for keeping thyroid levels consistent.

Short Stature

Overview

Short stature is defined as height measuring less than two standard deviations below the mean, or a distinct deviation from a previously established growth curve.[18] Short stature is also defined as a failure to achieve more than 4 cm of growth per year. Approximately 5% of the population is afflicted with short stature.

Proportional short stature may be caused by intrauterine growth retardation, maternal or fetal infection, chromosomal abnormalities, or a failure to thrive. Various endocrine conditions—including hypopituitarism, growth hormone deficiency, diabetes, and hypothyroidism—may also result in proportional short stature.[19] Disproportionate short stature commonly manifests as a result of dwarfism or rickets.

Presentation

Normal variants of the condition include a familial genetic variant and constitutional delay. The familial genetic variant is characterized by a normal linear growth rate with a short target height. Constitutional delay is marked by a consistency with bone age and height age; a slow growth rate is often seen for the first 2–3 years of life, followed by a low-normal growth rate. A family history of short stature and a delayed onset of puberty are often present in patients with constitutional delay.[1]

Workup

The presentation of short stature should warrant an assessment for chronic disease, neglect, and endocrine deficiencies. Proportion of short stature should first be determined, followed by investigation of underlying causes.

Tests for the condition include a complete blood count,[20] liver function tests, an electrolyte panel, a urinalysis, a thyroid function test, and an erythrocyte sedimentation rate. Bone age should be determined; a skeletal survey may be utilized if disproportionate features are present. Antiendomysial and antigliadin antibody tests should be performed to rule out celiac disease, and a sweat test is performed to rule out cystic fibrosis in cases of recurrent bronchitis. A stool test for ova and parasites may be ordered to determine an infectious cause. Growth hormone levels may also be checked.[20]

Treatment

Treatment for short stature depends on etiology; a referral to a sub-specialist may be warranted in some cases.

Family support, however, is healthy for management of all cases.[19]

References

1. Barkley TW Jr. Endocrine issues and disorders. In: Barkley TW Jr, ed. *Pediatric Primary Care Nurse Practitioner Certification Review/Clinical Update Continuing Education Course*. West Hollywood, CA: Barkley & Associates; 2015: 156–164.

2. Diabetes. A.D.A.M. Medical Encyclopedia. http://www.nlm.nih.gov/medlineplus/ency/article/001214.htm. Updated August 5, 2014. Accessed April 23, 2015.

3. Levitsky LL, Misra M. Epidemiology, presentation, and diagnosis of type 1 diabetes mellitus in children and adolescents. In: Basow DS, ed. *UpToDate*. Waltham, MA: UpToDate; 2015. http://www.uptodate.com/contents/epidemiology-presentation-and-diagnosis-of-type-1-diabetes-mellitus-in-children-and-adolescents. Last updated June 10, 2014. Accessed April 23, 2015.

4. American Diabetes Association. Standards of medical care in diabetes. *Diabetes Care*. 2011; 34(Suppl 1); S11–S61. doi: 10.2337/dc11-S011

5. Laffel LMB, Wood JRS. Diabetes mellitus in children and adolescents. In: Bope ET, Kellerman RD, eds. *Conn's Current Therapy 2012*. Philadelphia, PA: Elsevier Saunders; 2012: 1063–1070.

6. Mayo Clinic Staff. Type 2 diabetes. Mayo Clinic web site. http://www.mayoclinic.com/health/type-2-diabetes/DS00585. Updated July 24, 2014. Accessed April 23, 2015.

7. Diabetes symptoms. American Diabetes Association web site. http://www.diabetes.org/diabetes-basics/symptoms/?loc=DropDownDB-symptoms&print=t. Last reviewed August 1, 2013. Last edited September 12, 2014. Accessed April 23, 2015.

8. Barber TM, Franks S. The link between polycystic ovary syndrome and both type 1 and type 2 diabetes mellitus. *Womens Health*. 2012; 8(2): 147–154. doi: 10.2217/whe.11.94

9. United States Department of Health and Human Services, National Institutes of Health, National Institute of Diabetes and Digestive and Kidney Diseases. Diagnosis of diabetes and prediabetes. http://diabetes.niddk.nih.gov/dm/pubs/diagnosis/#3 . Published June 2014. Last updated September 10, 2014. Accessed April 23, 2015.

10. McCulloch DK. Patient information: Diabetes mellitus type 2: Treatment (Beyond the Basics). In: Basow DS, ed. *UpToDate*. Waltham, MA: UpToDate; 2015. http://www.uptodate.com/contents/diabetes-mellitus-type-2-treatment-beyond-the-basics. Last updated March 14, 2014. Accessed April 23, 2015.

11. LaFranchi S. Clinical manifestations and diagnosis of hyperthyroidism in children and adolescents. In: Basow DS, ed. *UpToDate*. Waltham, MA: UpToDate; 2015. http://www.uptodate.com/contents/clinical-manifestations-and-diagnosis-of-hyperthyroidism-in-children-and-adolescents. Last updated April 1, 2015. Accessed April 23, 2015.

12. Sinha S. Pediatric hyperthyroidism clinical presentation. In: Kemp S, ed. Medscape. http://emedicine.medscape.com/article/921707-clinical#showall. Updated June 3, 2013. Accessed April 23, 2015.

13. Sinha S. Pediatric hyperthyroidism workup. In: Kemp S, ed. Medscape. http://emedicine.medscape.com/article/921707-workup#showall. Updated June 3, 2013. Accessed April 23, 2015.

14. Lee SL, Ananthakrishnan S. Hyperthyroidism treatment & management: Thyroidectomy. In: Khardori R, ed. Medscape. http://emedicine.medscape.com/article/121865-treatment#showall. Updated September 4, 2014. Accessed April 23, 2015.

15. Mayo Clinic Staff. Hypothyroidism (underactive thyroid) - causes. Mayo Clinic web site. http://www.mayoclinic.org/diseases-conditions/hypothyroidism/basics/causes/con-20021179. Updated December 1, 2012. Accessed April 23, 2015.

16. Mayo Clinic Staff. Hypothyroidism (underactive thyroid): Symptoms. http://www.mayoclinic.com/health/hypothyroidism/DS00353/DSECTION=symptoms. Updated December 1, 2012. Accessed April 23, 2015.

17. Gaitonde DY, Rowley KD, Sweeney LB. Hypothyroidism: An update. *Am Fam Physician.* 2012; 86(3): 244–251. http://www.aafp.org/afp/2012/0801/p244.html

18. Rogol AD. Diagnostic approach to children and adolescents with short stature. In: Basow DS, ed. *UpToDate*. Waltham, MA: UpToDate; 2015. http://www.uptodate.com/contents/diagnostic-approach-to-children-and-adolescents-with-short-stature. Last updated September 11, 2014. Accessed April 23, 2015.

19. Short stature. A.D.A.M. Medical Encyclopedia. http://www.nlm.nih.gov/medlineplus/ency/article/003271.htm. Updated August 22, 2013. Accessed April 23, 2015.

20. Sinha S. Short stature workup. In: Kemp S, ed. Medscape. http://emedicine.medscape.com/article/924411-workup#showall . Updated August 1, 2014. Accessed April 23, 2015.

Chapter 18

Genitourinary Disorders

QUESTIONS

1. In male infants, cryptorchidism occurs in 20%–30% of which specific population?

   a. Infants 6 months of age

   b. Brothers of males who experienced cryptorchidism

   c. Premature infants

   d. Sons of males who experienced cryptorchidism

2. What is the preferred over-the-counter analgesic for the treatment of dysmenorrhea?

   a. Aspirin

   b. Acetaminophen

   c. Ibuprofen

   d. Indomethacin

3. In which of the following age groups is primary dysmenorrhea most commonly seen?

   a. Early adolescence in individuals with precocious puberty

   b. Women over the age of 30

   c. Late adolescence

   d. Pre-menopausal women

4. A 1-month-old male is brought to the clinic for a regular check-up. He exhibits irritability and a fever of 100.2°F, and shows signs of dehydration and documented weight loss. A urinalysis is positive for leukocytes and nitrites. Given the most likely diagnosis, what is the first step that should be taken in treating his underlying condition?

   a. Home course of oral cephalosporins

   b. Surgical intervention

   c. Oral desmopressin

   d. Hospitalization

5. Which of the following medications is least recommended for the treatment of enuresis?

   a. Desmopressin

   b. Oxybutynin

   c. Flavoxate

   d. Nitrofurantoin

6. Michael, a 5-year-old patient, is experiencing involuntary urination during waking hours. His parents point out that Michael historically exhibited bladder control until 2 weeks ago. As he does not demonstrate any signs of psychological distress, you suspect Michael's condition may be neurogenic in origin. How would you best classify Michael's enuresis?

   a. Primary enuresis

   b. Nocturnal enuresis

   c. Functional enuresis

   d. Diurnal enuresis

7. Which of the following conditions is least likely to present as asymptomatic in males?

   a. Gonorrhea

   b. Cryptorchidism

   c. Chlamydia

   d. Testicular torsion

8. Why must circumcision not be performed on patients with hypospadias?

   a. It makes the patient susceptible to infection.

   b. There is no foreskin to remove.

   c. The foreskin is used in repair.

   d. Complications often cause death.

9. Concerned parents bring their 2-month-old son with hypospadias to the clinic. They say they wish to learn more about the likelihood of other genitourinary anomalies that may occur alongside hypospadias. The nurse practitioner should explain that all of the following disorders may potentially present in conjunction with hypospadias except:

   a. Undescended testicles

   b. Urinary tract infection

   c. Inguinal hernia

   d. Hydrocele

10. You determine that a 12-year-old male presents with testicular torsion. Your treatment priorities should include:

    a. Recommend cilostazol to improve blood flow

    b. Write release from physical education for the next 5 days

    c. Advise to make appointment with urology

    d. Refer to the emergency department for immediate surgical evaluation

RATIONALES

1. c

Cryptorchidism occurs in about 20%–30% of all premature male newborns. About 3% of all male infants are born with the condition, but by 1 year of age, the rate drops to 1%. Heritability in first-degree male relatives is estimated to be 7%, with about 2% of fathers of patients with cryptorchidism experiencing the condition themselves.

2. c

Ibuprofen is the preferred over-the-counter analgesic for the treatment of dysmenorrhea due to its fast onset, ability to rapidly achieve peak serum concentrations, and low cost as a generic drug. Ibuprofen tablets have been shown to reduce elevated levels of prostaglandin activity during the menstrual cycle. Aspirin is generally less effective in treating dysmenorrhea than other non-steroidal anti-inflammatory drugs. Acetaminophen may only be useful as an adjunct treatment for mild menstrual pain, whereas indomethacin is often avoided due to the high incidence of adverse effects.

3. c

Primary dysmenorrhea is most commonly seen in late adolescence and early adulthood. Young adolescents with precocious puberty do not yet fall into this category, and women in older populations typically experience decreasing incidence of dysmenorrhea with age.

4. d

The patient's irritability, fever, dehydration, weight loss, and a urinalysis positive for leukocytes and nitrites all indicate a urinary tract infection (UTI); children under the age of 2 months who present with a UTI should be considered for hospitalization and treatment with parenteral antibiotics. A course of oral cephalosporins is recommended by national guidelines as the preferred oral course of treatment in older populations. Surgical intervention is recommended for hypospadias and testicular torsion, and oral desmopressin is a common course of treatment for enuresis.

5. d

Nitrofurantoin is an antibiotic commonly recommended for treatment of urinary tract infections, not enuresis. Desmopressin is often the treatment of choice for enuresis, with oxybutynin and flavoxate typically recommended for children who also experience daytime symptoms. Other methods of management, such as an enuresis alarm, positive reinforcement, and bladder control training, are often recommended before using medication.

6. d

Involuntary urination during waking hours is known as diurnal enuresis. In a child who has previously had control, evaluation for the presence of a urinary tract infection or constipation as a contributing factor may be indicated, as treatment may ameliorate symptoms. Primary enuresis, on the contrary, is only applicable to children who have never established bladder control. Nocturnal enuresis refers to incontinence during sleep, whereas functional enuresis refers to enuresis that has no neurogenic or anatomic cause.

7. d

Testicular torsion is not likely to present as asymptomatic, and is often heralded by sudden, severe pain in one testicle. Gonorrhea, cryptorchidism, and chlamydia are all often asymptomatic in males.

8. c

Circumcision should not be performed on patients born with hypospadias because the foreskin may be needed in correcting the condition. Hypospadias repair is usually performed when the child is between 6–24 months old. Susceptibility to infection and complications that can cause death are not common reasons to avoid circumcising patients with hypospadias. Lastly, patients born with hypospadias are typically born with foreskin; however, the foreskin may be incompletely formed in some cases.

9. b

A urinary tract infection is not known to accompany hypospadias, although patients who have undergone hypospadias corrective surgery are at an increased risk for urinary tract infections, especially if hair-bearing skin was used in the operation. Undescended testicles, inguinal hernia, and hydrocele are genitourinary anomalies that may potentially occur alongside hypospadias.

10. d

In patients with testicular torsion, acute pain occurs as a result of an interruption of vascular flow; this interruption warrants a referral for immediate urological surgery to return the blood flow. Although cilostazol dilates arteries and improves blood flow and oxygen, this medication is typically purposed for peripheral vascular disease and improving blood flow to the legs. Testicular torsion is not a self-resolving condition; thus, a temporary withdrawal from physical activity will not properly treat it. Recommending an appointment to be made with urology may take days and the testicular tissue would most likely be dead from a lack of blood flow.

DISCUSSION

Enuresis

Overview

Enuresis is a disorder of involuntary urination that presents at an age when voluntary control is typically present. Enuresis is classified as diurnal if it occurs during waking hours, or nocturnal if it occurs at night. The disorder is further divided into primary and secondary forms: Primary enuresis is the involuntary passage of urine in children who have never established control; secondary enuresis occurs when children begin wetting after being dry for at least 6 months.[1]

Although the rate of enuresis amongst the general population is difficult to determine, the condition is common in children younger than 5 years of age.[2] Physical, psychological, and emotional problems rarely cause enuresis; rather, the great majority of cases of enuresis are functional.[3,4,5] Functional enuresis involves involuntary voiding of urine without a neurogenic or anatomic cause.

Presentation

The evaluation of the patient should be aimed at isolating the source of the patient's bed wetting through the process of exclusion. A thorough history is a key component of the evaluation, which should include a review of present illnesses and therapy, the patient's history of voiding patterns, and symptoms that may suggest a neurogenic or anatomic etiology.[5,6]

Workup

The patient's history and a physical examination may help rule out physical causes of enuresis (e.g., spinal defects or obstructive sleep apnea).[7] The most important test is urinalysis, which can screen for various indications. Abnormal urinalysis findings may show the presence of white blood cells (WBCs), which may indicate cystitis as the underlying disorder. Findings of red blood cells (RBCs) may indicate urinary obstruction, and the presence of glucose may indicate diabetes mellitus.[4]

Treatment

Parent education is the most important aspect of enuresis treatment.[6] Preliminary management is aimed at behavior modification and helped by positive reinforcement measures.[4,5] Once behavioral training techniques are implemented, an enuresis alarm helps to optimize treatment of bedwetting.[3] Bladder control training also aids in treatment by conditioning the patient's bladder to hold more urine.[8]

When pharmacological treatment is necessary, the preferred medication is desmopressin, which may be administered orally or by nasal spray.[4] Tricyclic medications, such as imipramine, may help to decrease bladder contractility and increase outlet resistance, aiding in urine storage.[4] Anticholinergics with antispasmodic activity are also useful in treating patients with diurnal enuresis due to voiding dysfunction.[6,7] This category of medications includes oxybutynin, which is administered to patients 6 years of age and older in order to manage detrusor muscle hyperactivity, which commonly stems from neurological disorders such as spina bifida.[9] Oxybutynin is typically administered orally in 5 mg doses twice per day, but may be administered up to three times per day if required.[5]

Alternative methods of treatment used in place of medications include hypnosis and self-hypnosis; some practitioners believe that hypnosis methods are more effective than medications despite the lack of data to definitively assess the effectiveness of such alternative treatments.[3,5] Additional treatment or therapy may be required if secondary conditions such as urinary tract infections (UTIs) are detected.

Urinary Tract Infection

Overview

UTIs are common during childhood and may involve both the kidneys and the bladder, which can possibly lead to other complications.[10,11] Children with vesicoureteral reflux (VUR), which may result in renal scarring, hypertension, and kidney failure, are also at an increased risk of developing a UTI.[12]

UTIs are most frequently caused by infections due to bacteria residing in the bowels. The most common bacterium is *Escherichia coli*, although other types include *Staphylococcus aureus*. In the first year of life, bacterial UTIs are more common in uncircumcised males.[13] In the general population, however, UTIs occur more frequently in females.[14,15] Predisposing factors include urinary stasis and congenital or acquired obstructive lesions, as well as non-obstructive causes such as neurogenic bladder, constipation, poor hygiene, and sexual intercourse.[5] Sexual abuse and neglect should also be considered as potential causes of UTIs.[16]

Presentation

Infants with UTIs may be asymptomatic. Presenting symptoms that may appear in infants include failure to thrive, irritability, dehydration, and weight loss.[5,13] Older children may present with poor weight gain.[17] Other presenting indications in children and adolescents include dysuria, frequency, urgency, nocturia, suprapubic and lower abdominal discomfort, hematuria, and fever.[5,11] As UTIs may produce sepsis in younger patients, patients presenting with fever and chills should be assessed for the disease.

Workup

Diagnosis of a UTI is determined by collecting and analyzing a sample of the patient's urine for indications of pyuria or bacteriuria.[13] The method of urine collection depends on the child's age.[18] For children who can void voluntarily, a clean-catch specimen often sees use in cases with mild symptoms and follow-up examinations.[5,13] For infants and toddlers still wearing diapers, a plastic collection bag may be used.[18] A straight catheter is indicated for culture and sensitivity in those who cannot void voluntarily. Urinalysis findings indicative of a UTI include leukocytes, nitrites, WBCs, RBCs, and increased pH, among others.[19]

A urine culture may be indicated to determine the type of bacterium causing the UTI and can also aid in determining the most appropriate method of treatment.[15] Although not required, additional diagnostic methods may include blood studies, evaluation of renal function, and imaging studies.[13]

Treatment

Patients with UTIs who do not present with findings indicative of sepsis may be treated initially with oral antibiotics such as amoxicillin, ciprofloxacin, and nitrofurantoin.[13,15] The nurse practitioner (NP) should follow up with the patient in 2 days and change the patient's antibiotics if no improvement is seen; subsequently, the NP should follow up in 1–2 weeks, then every 1–3 months for 1 year.[5] Children younger than 2 months of age who present with a UTI should undergo hospitalization and a course of treatment with parenteral antibiotics. Parenteral antibiotics are also recommended for children with a presentation indicative of sepsis or those who are unable to retain oral intake.[11]

A voiding cystourethrography (VCUG) is indicated if ultrasound findings are reflective of recurrent UTIs, as well as bladder or renal abnormalities. A VCUG and antimicrobial prophylaxis are not indicated after first febrile UTI; furthermore, antimicrobial prophylaxis is not indicated for prevention of UTI recurrences.[20]

Frequent bladder emptying and proper wiping is also important in the treatment of UTIs.[21] Fluid intake should be encouraged; studies have shown that cranberry juice may help prevent symptomatic recurrence of UTIs in children and may prevent bacteria from adhering to uroepithelial cells.[5,22]

Hypospadias

Overview

Hypospadias is a relatively common congenital abnormality in males where the urethral opening forms on the underside, or ventral surface, of the penis rather than at the tip.[23] The cause of hypospadias is unknown, but the condition is often inherited. Current hypotheses hold hypospadias to be a deformity rather than a malformation; regardless, the condition is considered to be one of the most common congenital abnormalities in infants and live births. Hypospadias usually begins developing when the male fetus is in the ninth week of gestation as the external genitalia begin to differentiate between sexes.[24] The condition is also linked to an increased likelihood of other genitourinary (GU) abnormalities, such as undescended testicles, inguinal hernia, and hydrocele.[5]

Presentation

The characteristic findings of hypospadias include presentation of a dorsally hooded foreskin, downward aim of the patient's urinary stream, and ventral bowing of the penis (i.e., chordee).[25]

Workup

Diagnosis is made by clinical findings; evaluation of the patient should include a history, examining the patient's genitalia, and identifying other congenital anomalies.[24] Imaging tests are only required if the patient presents with anomalies in other organ systems, such as the renal system.[26]

Treatment

Patients with hypospadias should be referred to a urologist at birth. Surgery should be performed between 6 and 12 months of age, and involves straightening and correcting the opening by using tissue grafts from the foreskin.[5,23] Because the foreskin is used in repair, circumcision should not be done prior to surgery.[26]

Cryptorchidism (Undescended Testes)

Overview

Cryptorchidism is the failure of one or both testes to descend from the abdomen into the scrotal sac in utero. Since testes normally descend during the last trimester, the majority of cases of cryptorchidism are diagnosed at birth.[5,27] Although cryptorchidism occurs rarely in newborn males, it is the most common congenital abnormality of the genitourinary tract and is found in up to 30% of all premature male newborns.[5,28,29]

Presentation

The main sign of cryptorchidism is inability to palpate a testicle where it is expected; this sign is often described as an empty scrotum.[30,31] Cryptorchidism typically presents with no additional signs or symptoms.[32]

Workup

Cryptorchidism does not typically require laboratories or diagnostics to confirm a diagnosis if the patient presents with unilateral undescended testes.[5] For patients with bilateral undescended testes, however, consultation with an endocrinologist or a geneticist is recommended for diagnosis. An ultrasound and karyotyping for chromosomal abnormalities, such as prune belly syndrome, may also be ordered.[5,28]

Treatment

In most cases of cryptorchidism, the testes descend into the scrotum by 1 year of age.[31] If the testes are undescended at 1 year of age, the NP should refer the patient to a urologist. If the testes are palpable and undescended, surgical repair may be necessary. Surgical repair is recommended by 3–6 months of age in order to improve fertility potential and reduce risk of testicular cancer later in life.[27] Post-surgery, the surgeon should monitor the patient via a physical exam, ultrasound, or assessing hormone levels. Parents should monitor testicular development by regularly checking testicular positioning. Later in life, especially as the patient reaches puberty, the patient should be taught how to perform a testicular self-examination to ensure early detection of tumors.[30]

Testicular Torsion

Overview

Testicular torsion is the twisting and strangulation of the spermatic cord, which interrupts the vascular flow and produces acute pain. When the condition presents, it necessitates emergency surgical intervention with the goal of preventing necrotic testicles and infertility. Testicular torsion occurs primarily in neonates and adolescents, and is most often observed in patients between 10 and 20 years of age.[5,33]

Presentation

The most common signs of testicular torsion include sudden, severe pain in one testicle; redness and swelling within one side of the scrotum; and one testicle that rests higher than the other.[34] Additional signs and symptoms include lightheadedness, nausea and vomiting, a testicular lump, and presence of blood in the semen.[35] Testicular torsion does not present with a fever, irritative voiding symptoms, or systemic symptoms.[5]

Workup

Testicular torsion can often be treated on the basis of a clinical diagnosis alone and does not usually require laboratories or diagnostics to confirm.[36] In uncertain cases, an ultrasonography with Doppler color flow is the imaging test of choice. Radionuclide scans and magnetic resonance imaging may also be useful.[37]

Treatment

Patients with testicular torsion usually require immediate surgical intervention.[34] The success rate of surgical treatment of testicular torsion is approximately 95% if it is performed within 6 hours of onset but declines to 20% after 24 hours.[38]

Dysmenorrhea

Overview

Dysmenorrhea is pain and cramping associated with menstruation. Dysmenorrhea can be either primary or secondary, depending on its presentation and underlying cause. Primary dysmenorrhea has an absence of any pelvic pathology and is currently considered to be hormonal and endocrine-related in nature. Primary dysmenorrhea commonly starts to manifest 6–12 months after menarche, with symptoms gradually presenting more often until patients are in their mid-20s.[5] Secondary dysmenorrhea is commonly caused by organic underlying conditions such as pelvic inflammatory disease (PID), pregnancy, and endometriosis.[5,39] Secondary dysmenorrhea usually presents in adulthood, except in cases that are caused by congenital malformations such as bicornuate uterus.[40]

Presentation

Dysmenorrhea typically presents with dull, throbbing, or cramping pain in the lower abdomen that may radiate to the back and is typically strongest during the first few days of bleeding.[5,40,41] Additional signs and symptoms of dysmenorrhea include nausea, fatigue, headaches, and diarrhea.[42]

Workup

Primary dysmenorrhea is diagnosed clinically. Laboratory tests are useful in determining the underlying cause of secondary dysmenorrhea.[5] Imaging studies may include a pelvic ultrasound to determine the presence of comorbid conditions such as uterine fibroids, adenomyosis, and endometriosis.[43]

Treatment

Pharmacotherapy is the most effective method of relieving dysmenorrhea.[39] Non-steroidal anti-inflammatory drugs (NSAIDs) are recommended for moderate to severe dysmenorrhea and are very effective in reducing pain associated with the condition.[5,43] Patients may also be given oral contraceptives or other forms of hormonal birth control as needed to reduce the severity of menstrual cramps, prevent ovulation, and diminish the uterine contractions and menstrual bleeding that contribute to discomfort associated with dysmenorrhea.[41,43] Less severe cases of dysmenorrhea may necessitate over-the-counter analgesics as a support measure, preferably ibuprofen. Ibuprofen is given in doses of 400 mg every 4–6 hours, starting with the onset of the menstrual cycle and continuing for 24–72 hours.[5]

Additional support measures include heat application, psychological support, and referral as needed. Dysmenorrhea patients should be educated about menstruation and proper diet, as diets high in vitamin E and fish oil may decrease symptoms of dysmenorrhea.[39] It is also important for patients to get adequate exercise and sleep.[40]

Chlamydia

Overview

Chlamydia is a parasitic sexually transmitted infection (STI) that is caused by the bacteria *Chlamydia trachomatis* and may result in severe reproductive tract complications in both males and females. Chlamydiae are intracellular obligates that closely resemble gram-negative bacteria and cause diseases such as STIs and pneumonias.[5,44] Furthermore, chlamydia is the most common bacterial STI in the United States and is also the leading cause of urethritis and cervicitis in adolescents.[5,45]

Presentation

Although signs and symptoms may vary among males and females, both sexes are often asymptomatic.[46] Symptoms that may appear in female chlamydia patients include abnormal vaginal discharge after intercourse, dysuria, dyspareunia, intermenstrual spotting, postcoital bleeding, and lower abdominal or pelvic pain.[5,45] Males may present with dysuria and a thick, cloudy penile discharge. Testicular pain and swelling may also present, but these findings are less common.[47]

Workup

Although a diagnosis of chlamydia can sometimes be made solely on the basis of a clinical evaluation, testing is recommended for patients at risk for STIs because many chlamydia patients are asymptomatic.[44] Urine checks are recommended for adolescent patients. A culture is the most definitive diagnostic of chlamydia but results may take 3–9 days. An enzyme immunoassay, on the other hand, yields results in 30–120 minutes and can be performed at a low cost.[5]

Treatment

Antibiotics are the usual treatment for chlamydia.[45] *C. trachomatis* is particularly susceptible to tetracyclines and macrolides, the first-line agents of which are azithromycin (Zithromax) and doxycycline, respectively.[49] Azithromycin is given to chlamydia patients in a single dose of 1 gram orally, whereas doxycycline is given in doses of 100 mg orally twice a day for 7 days.[49] Additionally, it is recommended by the Centers for Disease Control and Prevention (CDC) that all confirmed cases of *C. trachomatis* infection be reported to the health department.[49]

Gonorrhea

Overview

Gonorrhea is a bacterial STI caused by *Neisseria gonorrhoeae*, which may be spread by sexual contact or by transmission during childbirth.[50] *N. gonorrhoeae* is a gram-negative diplococcus that may take root in the genitourinary tract, oropharynx, conjunctiva, or anorectum. Gonorrhea is the second most common communicable disease in the United States and is a major cause of cervicitis in women and urethritis in men.[51] Moreover, gonorrhea is also the leading cause of infertility among females.[52]

Presentation

Gonorrhea is often asymptomatic, especially in females.[5] Both males and females, however, may present with dysuria and urinary frequency, among other signs and symptoms. Additional signs and symptoms in men include testicular pain and penile discharge, which may be white, yellow, or green in color.[53] Female gonorrhea patients, on the other hand, may present with mucopurulent vaginal discharge, labial pain and swelling, lower abdominal pain, or dysmenorrhea.[54] Fever, chills, nausea, and vomiting may also appear in female patients with gonorrhea who develop PID, although these findings are less common.[50]

Workup

A diagnosis of gonorrhea may be confirmed when gonococci are detected by a Gram stain or culture.[55] Urine checks should be performed in adolescent patients, with these urine samples often serving as the base for cultures. A Gram stain is a rapid and inexpensive test and may show gram-negative diplococci and WBCs in the patient's discharge.[5,50] Cervical cultures for *N. gonorrhoeae* are processed using Thayer-Martin or Transgrow media and are particularly useful in isolating the bacteria from any site.[5,51]

Treatment

For antibiotic treatment of gonorrhea, uncomplicated cases should be treated with ceftriaxone in combination with azithromycin or doxycycline.[54] Patients should also be co-treated for chlamydia, as about half of all female gonorrhea patients experience a concomitant chlamydial infection. Ceftriaxone, distributed under the brand name Rocephin, is given intramuscularly in a 250 mg single dose. This dose should be given in combination with either azithromycin (Zithromax) 1 gram orally in a single dose or doxycycline 100 mg by mouth twice a day for 7 days, in order to cover concomitant chlamydial infection.[50] Additionally, all gonorrhea patients should be contacted and tested by the health department.[53]

Syphilis

Overview

Syphilis is an STI that is caused by the spirochete bacteria *Treponema pallidum* and involves multiple organ systems. Syphilis infections usually result from sexual contact, although *T. pallidum* may be transmitted by skin contact or through the placental barrier.[55]

Presentation

There are four clinical stages of syphilis. In the primary stage, the first sign of syphilis is a chancre that appears at the site of transmission.[56] The secondary stage presents with flu-like symptoms as well as a generalized maculopapular rash that appears on various parts of the body, especially the palms and soles.[57] Latent syphilis is seropositive, but asymptomatic.

The latent stage may persist indefinitely or be followed by late-stage syphilis (i.e., tertiary syphilis).[55] Approximately one-third of all untreated cases of the disease develop into tertiary syphilis, which often presents with leukoplakia and cardiac insufficiencies such as aortitis, aneurysms, and aortic regurgitation.[5] At the tertiary stage, the condition may damage parts of the body, such as the bones and liver, and may produce central nervous system disorders such as meningitis, hemiparesis, and hemiplegia, among others.[5,56]

Workup

Syphilis is most commonly diagnosed by serologic testing, the two primary methods of which are treponema-specific tests and non-treponemal reaginic tests.[58,59] Non-treponemal antibody tests such as the Venereal Disease Research Laboratory test or the rapid plasma reagin test are given first. A diagnosis is then confirmed with treponemal tests such as a fluorescent treponemal antibody absorption test or a microhemagglutination assay for antibody to *T. pallidum*.[5]

In addition to serologic testing, spirochetes can be directly identified through darkfield microscopy, which will show treponemes in almost all chancres that appear in primary syphilis.[58] Primary syphilis can also be diagnosed by a typical lesion or newly positive syphilis screen. Furthermore, a syphilis screen will typically be strongly reactive in cases of secondary syphilis, whereas the screen will show serologic evidence of untreated syphilis in the latent and tertiary stages.[5]

Treatment

Penicillin is the preferred treatment in all stages of syphilis.[60] Most syphilis infections are treated by benzathine penicillin G, which is given in a single dose of 2.4 million units intramuscularly.[55] For patients who are allergic to penicillin, the NP may prescribe alternatives such as doxycycline or tetracycline.[49] Patients with tertiary syphilis will likely also require surgical care for treatment of complications such as aortitis. In addition to antibiotic treatment, the NP should report all cases of syphilis to the health department.

Bacterial Vaginosis

Overview

Bacterial vaginosis is a vaginal infection in which "harmful" species of bacteria produce an alteration in the normal functioning of vaginal flora. In this alteration, lactobacilli decrease and anaerobic pathogens overgrow.[62] Bacterial vaginosis is not considered an STI; however, it manifests more often in women who are sexually active, and the development of this condition is associated with sexual activity.[5,63] Although the cause of bacterial vaginosis is unknown, it is the most common type of infectious vaginitis, as well as the most common cause of vaginal discharge in women of childbearing age.[6,62]

Presentation

A large percentage of patients with bacterial vaginosis are asymptomatic.[64] Symptomatic patients often present with an increased milky discharge that is thin and grayish white.[65] A malodorous, "fishy" discharge is also usually present and is most evident after sexual intercourse, when the discharge is more alkaline.[62] Other physical findings may include pain during urination as well as pruritus around the vagina.[66] On a physical exam, the patient's cervix, uterus, and adnexa will usually appear normal.[5,63]

Workup

Bacterial vaginosis is diagnosed upon detection of clue cells—epithelial cells covered with bacteria that appear with poorly defined borders and small dots or specks.[63] Clue cells are detected by microscopic examination of a saline wet mount, which also detects decreasing or absent lactobacilli as well as few or absent white blood cells.[5,62] A positive amine "whiff" test detects a fishy odor when potassium hydroxide is added to the slide.[67]

Treatment

Antibiotics are the mainstay of bacterial vaginosis treatment.[63] Medications that may be used in treatment include metronidazole; common preparations include 500 mg oral doses administered twice a day for 7 days, or a 0.75% gel administered in 5 gram doses inserted intravaginally once a day for 5 days. Clindamycin cream (2%) may be given in 5 gram doses intravaginally at bedtime for 7 days.[49]

Herpes

Overview

Herpes is a recurrent, viral STI that is associated with painful lesions and caused by two types of herpes simplex virus (HSV), known as types 1 and 2. HSV type 1 is found on the lips, face, and mucosa, whereas HSV type 2 is found on the genitalia.[68] Transmission of herpes occurs by direct contact with the virus across broken skin or intact mucosa.[69]

Presentation

Presentation of herpes varies depending on the clinical designation of the patient's condition. The three clinical designations of herpes are primary, non-primary first episode, and recurrent.[70] Initial signs and symptoms of herpes include fever, malaise, and dysuria, as well as painful and pruritic ulcers lasting for approximately 12 days. Non-primary first episodes follow the same pattern of symptoms, but tend to present with fewer lesions and less systemic symptoms. Recurrent herpes also presents with ulcers, but these ulcers are less painful and pruritic than those of primary herpes and usually last for only 5 days.[5]

Workup

A diagnosis of herpes can often be made clinically based on the appearance of characteristic lesions.[71] The most definitive laboratory test to confirm an HSV infection is a tissue culture, which isolates the virus.[72]

Additionally, HSV may be detected by a Papanicolaou or Tzanck stain.[5]

Treatment

There is no curative treatment for herpes, and the patient's symptoms may disappear without treatment in 1–2 weeks.[73] Patients may be given drying and antipruritic agents for symptomatic treatment. Medication options include acyclovir (Zovirax), given orally at 400 mg three times a day for 7–10 days or 200 mg orally five times a day for 7–10 days. Valacyclovir, 1 gram orally twice a day for 7–10 days, may also be used. Treatment may be extended if healing is incomplete after the recommended length of therapy.[49]

Acquired Immune Deficiency Syndrome (AIDS)

Overview

AIDS is the final stage of HIV infection. This stage occurs the patient's immune system becomes damaged, leaving the patient vulnerable to opportunistic infections.[74] AIDS is typically transmitted prenatally by perinatal transmission from mother to child by shared blood circulation; postnatally, breastfeeding is the primary vertical route in infants and neonates.[5,75]

Presentation

Neonates with AIDS present with a low birth weight. Such patients also typically demonstrate a falling ratio of head circumference to height and weight. Additional signs and symptoms of AIDS in pediatric patients may include recurrent infections, diminishing activity, developmental delays, hepatosplenomegaly, and generalized lymphadenopathy.[5]

Workup

HIV polymerase chain reaction testing is used to test for the genetic material of the virus and is particularly recommended for children born to HIV-positive mothers.[76] Older children are screened with the ELISA test, which is the most common type of HIV test and has greater than 99.9% sensitivity.[5,77] If the HIV patient shows progress towards AIDS, the western blot test confirms this diagnosis.[76]

The patient's CD4 lymphocyte percentage of white blood cells should be assessed to confirm a diagnosis of AIDS. The risk of progression to AIDS is high if the patient's CD4 lymphocyte count is below 20%, whereas a normal absolute CD4 lymphocyte count is greater than 800 cells/µL.[5] Ideally, the patient's viral load should be less than 5,000 copies, which may be described as "zero" or "undetectable."[78]

Treatment

The patient should be referred to an HIV infectious disease specialist for care. Although there is no available cure for AIDS, a number of treatments can help improve the patient's quality of life and diminish signs and symptoms.[75] To help prevent pneumocystic pneumonia, Bactrim may be given to treat *Pneumocystis jiroveci*. The patient should also be monitored for cytomegalovirus. Antiretroviral therapy includes combination treatment; although decisions on when to start antiretroviral therapy typically vary based on age and presentation of symptoms, various studies indicate that treatment should ideally be started by the time the patient has a CD4 of 350 cells/µL.[5,79] Because drug resistance may develop rapidly, the patient should be taught to take medications exactly as prescribed and at the same time every day.[80]

References

1. Knott L, Tidy C. Nocturnal enuresis in children. Patient.co.uk web site. http://www.patient.co.uk/doctor/nocturnal-enuresis-in-children. Last updated March 26, 2014. Accessed April 23, 2015.

2. Tu ND, Baskin LS. Nocturnal enuresis in children: Management. In: Basow DS, ed. *UpToDate*. Waltham, MA: UpToDate; 2015. http://www.uptodate.com/contents/nocturnal-enuresis-in-children-management. Last updated August 13, 2014. Accessed April 23, 2015.

3. Drutz JE, Tu ND. Patient information: Bedwetting in children (Beyond the Basics). In: Basow DS, ed. *UpToDate*. Waltham, MA: UpToDate; 2015. http://www.uptodate.com/contents/bedwetting-in-children-beyond-the-basics. Last updated January 9, 2013. Accessed April 23, 2015.

4. Robson WML. Enuresis. In: Cendron M, ed. Medscape. http://emedicine.medscape.com/article/1014762-overview. Updated February 19, 2014. Accessed April 23, 2015.

5. Barkley TW Jr. *Pediatric Primary Care Nurse Practitioner Certification Review/Clinical Update Continuing Education Course*. West Hollywood, CA: Barkley and Associates; 2015.

6. Figueroa TE. Incontinence in children. In: Porter RS, Kaplan JL, eds. The Merck Manual Online. http://www.merckmanuals.com/professional/pediatrics/incontinence_in_children/urinary_incontinence_in_children.html?qt=enuresis&alt=sh. Last reviewed October 2014. Accessed April 23, 2015.

7. Bedwetting. A.D.A.M. Medical Encyclopedia. http://www.nlm.nih.gov/medlineplus/ency/patientinstructions/000703.htm. Updated March 19, 2014. Accessed April 23, 2015.

8. Urinary incontinence (Enuresis). Lucile Packard Children's Hospital at Stanford web site. http://www.lpch.org/DiseaseHealthInfo/HealthLibrary/growth/enuresis.html. Accessed April 23, 2015.

9. Oxybutynin. A.D.A.M. Medical Encyclopedia. http://www.nlm.nih.gov/medlineplus/druginfo/meds/a682141.html. Last revised May 15, 2014. Accessed April 23, 2015.

10. Shaikh N, Hoberman A. Urinary tract infections in children: Epidemiology and risk factors. In: Basow DS, ed. *UpToDate*. Waltham, MA: UpToDate; 2015. http://www.uptodate.com/contents/urinary-tract-infections-in-children-epidemiology-and-risk-factors. Last updated December 8, 2014. Accessed April 23, 2015.

11. Weinberg GA. Urinary tract infection in children (UTI). In: Porter RS, Kaplan JL, eds. The Merck Manual Online. http://www.merckmanuals.com/professional/pediatrics/miscellaneous_infections_in_infants_and_children/urinary_tract_infection_in_children_uti.html?qt=urinary%20tract%20infection&alt=sh. Last reviewed March 2010. Accessed April 23, 2015.

12. United States Department of Health and Human Services, National Institutes of Health (NIH), National Institute of Diabetes and Digestive and Kidney Diseases (NIDDK), National Kidney and Urologic Diseases Information Clearinghouse (NKUDIC). Vesicoureteral reflux. http://kidney.niddk.nih.gov/kudiseases/pubs/vesicoureteralreflux. Published September 2011. Last updated June 29, 2012. Accessed April 23, 2015.

13. Fisher DJ. Pediatric urinary tract infection. In: Steele RW, ed. Medscape. http://emedicine.medscape.com/article/969643-overview#aw2aab6b2b. Updated August 18, 2014. Accessed April 23, 2015.

14. Mersch J. Urinary tract infections (UTIs) in children. In: Stöppler MC, ed. MedicineNet. http://www.medicinenet.com/urinary_tract_infections_in_children/article.htm. Reviewed February 5, 2015. Accessed April 23, 2015.

15. Mayo Clinic Staff. Urinary tract infection (UTI). Mayo Clinic web site. http://www.mayoclinic.org/diseases-conditions/urinary-tract-infection/basics/definition/con-20037892. Updated August 29, 2012. Accessed April 23, 2015.

16. Pediatric urinary tract infections. American Urological Association web site. http://www.auanet.org/education/pediatric-urinary-tract-infections.cfm. Accessed April 23, 2015.

17. Shaikh N, Hoberman A. Urinary tract infections in infants and children older than one month: Clinical features and diagnosis. In: Basow DS, ed. *UpToDate*. Waltham, MA: UpToDate; 2015. http://www.uptodate.com/contents/urinary-tract-infections-in-infants-and-children-older-than-one-month-clinical-features-and-diagnosis. Last updated March 17, 2015. Accessed April 23, 2015.

18. United States Department of Health and Human Services, NIH, NIDDK, NKUDIC. Urinary tract infections in children. http://kidney.niddk.nih.gov/kudiseases/pubs/utichildren. Published November 2011. Last updated November 16, 2011. Accessed April 23, 2015.

19. Bates BN. Interpretation of urinalysis and urine culture for UTI treatment. *US Pharm.* 2013; 38(11): 65–68. http://www.uspharmacist.com/content/c/44877/?t=men%27s_health,urology

20. Voiding cystourethrogram. A.D.A.M. Medical Encyclopedia. http://www.nlm.nih.gov/medlineplus/ency/article/003784.htm. Updated October 9, 2012. Accessed April 23, 2015.

21. Minnesota Department of Public Health and Human Services. Best practice guidelines: Urinary tract infections. https://dphhs.mt.gov/Portals/85/dsd/documents/DDP/MedicalDirector/UrinaryTractInfections.pdf. Published 2010. Accessed April 23, 2015.

22. Jepson R, Williams GJ, Craig JC. Cranberries for preventing urinary tract infections. *Cochrane Database Syst Rev.* 2012; 10: CD001321. doi: 10.1002/14651858.CD001321.pub5

23. Hypospadias. A.D.A.M. Medical Encyclopedia. http://www.nlm.nih.gov/medlineplus/ency/article/001286.htm. Updated October 9, 2012. Accessed April 23, 2015.

24. Baskin LS. Hypospadias. In: Basow DS, ed. *UpToDate*. Waltham, MA: UpToDate; 2015. http://www.uptodate.com/contents/hypospadias. Last updated April 20, 2015. Accessed April 23, 2015.

25. Mayo Clinic Staff. Hypospadias. Mayo Clinic web site. http://www.mayoclinic.org/diseases-conditions/hypospadias/basics/definition/con-20031354. Updated October 1, 2013. Accessed April 23, 2015.

26. Gatti JM, Kirsch AJ, Snyder HM III. Hypospadias. In: Cendron M, ed. Medscape. http://emedicine.medscape.com/article/1015227-workup. Updated May 2, 2013. Accessed April 23, 2015.

27. Rabinowitz R, Cubillos J. Congenital renal and genitourinary anomalies. In: Porter RS, Kaplan JL, eds. The Merck Manual Online. http://www.merckmanuals.com/professional/pediatrics/ congenital_renal_and_genitourinary_anomalies/penile_and_urethral_anomalies.html?qt=hypospadias&alt=sh. Last reviewed May 2013. Accessed April 23, 2015.

28. Sumfest JM, Kolon TF, Rukstalis DB. Cryptorchidism. In: Kim ED, ed. Medscape. http://emedicine.medscape.com/article/438378-overview#a0199. Updated November 19, 2014. Accessed April 23, 2015.

29. Kolon TF, Herndon CD, Baker LA, et al. Evaluation and treatment of cryptorchidism: AUA guideline. *J Urol.* 2014; 192(2): 337–345. doi: 10.1016/j.juro.2014.05.005.

30. Mayo Clinic Staff. Undescended testicle (cryptorchidism). Mayo Clinic web site. http://www.mayoclinic.com/health/undescended-testicle/DS00845/DSECTION=symptoms. Updated April 11, 2013. Accessed April 23, 2015.

31. Undescended testicle. A.D.A.M. Medical Encyclopedia. http://www.nlm.nih.gov/medlineplus/ency/article/000973.htm. Updated October 2, 2013. Accessed April 23, 2015.

32. Undescended testicle – topic overview. WebMD web site. http://www.webmd.com/parenting/baby/tc/undescended-testicle-topic-overview. Last updated December 28, 2012. Accessed April 23, 2015.

33. Ogunyemi OI, Weiker M, Abel EJ. Testicular torsion. In: Kim ED, ed. Medscape. http://emedicine.medscape.com/article/2036003-overview#a0101. Updated November 17, 2014. Accessed April 23, 2015.

34. Testicular torsion repair. A.D.A.M. Medical Encyclopedia. http://www.nlm.nih.gov/medlineplus/ency/article/002994.htm. Updated October 2, 2013. Accessed April 23, 2015.

35. Testicular torsion. A.D.A.M. Medical Encyclopedia. http://www.nlm.nih.gov/medlineplus/ency/article/000517.htm. Updated October 2, 2013. Accessed April 23, 2015.

36. Shenot PJ. Penile and scrotal disorders. In: Porter RS, Kaplan JL, eds. The Merck Manual Online. http://www.merckmanuals.com/professional/genitourinary_disorders/penile_and_scrotal_disorders/testicular_torsion.html?qt=testicular%20torsion&alt=sh. Last reviewed December 2012. Accessed April 23, 2015.

37. Hittelman AB. Neonatal testicular torsion. In: Basow DS, ed. *UpToDate*. Waltham, MA: UpToDate; 2015. http://www.uptodate.com/contents/neonatal-testicular-torsion. Last updated January 14, 2014. Accessed April 23, 2015.

38. Mayo Clinic Staff. Testicular torsion. Mayo Clinic web site. http://www.mayoclinic.com/health/testicular-torsion/DS01039. Updated March 12, 2015. Accessed April 23, 2015.

39. Calis KA, Popat V, Dang DK, Kalantaridou SN, Erogul M. Dysmenorrhea. In: Rivlin ME, ed. Medscape. http://emedicine.medscape.com/article/253812-overview. Updated December 1, 2014. Accessed April 23, 2015.

40. Pinkerton JV. Dysmenorrhea. In: Porter RS, Kaplan JL, eds. The Merck Manual Online. http://www.merckmanuals.com/professional/gynecology_and_obstetrics/menstrual_abnormalities/dysmenorrhea.html?qt=dysmenorrhea&alt=sh. Last reviewed August 2012. Accessed April 23, 2015.

41. Mayo Clinic Staff. Menstrual cramps. Mayo Clinic web site. http://www.mayoclinic.com/health/menstrual-cramps/DS00506/DSECTION=symptoms. Updated May 8, 2014. Accessed April 23, 2015.

42. Painful periods (dysmenorrhea) – Symptoms. NHS Choices web site. http://www.nhs.uk/Conditions/Periods-painful/Pages/Symptoms.aspx. Last reviewed November 5, 2014. Accessed April 23, 2015.

43. Smith RP, Kaunitz AM. Patient information: Painful menstrual periods (dysmenorrhea) (Beyond the basics). In: Basow DS, ed. *UpToDate*. Waltham, MA: UpToDate; 2015. http://www.uptodate.com/contents/painful-menstrual-periods-dysmenorrhea-beyond-the-basics. Last updated April 13, 2015. Accessed April 23, 2015.

44. Hammerschlag MR. Chlamydia. In: Porter RS, Kaplan JL, eds. The Merck Manual Online. http://www.merckmanuals.com/professional/infectious_diseases/chlamydia_and_mycoplasmas/chlamydia.html?qt=chlamydia&alt=sh. Last reviewed February 2014. Accessed April 23, 2015.

45. Chlamydia. A.D.A.M. Medical Encyclopedia. http://www.nlm.nih.gov/medlineplus/ency/article/001345.htm. Updated June 11, 2014. Accessed April 23, 2015.

46. Marrazzo J. Clinical manifestations and diagnosis of chlamydia trachomatis infections. In: Basow DS, ed. *UpToDate*. Waltham, MA: UpToDate; 2015. http://www.uptodate.com/contents/clinical-manifestations-and-diagnosis-of-chlamydia-trachomatis-infections. Last updated March 13, 2015. Accessed April 23, 2015.

47. United States Department of Health and Human Services, Centers for Disease Control and Prevention. Chlamydia – CDC fact sheet. http://www.cdc.gov/std/chlamydia/STDFact-chlamydia-detailed.htm. Last reviewed November 29, 2012. Last updated December 16, 2014. Accessed April 23, 2015.

48. Marrazzo J. Treatment of Chlamydia trachomatis infection. In: Basow DS, ed. *UpToDate*. Waltham, MA: UpToDate; 2015. http://www.uptodate.com/contents/treatment-of-chlamydia-trachomatis-infection. Last updated December 23, 2014. Accessed April 23, 2015.

49. Workowski KA, Bolan GA. Sexually transmitted diseases treatment guidelines, 2015. *MMWR Morb Mortal Wkly Rep.* 2015; 64(3): 1–137. http://www.cdc.gov/std/tg2015/tg-2015-print.pdf

50. Wong B. Gonorrhea. In: Chandrasekar PH, ed. Medscape. http://emedicine.medscape.com/article/218059-overview. Updated April 16, 2014. Accessed April 23, 2015.

51. Leone PA. Epidemiology, pathogenesis, and clinical manifestations of Neisseria gonorrhoeae infection. In: Basow DS, ed. *UpToDate*. Waltham, MA: UpToDate; 2015. http://www.uptodate.com/contents/epidemiology-and-pathogenesis-of-neisseria-gonorrhoeae-infection. Last updated June 26, 2014. Accessed April 23, 2015.

52. Crosta P. What is gonorrhea? What causes gonorrhea? Medical News Today web site. http://www.medicalnewstoday.com/articles/155653.php. Last updated September 26, 2014. Accessed April 23, 2015.

53. Gonorrhea. A.D.A.M. Medical Encyclopedia. http://www.nlm.nih.gov/medlineplus/ency/article/007267.htm. Updated April 25, 2013. Accessed April 23, 2015.

54. Mayo Clinic Staff. Gonorrhea. Mayo Clinic web site. http://www.mayoclinic.com/health/gonorrhea/DS00180/DSECTION=symptoms. Updated January 2, 2014. Accessed April 23, 2015.

55. McCutchan JA. Overview of sexually transmitted diseases. In: Porter RS, Kaplan JL, eds. The Merck Manual Online. http://www.merckmanuals.com/professional/infectious_diseases/sexually_transmitted_diseases_std/overview_of_sexually_transmitted_diseases.html. Last reviewed September 2013. Accessed April 23, 2015.

56. Mayo Clinic Staff. Syphilis. Mayo Clinic web site. http://www.mayoclinic.org/diseases-conditions/syphilis/basics/definition/con-20021862. Updated January 2, 2014. Accessed April 23, 2015.

57. United States Department of Health and Human Services, Centers for Disease Control and Prevention. Syphilis – CDC fact sheet. http://www.cdc.gov/std/syphilis/std-fact-syphilis.htm. Last reviewed January 29, 2014. Last updated July 8, 2014. Accessed April 23, 2015.

58. Hicks CB. Diagnostic testing for syphilis. In: Basow DS, ed. *UpToDate*. Waltham, MA: UpToDate; 2015. http://www.uptodate.com/contents/diagnostic-testing-for-syphilis. Last updated October 16, 2014. Accessed April 23, 2015.

59. Waseem M, Aslam M. Pediatric syphilis. In: Steele RW, ed. Medscape. http://emedicine.medscape.com/article/969023-workup#showall. Updated April 1, 2013. Accessed April 23, 2015.

60. Mayo Clinic Staff. Syphilis. Mayo Clinic web site. http://www.mayoclinic.com/health/syphilis/DS00374/DSECTION=treatments-and-drugs. Updated January 2, 2014. Accessed April 23, 2015.

61. Healthwise Staff. Antibiotics for syphilis. WebMD web site. http://www.webmd.com/sexual-conditions/antibiotics-for-syphilis. Last updated October 8, 2013. Accessed April 23, 2015.

62. Soper DE. Bacterial vaginosis. In: Porter RS, Kaplan JL, eds. The Merck Manual Online. http://www.merckmanuals.com/professional/gynecology-and-obstetrics/vaginitis-cervicitis-and-pelvic-inflammatory-disease-pid/bacterial-vaginosis?qt=bacterialvaginosis&alt=sh. Last reviewed January 2015. Accessed April 23, 2015.

63. Girerd PH. Bacterial vaginosis. In: Rivlin ME, ed. Medscape. http://emedicine.medscape.com/article/254342-overview#aw2aab6b2b2aa. Updated March 27, 2014. Accessed April 23, 2015.

64. Sobel JD. Bacterial vaginosis. In: Basow DS, ed. *UpToDate*. Waltham, MA: UpToDate; 2015. http://www.uptodate.com/contents/bacterial-vaginosis. Last updated March 18, 2015. Accessed April 23, 2015.

65. Mayo Clinic Staff. Bacterial vaginosis. Mayo Clinic web site. http://www.mayoclinic.com/health/bacterial-vaginosis/DS01193/DSECTION=symptoms. Updated April 20, 2013. Accessed April 23, 2015.

66. United States Department of Health and Human Services, NIH, National Institute of Allergy and Infectious Diseases. Bacterial vaginosis. http://www.niaid.nih.gov/topics/bacterialvaginosis/Pages/default.aspx. Last updated January 31, 2013. Accessed April 23, 2015.

67. Healthwise Staff. Tests for bacterial vaginosis. WebMD web site. http://www.webmd.com/sexual-conditions/tests-for-bacterial-vaginosis. Last updated March 12, 2014. Accessed April 23, 2015.

68. Herpes simplex: Herpes types 1 and 2. WebMD web site. http://www.webmd.com/genital-herpes/pain-management-herpes. Last updated September 30, 2014. Accessed April 23, 2015.

69. Straface G, Selmin A, Zanardo V, De Santis M, Ercoli A, Scambia G. Herpes simplex virus infection in pregnancy. *Infect Dis Obstet Gynecol.* 2012; 2012: 385697. doi: 10.1155/2012/385697

70. Albrecht MA. Epidemiology, clinical manifestations, and diagnosis of genital herpes simplex virus infection. In: Basow DS, ed. *UpToDate*. Waltham, MA: UpToDate; 2015. http://www.uptodate.com/contents/epidemiology-clinical-manifestations-and-diagnosis-of-genital-herpes-simplex-virus-infection. Last updated July 2, 2014. Accessed April 23, 2015.

71. Kaye KM. Herpes simplex viruses (HSV) infections. In: Porter RS, Kaplan JL, eds. The Merck Manual Online. http://www.merckmanuals.com/professional/infectious_diseases/herpesviruses/herpes_simplex_virus_hsv_infections.html?qt=herpes&alt=sh. Last updated April 2013. Accessed April 23, 2015.

72. Salvaggio MR, Lutwick LI, Seenivasan M, Kumar S. Herpes simplex. In: Bronze MS, ed. Medscape. http://emedicine.medscape.com/article/218580-overview. Updated November 14, 2014. Accessed April 23, 2015.

73. Oral herpes (cold sore). A.D.A.M. Medical Encyclopedia. http://www.ncbi.nlm.nih.gov/pubmedhealth/PMH0001631. Accessed April 23, 2015.

74. United States Department of Health and Human Services. HIV/AIDS 101: What is HIV/AIDS? AIDS.gov web site. https://aids.gov/hiv-aids-basics/hiv-aids-101/what-is-hiv-aids. Last revised April 29, 2014. Accessed April 23, 2015.

75. HIV/AIDS. A.D.A.M. Medical Encyclopedia. http://www.ncbi.nlm.nih.gov/pubmedhealth/PMH0001620. Accessed April 23, 2015.

76. United States Department of Health and Human Services. HIV testing: Get the basics. AIDS.gov web site. http://aids.gov/hiv-aids-basics/prevention/hiv-testing/hiv-test-types. Last revised March 27, 2015. Accessed April 23, 2015.

77. Lancaster JB. HIV testing resources. TeensHealth web site. http://kidshealth.org/teen/sexual_health/stds/hiv_tests.html#. Reviewed November 2013. Accessed April 23, 2015.

78. HIV viral load testing. WebMD web site. http://www.webmd.com/hiv-aids/hiv-viral-load-what-you-need-to-know?page=2. Reviewed April 17, 2014. Accessed April 23, 2015.

79. United States Department of Health and Human Services. Guidelines for the use of antiretroviral agents in pediatric HIV infection. http://aidsinfo.nih.gov/guidelines/html/2/pediatric-arv-guidelines/70/when-to-initiate-therapy-in-antiretroviral-naive-children. Last updated April 27, 2015. Accessed April 28, 2015.

80. AIDS treatment. University of California San Francisco Medical Center web site. http://www.ucsfhealth.org/conditions/aids/treatment.html. Accessed April 23, 2015.

Index

A

abdominal 19, 20, 44, 45, 50, 66, 96, 122, 128, 130, 132-138, 219, 233, 235, 236, 238, 257, 261
Achenbach Behavior Checklist 97
acne 143, 145, 149-150, 150f
acquired immune deficiency syndrome (AIDS) 93, 264
acute otitis media (AOM) 170-173, 177, 178
acyanotic defects 117, 119-120, 121
acyanotic lesions 119
adenovirus 132, 134, 179
adolescence 7, 17, 18, 21, 65, 96, 104-108, 110, 111, 206, 232, 253, 255
adolescent 5, 7, 17, 21, 31, 53, 65, 90, 105-112, 149, 153, 158, 159, 194, 200, 203-206, 218-220, 228, 230-234. 249, 255, 257, 259-261)
Adolescent Preventive Services (GAPS) 105, 107, 108
afebrile 173, 204, 214, 216
aganglionic megacolon 135
Ages and Stages Questionnaire (ASQ) 18, 62, 64, 65, 67, 77, 80,
alkaline phosphatase 95, 136
allergic contact dermatitis 153, 153f
American Academy of Pediatrics (AAP) 7, 8, 17, 65, 67, 68, 77, 80, 92, 93
American Medical Association 108
amphetamines 97, 98, 222
ampicillin 182
analgesia 8, 47
analgesic 204, 219, 235, 253, 255, 260)
anemias 8, 36, 38, 55, 67, 76, 77, 92, 104, 106, 108, 111, 117, 123, 130, 220, 228-236, 238, 239, 250
animism 16, 77, 79
ankle sprain 201, 208
annular 149, 156, 209
anorexia 98, 105, 111-112, 130, 132, 135, 136, 138, 155, 157, 236
anorexia nervosa 105, 111-112
antiendomysial 250
antigliadin 250
aortic regurgitation 39, 121, 262
aortic stenosis 118, 120, 121
APGAR score 47, 47t
apnea 94, 256
appendicitis 129, 130, 135-136, 216
areola 109
arthralgia 123, 156, 159, 243, 250
ascites 53, 250
Ashkenazic 37, 38, 40
Asperger's Syndrome 73, 75, 82, 83
asthma 145, 152, 187-192, 192t, 193t, 194
atopic dermatitis (eczema) 20, 143, 152, 175
atrial fibrillation 249
atrial septal defect (ASD) 119, 121
atrioventricular septal defect AVSD 121
Attention Deficit Hyperactivity Disorder (ADHD) 5, 6, 40, 87, 88, 90, 96-98, 97t, 222
autism 55, 67, 80, 82, 83, 158
autistic 73, 75, 82, 83
autonomy versus shame and doubt 16, 77, 79, 80

B

Babinski 44, 46, 51t, 218
bacteremia 62, 63
bacterial vaginosis 263
basic metabolic panel (BMP) 122, 219
Bayley Infant Neurodevelopmental Screener (BINS) 62, 64, 67, 80
BAYLEY-III 80
Beckwith-Wiedemann syndrome 48, 49
bicuspid 52, 88, 90, 121
bilirubin 138, 233, 234, 249
biventricular hypertrophy 119-120
blood urea nitrogen (BUN) 115, 117, 132, 247
body mass index (BMI) 17, 78, 92, 94, 108
body surface area (BSA) 4-6, 19, 20, 147, 148t
bradycardia 52, 249
brain stem auditory evoked response test (BSAER) 54
brain tumor 176, 214-218, 220
BRAT diet 132
bronchiolitis 187, 191
Brudzinski's sign 217
bulimia nervosa 104, 105, 111, 112
burns 19t, 68, 89, 95, 144, 147-149, 148f, 148t

C

Campylobacter 132
capital epiphysis *See slipped capital femoral epiphysis (SCFE)*
cardiopulmonary disease 181
cataracts 46, 68, 172, 175-176
CD4 count 264
cefotaxime 175t, 217
ceftriaxone 61, 63, 175t, 217, 262
celiac disease (Sprue) 134, 136, 137, 243, 245, 250
Centers for Disease Control and Prevention (CDC) 7, 17, 29, 30, 77, 79, 106, 261
central incisors 8, 90
central nervous system (CNS) 46, 52, 82, 90, 96, 97, 122, 235, 236, 238, 239, 262
cerebral palsy 96, 176
cerebrospinal fluid (CSF) 217
cervical adenopathy 180
cervical lymphadenopathy 117, 123
chalazion 171, 172, 174
chalmydial 173, 175, 175t, 262
Checklist for Autism in Toddlers (CHAT) 83
child abuse 87, 89, 95-96, 108, 228, 230, 257
child protective agency 229
childhood disintegrative disorder 73, 75, 82
chlamydia 254, 255, 260-262
Chlamydia trachomatis 170, 172, 180, 260
chorionic villus sampling (CVS) 234
ciprofloxacin 258

clonidine (Catapres) 222
coagulopathies 55, 239
coarctation 53, 115, 117, 118, 120, 121
common cold 179-180, 182
complete blood count 70, 95, 122, 123, 132, 133, 138, 156, 202, 203, 204, 219, 220, 228, 230, 232, 233, 235, 238, 250
computed axial tomography (CAT) scan 218
computed tomography (CT) scan 96, 128, 130, 136, 137, 172, 178, 182, 200, 218-220, 222
concrete operational thinking 16, 89, 91, 92
confluent 149
confusional migraine 214, 215, 218-219
congenital heart defects 38-40, 53-55, 115-119, 121, 158
congenital rubella 158-159
congenital syphilis 262
congestive heart failure (CHF) 118, 121
conjunctivitis 117, 123, 157, 170-175, 175t
conotruncal defects 121
conotruncal region of the heart 40
coxsackie virus (hand, foot, and mouth disease) 160-161
cranial nerve palsy 217-218
cranial nerves 50, 178, 213
creatine kinase (CK) 200, 202, 207
croup 170-173, 181
cryptorchidism 253-255, 259
cyanosis 121, 181, 191, 192
cyanotic 220
cyanotic defects 116-118, 120
cyanotic heart disease 49, 121
cyanotic lesions 119
cyst 44, 46, 52, 144-146, 149, 174
cystic fibrosis 54, 55, 134, 136, 137, 187-189, 191, 195, 250
Cytomegalovirus 264

D

Dawn Phenomenon 245, 247-248
decibel threshold 178
deep tendon reflexes (DTRs) 243, 247, 249, 250
dehydrated 134, 147, 195
dehydration 51, 104, 106, 112, 129, 132, 132t, 216, 235, 247, 248, 253, 255, 257
dental development 8
dental health 68, 80, 93, 112
Denver Developmental Screening (Denver II) 3, 5, 17, 18, 62, 64, 65, 67, 77, 80
detachment issues 67
developmental delay 38, 55, 65, 73, 75, 80, 83, 89, 95, 158, 264
developmental dysplasia of the hip (DDH) 43, 45, 48, 54, 64, 66, 201, 202, 206-207
developmental milestones 4, 6, 9t-15t, 17, 63, 79, 82, 92, 218, 237
developmental warning signs 7, 9t-15t, 63, 68, 69t, 75, 80, 81t, 88, 89, 93, 112
diabetes mellitus 94, 175, 220, 243-248, 257
diabetic ketoacidosis 247, 248
Diagnostic and Statistic Manual of Mental Disorders-5 (DSM-5) 82, 83, 96
diastole 117, 119
DiGeorge (Velocardiofacial) syndrome 34, 36, 37, 40, 121
diphtheria 27, 29, 33t, 91, 104, 106, 108
discrete 149, 151
DTaP vaccine 27, 29, 33t, 106
Dubowitz/Ballard exam see New Ballard Score
dwarfism 250
dysfluency 80
dysmenorrhea 243, 245, 253, 255, 260, 261
dysrhythmia 52

E

ecchymoses 199, 201, 208
ectopia lentis 40
eczema 20, 152
edema 51, 52, 78, 117, 121, 146, 147, 156, 172, 173, 176, 177, 192, 199, 201, 208, 250
egocentrism 16, 77, 79
elbow fracture 201, 208-209
electrocardiogram (ECG) 35, 37, 52, 115, 117, 119-121, 123, 207, 247
encephalopathy/encephalitis 146, 156-158, 216, 220, 236
enteroviral meningitis 217
enuresis 91, 247, 254-257
epicanthal folds 38, 51
epiglottitis 170-173, 181
epistaxis (nosebleed) 122, 180
Erb's point 119
Erikson, Erik 16, 77, 79, 87, 89, 91, 92, 110
erythema 43, 45, 49, 53, 117, 123, 146, 152-154, 156, 159, 176
erythema infectiosum (Fifth disease) 159
erythema marginatum 123
erythematous 150, 151, 157, 158, 160, 177, 180
erythrocyte sedimentation rate (ESR) 115, 117, 123, 136, 156, 200, 202, 204, 219, 250
Escherichia coli (*E. coli*) 132, 133, 194, 217, 257

F

failure to thrive (FTT) 38, 116, 118, 133, 135-137, 189, 195, 214, 215, 218, 250, 257
famotidine 134
febrile seizure 132, 158, 159, 213, 215, 221
femoral anteversion 79
fever 30, 61-64, 68, 70, 115, 117, 122-124, 132, 135, 136, 138, 151, 155-161, 170, 171, 173, 177, 180-182, 191, 194, 204, 213, 215-217, 219, 221, 228, 234, 238, 253, 255, 257, 258, 259, 261, 263
first molars 8, 90, 157
first-degree burns 147
fluoride 8, 66, 68, 78
fluoride supplements 8, 68
food jags 76, 80
forced expiratory volume (FEV1) 192t, 193t
forced vital capacity (FVC) 193t
fourth intercostal space 52, 78, 119
Fragile X Syndrome (Martin-Bell Syndrome/Marker X Syndrome) 37
Freud, Sigmund 16-17, 91
fungal infections 145, 150-151, 154, 176, 194, 239

G

galactorrhea 61, 63, 66
galactosemia 38, 54, 55
Galeazzi's sign 62, 64, 66, 199, 201, 206
gastroenteritis 64, 128-133
gastroesophageal reflux disease (GERD) 129, 131, 133-134
genetic evaluation 34-40
genetic testing 38, 199, 201

prothrombin time 95, 138, 236
pruritic 143, 145, 154, 155, 158, 263, 264
pruritus 145, 150-156, 159, 176, 248, 263
PS23/PPSV23 25, 27, 29-30, 33t
psoriasis 143, 145, 149, 154
pulmonary atresia 55
pulmonary stenosis 115, 117, 118, 120, 121
pulse in school age children 92
purified protein derivative test 25, 27, 77, 88, 90, 92
pyloric stenosis 128-130, 133, 134

Q

quadrivalent inactivated influenza vaccine 26, 28, 30, 31
QT intervals 124

R

radiographic studies 70, 92, 120, 121, 135, 181, 188, 190, 194, 195, 199-203, 205-209
rapid decelerating growth 7
reflexes 44, 46, 50, 51, 67, 243, 247
renovascular disease 122
respiration 47, 92, 220
restrictive disease 180, 190, 191
retinoblastoma 44, 46
Rett's disorder 73, 75, 82
Reye's syndrome 151
rheumatic fever/heart disease 115, 117, 122, 123
rhinosinusitis 182
rickets 250
right lower quadrant (RLQ) 129, 130, 135, 136
right upper quadrant (RUQ) 138
right upper sternal border (RUSB) 119, 120, 122
roseola infantum (Sixth disease) 144, 146, 159, 160
rotavirus 29, 33, 131, 132, 133
rotavirus vaccine (Rota) 29
rubella 144, 146, 158, 159
rubeola 144, 146, 157, 158, 216
rugae 48, 104, 106, 109, 110
Rule of Nines 147

S

SAFETEENS format 105, 107, 109
Salmonella 132
scabies 145, 155, 156
school age 6, 7, 26, 87-103, 107, 222
scoliosis 36, 37, 39, 82, 92, 105, 107, 108, 199, 201, 206
secondary lesions 149
secondary sexual characteristics 38, 108, 109
second-degree burns 144, 147
seizure disorder 219
sensorineural hearing loss 178
sepsis 55, 70, 257, 258
septic arthritis 203, 204
sequelae 19, 133
serotype (HLA DR3) 246
serous otitis media 177
serum antinuclear antibodies (ANA) 243, 244, 246, 249
serum T3 243
severe malnutrition 106, 112
sexual maturity rating (SMR) 104, 106, 109
sexuality 73, 107, 109, 112
sexually transmitted diseases (STDs)/sexually transmitted infections (STIs) 31, 93, 108, 260
Shigella 132, 133
short palpebral fissures 40
short philtrum 40
short stature 38, 205, 243, 245, 250
sickle cell anemia 36, 38, 228, 229, 233, 234, 235
sickle cell disease 37, 54, 55, 229, 233, 234
single palmar crease 38, 54
sinusitis 170, 172, 173, 180, 182, 216, 238
skin lesions 149
slipped capital femoral epiphysis (SCFE) 200-204
small gestational age (SGA) 49
solitary 149, 150
Somogyi effect 245, 247
spermarche 105, 107, 109, 112
standard deviation 50, 51, 232, 250
Staphylococcal abscess 173
Staphylococcus 155, 181, 194, 217, 257
Still's murmur 117, 118, 122
stimulants 90, 97, 98
strabismus 39, 68, 78, 171, 172, 176
Streptococcus 68, 123, 171, 172, 177, 188, 190, 194, 217
Streptococcus pneumoniae 68, 171, 172, 173, 177, 188, 189, 190, 194, 217
stuttering 74, 76, 80, 82
stye 173, 174
subarachnoid hemorrhage 216
subcutaneous nodules 123
sudden infant death syndrome 68
swimmer's ear 176
synapse formation 20
syphilis 155, 219, 220, 262
systole 119
systolic 119-122, 192, 234
systolic ejection murmur 118, 120

T

tachycardia 52, 98, 130, 227, 229, 231, 235, 249
tachypnea 64, 121, 191, 194, 229, 231, 235
Tanner staging 92, 104-110, 110f
Tay-Sachs disease 34-38, 40
Td Vaccine 29
Tdap vaccine 25, 26, 28, 29, 33t, 91, 104, 108
teeth 8, 8f, 15t, 68, 78, 81t, 88, 90, 92, 93, 133, 216, 220
television 93, 94, 111
testicular self exam (TSE) 108, 249
testicular torsion 254-256, 259-260
tetanus 25-29, 33t, 91, 104, 106, 108
Tetanus (DTaP) 25, 27, 29, 33t, 106
Tetralogy of Fallot (TOF) 55, 115, 117, 118, 120, 121
thalassemia 55, 229, 231-233
third-degree burns 147, 149
thrombocytopenia 157, 158, 238, 239
thrombocytopenic 228, 230
thrombocytosis 123
thromboplastin time 95
thymus aplasia 35, 37
thyroid 243-246, 248-250
thyroid radioactive iodine 249
thyroid stimulating hormone 243-250
thyrotoxicosis 245, 248
thyrotropin 249
thyrotropin releasing hormone 249
thyroxine 244, 246, 248-250
tibia 203, 205
tibial torsion 79
tibial tubercle 199, 201, 203
tic disorders 214, 216, 222

tinea capitis 143, 145, 150
tinea corporis 150, 151
tinea cruris 150
tinea manuum 145, 150, 151
tinea pedis 145, 150, 151
tinea versicolor 150, 151
toddler 4, 6, 18, 21, 67, 73-83, 194, 205, 215, 228, 231, 232, 258
toilet training 75, 76, 80
tonsillitis 171-173, 180-181, 221
tonsils 66, 78, 170, 172, 180, 237
tooth eruption 8, 8f, 66, 77, 92
toxic synovitis 200-204
transient toxic synovitis 203-204
transposition of great arteries (TGA) 55, 115, 120
transposition of great vessels 115
tricuspid 55, 118, 119
tricuspid atresia 55
trigeminal 50
triiodothyronine (T3) 243-246, 248, 249
trimethoprim/sulfamethoxazole (TMP/SMX) 239
trisomies 36, 38, 46, 51, 54, 66, 121
trisomy 18 (Edward's syndrome) 46, 121
trisomy 21 (Down syndrome) 36, 38, 46, 51, 54
trochlear 50
truncus arteriosus 55, 121
tuberculosis 25, 27, 77, 88, 90, 92
tumor 137, 144, 146, 149, 176, 179, 213-222, 249, 259
Turner's Syndrome 34-37, 39, 52, 121
type 1 diabetes mellitus 243-248
type 2 diabetes mellitus 94, 244, 246, 248

U

ultrasonography 96, 133, 135, 200, 202, 203, 209, 259
ultrasound 35, 37, 129, 131, 134, 136, 199-202, 207, 258-260
urinary tract infection (UTI) 62, 64, 70, 254-258

V

vagus 50
Vanderbilt Assessment Tool 97
varicella vaccine 25, 27, 30, 33t, 151
varicella zoster virus (chickenpox) 30, 143, 145, 151, 158
vascular dilation 213, 215, 216
vascular headache 218-219
velocardiofacial syndrome (VCFS) 34, 36, 37, 40
Venereal Disease Research Laboratory test (VDRL) 219, 262
venous hum 115, 117, 118, 122
ventricular hypertrophy 119 (LVH - 121, 122; RVH - 120, 121)
ventricular septal defect (VSD) 116-121
verapamil (Calan) 219
vitamin B12 106
vitamin C 232, 233
vitamin E 233
vitamin K 138
vitamin supplementation 8, 67, 106, 137
Vonrecklinghausen disease 221-222

W

warts 31
weight 3-8, 10t, 17, 45, 47-49, 63, 65, 66, 68, 69t, 77, 78, 92-95, 98, 111, 112, 133, 134, 138, 151, 153, 208, 236, 243, 245, 247-250, 253, 255, 257, 264
well child check (WCC) 4, 5, 6, 17-18, 61, 65, 74, 77, 78, 91, 92, 105, 107, 108, 109, 207
wheal 144, 146, 149

X

XO karyotype (Turner's syndrome) 37, 39
x-ray 3, 5, 38, 116, 118-123, 135, 171-173, 181, 191, 192, 194, 199, 203, 204, 208

Z

zinc 106, 144, 146
Zithromax 261, 262

genu recurvatum 39
genu valgum (knock-knee) 79, 199-202, 206
genu varum (bowleg) 79, 200, 202, 205
gestational age 17, 48-49, 52
glossopharyngeal 50
glucosuria 247
gonorrhea 254, 255, 261-262
Gram-negative enteric organisms 68
Graves disease 248
Group B streptococcus (GBS) 62, 68, 188, 194, 217
grouped lesions 149
growth and development milestones 9t-15t, 17
growth hormone (GH) 243, 245, 248, 250
gynecomastia 39, 66

H

Haemophilus influenzae 25, 27, 29, 33t, 68, 171-173, 177, 181, 188, 190, 194, 195, 217, 235
Hashimoto's thyroiditis 249
headache 98, 122, 144, 146, 156, 159, 180, 182, 194, 213, 215-220, 231, 236, 260
hearing loss 54, 178-179, 179f
heart failure 116, 118, 121, 122
hematocrit 74, 76, 77, 92, 108, 115, 117, 228, 230-232, 234, 236
hematuria 234, 235, 257
hemoglobinopathies 49, 54, 55, 237
hemophilia 228, 230
hemophilia A 235-236
hepatitis A 26-28, 30-31, 33t, 137, 138, 138t
hepatitis A vaccine 26-28, 30-31, 33t, 138
hepatitis B 25, 27-29, 33t, 137-139, 138t, 235
hepatitis B antigen 29, 138, 138t
hepatitis B immune globulin (HBIG) 27, 29
hepatitis B vaccination 25, 27-29, 33t, 138-139, 235
hepatitis C 137, 138, 138t
hepatosplenomegaly 182, 195, 234, 264
hernias 44, 45, 53, 254, 256, 258
herpes 146, 220, 221, 263-264
herpes virus 159
Hib vaccine 29, 33t
Hirschsprung's disease 128-131, 135
HLA-DR4 246
holosystolic murmur 117
holosystolic thrill 116, 118
homeopathic 95
hordeolum (styes) 170-174
HPV vaccine 31, 33t, 91, 104, 106, 108
human immunodeficiency virus (HIV) 27, 30, 93, 202, 264
human leukocyte antigen system (HLA) 238, 243, 245, 246, 248
human papillomavirus vaccine 31, 33t, 91, 104, 106, 108, 202
hyperextension of joints 34, 36, 39
hyperglycemia 246-248
hypertension 47, 49, 53, 98, 117, 122, 216, 234, 243-246, 248, 257
hyperthyroid conditions 245
hyperthyroidism 66, 244, 248-249
hypocalcemia 36, 40, 220
hypoglossal 50
hypoglycemia 20, 216, 220, 244-246, 248, 250
hypoglycemic state 247
hypogonadism 39
hyponatremia 250
hypoparathyroidism 40
hypospadias 53, 62, 64, 66, 254-256, 258-259
hypothalamic thyrotropin-releasing hormone (TRH) 249
hypothyroidism 37, 38, 46, 51, 54, 78, 243, 245, 246, 249-250
hypotonia 35, 38, 249
hypovolemic shock 20

I

ibuprofen 63, 64, 70, 213, 215, 219, 253, 255, 260
identity 16, 105, 107-112
imipramine (Tofranil) 219, 257
immunocompetent 151, 152
immunocompromised 28, 151, 191, 194
impetigo 143, 145, 155
Inactivated Polio Vaccine 25, 30, 33t
inactivated poliovirus 26
increased intracranial pressure (ICP) 63, 66, 215, 216
industry vs. inferiority 16, 87, 89, 91, 92
infectious mononucleosis 170-173, 182
influenza 25, 26, 28, 30, 33t, 171, 173, 179, 180, 216, 235
influenza vaccine 25, 26, 28, 30, 33t
inner canthi 40
innocent murmurs 53, 116, 118, 121-122
interdisciplinary management 112
intracranial pressure 51, 63, 66, 215, 216
intraparenchymal hemorrhage 216
intrauterine growth restriction (IUGR) 45, 49, 51, 250
intussusception 128-131, 134-135
iodide deficiency 249
iridodonesis 40
iron deficiency anemia 67, 228-232, 236
irritant diaper dermatitis 146, 153-154, 153f

J

jaundice 111, 135, 138, 182, 233, 234
joints 34, 36, 38, 39, 122, 144, 146, 149, 156, 202, 235

K

Kawasaki disease 115, 117, 123-124
Kernig's sign 216, 217
ketonuria 247
Klinefelter Syndrome 34-37, 39
kyphoscoliosis 35-37, 39

L

lanugo 48, 104, 105, 111
large gestational age (LGA) 48
latency period 17, 91
lateral incisors 8
lead poisoning 76, 227-229, 231, 236-237
left lower sternal border (LLSB) 115-119, 122
left upper sternal border (LUSB) 115-117, 119, 120
left ventricular hypertrophy (LVH) 119, 121, 122
Legg-Calve Perthes Disease (LCPD) 199-202, 204
leukemia 26, 38, 61, 63, 228, 230, 237-240
leukocytosis 182, 238
level of consciousness (LOC) 247
linear statistical - 95, 250; patterns - 149, 155
live attenuated influenza vaccine (LAIV) 30, 33t
liver function tests 105, 107, 108, 136, 220, 250
low birth weight 47, 133, 264
Lund-Browder chart 147, 148, 148f, 148t
Lyme disease 144, 146, 156-157, 156f
lymphadenopathy 63, 117, 123, 143, 145, 151, 157, 158, 170, 172, 238, 264

M

magnetic resonance imaging (MRI) 96, 200, 202, 204, 205, 209, 218, 220, 222, 259
malabsorption 128, 130, 131, 136-137, 195
malformations 35, 37, 50, 119, 258, 260
malformed thorax 52
malnutrition 6, 45, 106, 112, 135
Marfan syndrome 34-37, 39-40, 121, 175
maternal rubella 158
measles 25-27, 30, 33t, 91, 104, 106, 146, 157-158
measles, mumps, rubella (MMR) 25-27, 30, 33t, 91, 104, 106, 158
meningitis 146, 156, 214-217, 220, 221, 262
meningococcal vaccine 26, 28, 31, 33t, 91, 104, 106, 108
metformin 244-246, 248
methimazole 249
methylphenidates 88, 90, 97, 98, 222
metronidazole 263
microcephaly 50, 66
microcytic anemias 229, 231-233
micrognathia 40
midclavicular line 52, 78
migraine headaches 213-216, 218-219, 249
miscarriages, stillbirths 34-36, 38, 39
mitral 39, 118, 119, 121
mitral valve prolapse 39, 121
Modified Checklist for Autism in Toddlers (MCHAT) 67, 80, 83
molars 8, 88, 90, 93, 157
molluscum contagiosum 151-152, 152f
motor skills 17, 21, 39, 67, 74, 76, 79, 92
muscular dystrophy 200-202, 207
musculoskeletal assessment 53-54, 96
musculoskeletal development 110
myelination 20
myopathic 207

N

narcissism 105, 107, 108
necrosis 204
necrotic 207, 259
neglect 95-96, 250, 257
Neisseria gonorrhoeae 171, 173, 180, 261
Neisseria meningitidis 217, 235
neonatal morbidity 40, 54
neonatal period 37, 38
neuroblastoma 128, 130, 137
neurofibromatosis (von Recklinghausen disease) 46, 50, 214, 215, 221-222
neuronal plasticity 20
newborn assessment/screening 46-55
Newborn Behavioral Assessment Scale (NBAS) 62, 64, 67
non-judgmental approach 4, 6, 18
Non-steroidal antiinflammatory drugs (NSAIDS) 176, 182, 192, 199, 201, 203, 205, 208, 209, 219, 255, 260
nursemaid elbow 201, 209

O

obese 8, 17, 94, 200, 203, 204, 248
obesity 6, 49, 78, 92, 94-95, 245, 247, 248
obstructive defects 118
obstructive disease 190, 191, 195
obstructive lesions 117, 119-121, 257
obstructive sleep apnea 256
ocular misalignment 172, 176
oculomotor 59
Oedipus complex 17
OLD CART system 216
olfactory 50
omeprazole (Prilosec) 134
Oral Polio Vaccine 30
oropharyngeal 222
oropharynx 3, 5, 31, 261
Ortolani's sign 45, 54, 62, 64, 66, 206, 207
Osgood-Schlatter disease 199, 201, 203
osteogenesis imperfecta 51, 96
otitis externa (swimmer's ear) 176-177
otitis media 62, 64, 133, 170-173, 177, 178
otitis media with effusion (OME) 177-178
Ottawa ankle rule 208
ova and parasites (O and P) 136, 250
oximetry 53, 55, 181, 194

P

PACES format 109
parainfluenza 172, 173, 179, 181, 191
parathyroid glands 40
parotid gland enlargement 104
patent ductus arteriosus (PDA) 53, 116, 117, 119-121
PCV13 25, 27, 29-30, 33t
peak height velocity 92, 107, 108, 110
pectus carinatum 39, 52, 66
pectus excavatum 39, 52, 66
pelvic exam 105, 107, 108
periorbital edema 78
pernicious anemia 231
pertussis 25-29, 33t, 91, 104, 106, 108
pervasive development disorders (PDD) 82-83
pharyngitis/tonsillitis 133, 170-173, 180-181, 221
phenylketonuria 38, 54, 55
phimosis 53, 62, 64, 66, 79
phosphorus 95, 136
physical exam 6, 17, 18, 34, 43, 48-54, 61, 65-67, 74, 76-79, 91-92, 95, 96, 104, 108-110, 121, 128, 130, 136, 144, 154, 170, 176-178, 180-182, 191, 194, 200, 205, 206, 208, 219, 221, 222, 227, 229, 236, 243, 247, 256, 259, 263
Piaget, Jean 16, 67, 77, 79, 87, 89, 91, 92, 110-111
pink eye 174
pityriasis rosea 143, 145, 154-155
pneumococcal vaccine 29-30, 33t, 177
pneumonia 52, 64, 70, 133, 157, 188-191, 194-195, 260, 264
point of maximal impulse 52, 78
polio vaccine (IPV) 25, 26, 30, 33t
polyarthritis 123
polycyclic 149
polydipsia 244, 246-248
polyphagia 247, 248
polyuria 189, 247, 248
Prader-Willi Syndrome 94
prenatal 34, 38, 43-55, 96, 97, 264
primary lesions 121, 149
primitive reflexes 44, 50, 51t
propanolol (Inderal) 219, 244, 246, 249
prophylactic 116, 118, 148, 213, 219, 235, 239
prophylaxis 138, 189, 191, 195, 215, 221, 236, 258
propylthiouracil 244, 246, 249
proteinuria 138, 228, 229